Introduction to **Epidemiology** for the **Health Sciences**

Dispelling the myth that epidemiology is intimidating, *Introduction to Epidemiology for the Health Sciences* is highly approachable from start to finish, providing foundational knowledge for students new to epidemiology. Its focus on critical thinking allows readers to become competent consumers of health literature, equipping them with skills that transfer to various health sciences and other professional workplaces.

The text is structured to take the reader on a journey: each chapter opens with a scientific question before exploring the epidemiological tools available to address it. A conversation tool with representative students clarifies common points of confusion in the classroom, encouraging learners to ask questions to deepen their understanding. Example boxes feature contemporary local and global cases, often with step-by-step workings, while explanation boxes provide further clarification of complex topics. Multiple-choice and short-answer questions at the end of each chapter allow students to test their knowledge.

Authored by epidemiology and public health educators, this engaging textbook provides all readers with the skills they need to critically evaluate epidemiological literature and develop their own epidemiology toolkit.

Emma Miller has held academic posts at Deakin University, La Trobe University, Flinders University and The University of Adelaide, where she is currently an adjunct associate professor within the Stretton Institute.

Stephen Begg is one of Australia's most experienced academics in the field of population health assessment and burden of disease analysis, a field he helped introduce to Australia in the 1990s and to which he has contributed through positions at Harvard University and the World Health Organization.

Patricia Lee is an associate professor specialising in epidemiology and public health. One of her major academic roles is the epidemiology subject lead within the Public Health discipline, Griffith University, leading the epidemiology curriculum development in different degree programs.

Introduction to

Epidemiology for the Health Sciences

Emma Miller

Stephen Begg

Patricia Lee

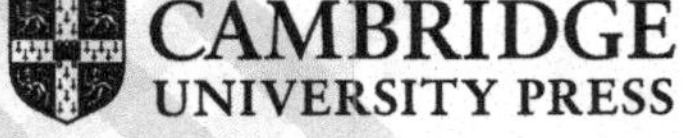

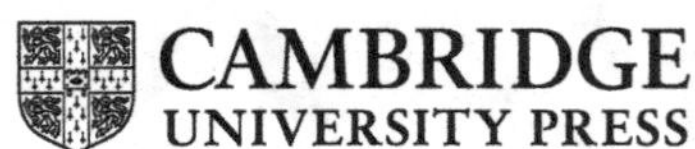

Shaftesbury Road, Cambridge CB2 8EA, United Kingdom

One Liberty Plaza, 20th Floor, New York, NY 10006, USA

477 Williamstown Road, Port Melbourne, VIC 3207, Australia

314–321, 3rd Floor, Plot 3, Splendor Forum, Jasola District Centre, New Delhi – 110025, India

103 Penang Road, #05–06/07, Visioncrest Commercial, Singapore 238467

Cambridge University Press is part of Cambridge University Press & Assessment, a department of the University of Cambridge.

We share the University's mission to contribute to society through the pursuit of education, learning and research at the highest international levels of excellence.

www.cambridge.org
Information on this title: www.cambridge.org/highereducation/isbn/9781009522366

First published 2025

Cover designed by Shaun Jury
Typeset by Integra Software Services Pvt. Ltd

A catalogue record for this publication is available from the British Library

A catalogue record for this book is available from the National Library of Australia

ISBN 978-1-009-52236-6 Paperback

Additional resources for this publication at www.cambridge.org/highereducation/isbn/9781009522366/resources

Contents

About the authors

Emma Miller is an epidemiologist with particular expertise in hepatitis C, sexually transmissible infections (STI) and substance use. She has extensive experience in the surveillance of communicable diseases and a long history of research in this area. Other streams of research interest include alcohol consumption and its links with cancer, and STI and associated risk behaviours. In various government and academic roles, including the state surveillance of influenza in Victoria and STI and blood-borne viruses in South Australia, she has worked extensively with priority populations primarily affected by substance use issues, including prisoners in the South Australian correctional system. The primary focus of her teaching has been in research methods and epidemiology at both undergraduate and postgraduate levels at multiple institutions. She has held academic posts at Deakin University, La Trobe University, Flinders University and The University of Adelaide, where she is currently an adjunct associate professor within the Stretton Institute.

Stephen Begg is an associate professor of public health at La Trobe University. He is one of Australia's most experienced academics in the field of population health assessment and burden of disease analysis, a field he helped introduce to Australia in the 1990s and to which he has contributed through positions at Harvard University and the World Health Organization. He is a trained epidemiologist with over 25 years' experience in international research and consultancy, and has led and managed teams in both academia and the public sector. Associate Professor Begg manages a diverse industry-driven research portfolio with a focus on rural and Indigenous health inequalities, and health system strengthening.

Patricia Lee is an associate professor specialising in epidemiology and public health. With expertise in biostatistics and mixed methods research, she has had the opportunity to work with various research teams in collaboration with government agencies and communities on public health/health promotion projects. She has contributed to many funded research projects and established partnerships with several international researchers in Taiwan, China and Vietnam. Her research interests include health risk modelling, infectious disease surveillance, climate change and health, and health promotion among disadvantaged populations. One of her major academic roles is as the epidemiology subject lead within the Public Health discipline at Griffith University, leading the epidemiology curriculum development in different degree programs (undergraduate and postgraduate). Recognised as an accomplished senior epidemiologist, Patricia has been invited to contribute to epidemiology-related chapters in several public health textbooks.

Acknowledgements

The authors would like to acknowledge the contribution of Barry Borman, who helped to structure the content and direction of this book. We would also like to acknowledge Lucy Russell, who deftly 'wrangled' the author team for an extended period during the development phase of the work, as well as the ongoing efforts of Emily Baxter and Lydia McClelland in bringing things to a successful conclusion. Mostly, the authors would like to thank their partners and families for their support, forbearance of grumpiness and sacrifice of time that could have been spent on far more leisurely pursuits.

Cambridge University Press and the authors would like to acknowledge the feedback provided by peer reviewers of the draft manuscript, including Shazia Shehzad Abbas, Catherine Bennett, Silvana Bettiol, R. Wesley Farr, Md Saiful Islam, Seana Gall, Danijela Gasevic, Matt McDaniel, William Mude, Linda Murray, Lisa Salazar, Linda Slack-Smith and Kido Uyamasi. Their feedback and comments were invaluable to the development of this edition.

The authors and Cambridge University Press would like to thank the following for permission to reproduce material in this book.

Cover image: © Getty Images/filo. **Figure 1.3**: Data from Australian Bureau of Statistics. Reproduced under Creative Commons Attribution 4.0 International, https://creativecommons.org/licenses/by/4.0/. **Figure 3.1**: © 2024 United Nations. Reproduced under Creative Commons Attribution 3.0 Intergovernmental Organization, https://creativecommons.org/licenses/by/3.0/igo/deed.en. **Figure 3.2**, **Figure 3.9** and **Figure 3.11**: © 2024 Institute for Health Metrics and Evaluation. Used with permission. All rights reserved. **Figure 3.5**: © 2023 OECD. https://doi.org/10.1787/data-00540-en, accessed on 9 November 2023. **Figure 3.6**: © 2023 OECD. https://doi.org/10.1787/7a7afb35-en, accessed on 9 November 2023. **Figure 3.7**: © 2023 Australian Institute of Health and Welfare. Reproduced under Creative Commons Attribution 4.0 International, https://creativecommons.org/licenses/by/4.0/. **Figure 3.8**: © 2023 OECD. https://doi.org/10.1787/193a2829-en, accessed on 12 November 2023. **Figure 4.3**: © Getty Images/Keystone-France. **Figure 5.1**: © 2019 State of Queensland (Queensland Health). Reproduced under Creative Commons Attribution 3.0 Australia, https://creativecommons.org/licenses/by/3.0/au/. **Figure 5.3**, **Figure 5.5**, **Figure 5.7**, **Figure 5.11** and **Figure 5.12**: © 2024 World Health Organization. Reproduced under Creative Commons Attribution 4.0 International, https://creativecommons.org/licenses/by/4.0/. **Figure 5.6:** created with MapChart. Reproduced under Creative Commons Attribution-Sharealike 4.0 International, https://creativecommons.org/licenses/by-sa/4.0/. **Figure 5.8**: © 2023 World Health Organization. Reproduced under Creative Commons Attribution 4.0 International, https://creativecommons.org/licenses/by/4.0/. **Figure 5.9** and **Figure 5.10**: © 2022 The Australian Institute of Health and Welfare. Reproduced under Creative Commons Attribution 4.0 International, https://creativecommons.org/licenses/by/4.0/. **Figure 5.13**: Data © 2024 World Health Organization. Reproduced under Creative Commons Attribution 4.0 International, https://creativecommons.org/licenses/by/4.0/.

Figure 5.14: © 2023 The Australian Institute of Health and Welfare. Reproduced under Creative Commons Attribution 4.0 International, https://creativecommons.org/licenses/by/4.0/. **Figure 5.15**: © 2022 World Health Organization. Reproduced with permission. **Figure 6.1**, **Figure 6.2** and **Figure 6.3**: people avatars © Getty Images/dejanj01. **Figure 6.5**: © 2022 Our World in Data. Reproduced under Creative Commons Attribution 4.0 International, https://creativecommons.org/licenses/by/4.0/. **Figure 12.1**: © 2014 Elsevier. Reprinted from *The Lancet*, Vol. 384, Rangaka MX, Wilkinson RJ, Boulle A, Glynn JR, Fielding K, van Cutsem G, et al., Isoniazid plus antiretroviral therapy to prevent tuberculosis: a randomised double-blind, placebo-controlled trial, p. 682–90, with permission from Elsevier.

Table 5.1: © 2020 World Health Organization. Reproduced under Creative Commons Attribution 4.0 International, https://creativecommons.org/licenses/by/4.0/. **Table 5.2**: © 2023 State of Queensland (Queensland Health). Reproduced under Creative Commons Attribution 3.0 Australia, https://creativecommons.org/licenses/by/3.0/au/. **Table 6.5**: © 2023 World Health Organization. Reproduced with permission. **Table 8.3**: © 1957 Sage Publications.

Extract of WG McBride 'Thalidomide and congenital abnormalities', *The Lancet*, 16 December 1961: © Elsevier. Reproduced with permission.

Every effort has been made to trace and acknowledge copyright. The publisher apologises for any accidental infringement and welcomes information that would redress this situation.

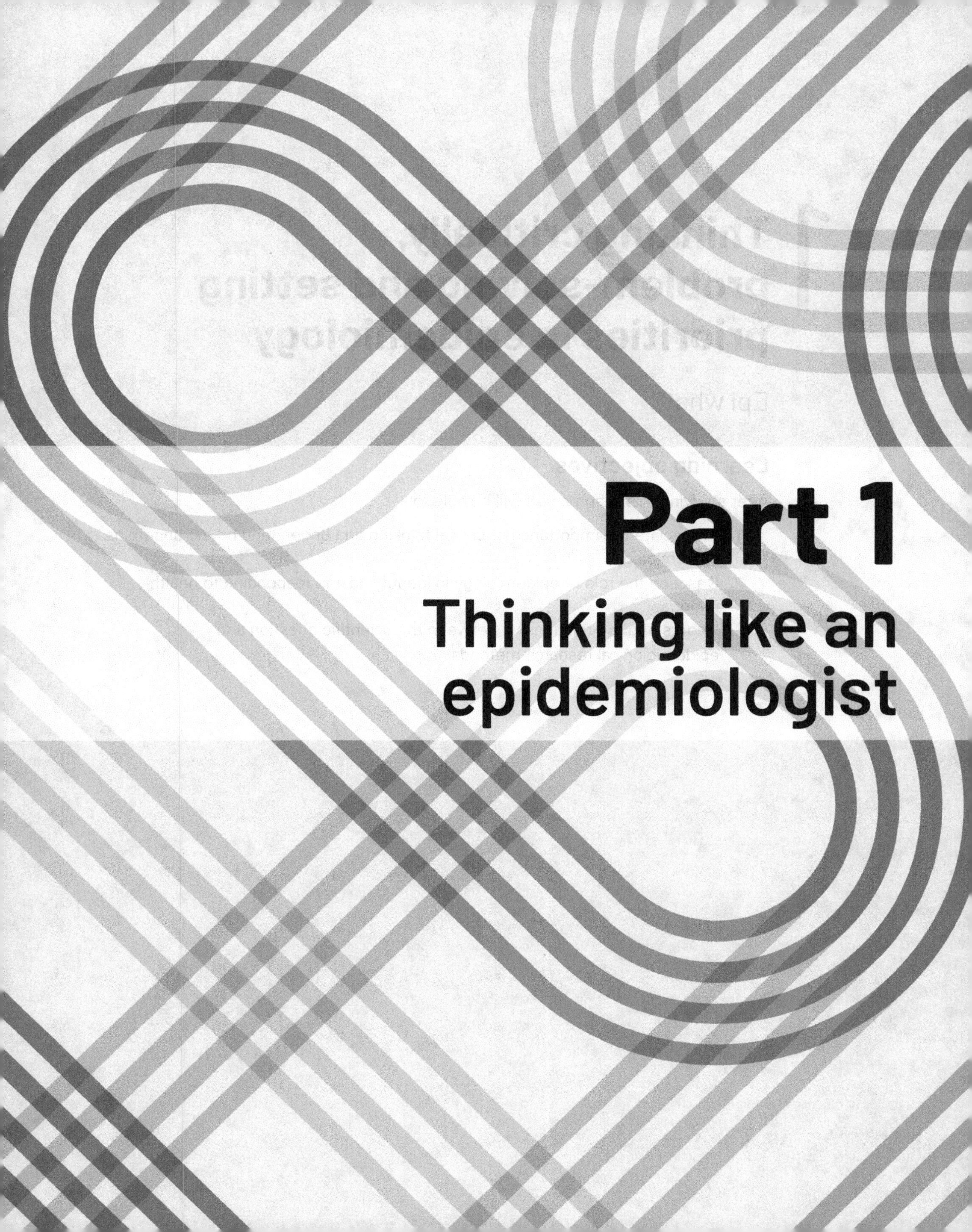

Part 1
Thinking like an epidemiologist

1 Thinking critically, problem-solving and setting priorities in epidemiology

Epi what?

Learning objectives

After studying this chapter, you will be able to:

1. Appreciate the importance of critical thinking and understand how it underpins epidemiology
2. Describe the role of epidemiology in identifying and responding to health priorities
3. Understand the relationship between the scientific question and epidemiological research methods

Introduction

If you are reading this book, you are either particularly interested in health and the field of epidemiology or you are undertaking a program of study in the health sciences. While you may have picked up this text out of interest, it is highly probable that you are undertaking a compulsory component in your study program and are now approaching the subject of epidemiology with some degree of trepidation. Perhaps some of you really enjoy this kind of thing, but others may be worried that this text will be heavy with daunting formulae and complicated calculations. Statistics (commonly referred to as *bio*statistics in the health sciences) is an incredibly important and intensely interesting field of endeavour; however, with apologies to those who may be disappointed, this book is *not* a text on statistics. Epidemiology is the study of patterns and determinants of disease and other health states in populations. It primarily uses quantitative methods (which deal with counting, measuring and comparing things) that definitely *use* statistics and include statistical methods, but in this book we will not be talking about performing any statistical acrobatics more complicated than completing a sudoku puzzle.

Rachael: That all sounds good – I haven't done a lot of maths, but I do like solving puzzles!

Hugo: Well, I hope they mean it. I'm scared of numbers and I'm not even sure I can manage a sudoku.

Author (Emma): Lots of people find numbers a little scary at first, but this is usually just the thought, rather than the reality, of them. I don't mind a number or two myself but remember that I am an epidemiologist and not a biostatistician. I like to solve health puzzles using numbers (and I'm sure you will too after reading this book!) but when serious statistical manoeuvres are called for, my most important solution involves calling the team biostatistician …

It is probably time to point out that you are not alone here. We'd like to introduce Rachael and Hugo, who will be coming along for the ride with you. Their role is to ask the questions you might think about asking and to keep us authors on track. Their contributions will be clearly signposted, so you should feel free to skip those bits if this is not your thing, but their questions (and author responses) might really help to clarify things along the way.

Other things that might be useful are the real-life examples that will be included in every chapter, along with explanation boxes where relevant. The examples will describe epidemiological concepts, often (though not always) in the form of studies or investigations that have been done in the real world. Most of these examples will involve large population trends and events, including the recent **COVID-19** pandemic. If those examples include them, you will get the opportunity to try to calculate some fancy-sounding measures for yourself and the explanation boxes will show you how to do them in clear terms. At the end of each chapter, you can have a go at the review questions and keen readers can access further review questions online.

COVID-19: Coronavirus disease 2019, a disease caused by infection with the SARS-CoV-2 virus, first noted in 2019.

Now, let's set the scene by beginning to address the main question of this chapter – 'Epi what?'

Epidemic: (synonym 'outbreak') An increase in the number of cases, which is beyond that normally expected for a particular region during a particular period of time.

Risk factor: In the context of epidemiology, a factor/variable that increases the chance of having a particular disease or health condition among the people who are exposed to this factor.

Surveillance: Continuous monitoring of diseases or health conditions in a defined population or geographic location. Involves systematic and ongoing data collection, analysis, interpretation and dissemination to detect potential outbreaks and inform timely control measures.

Epidemiology

If asked to describe the principal purpose of the health sciences, a reasonable starting point might be to suggest that it is to prevent illness and maintain good health in the population. One might then extend this to enhancing quality of life, curing those with disease and minimising complications in those with illnesses that can't be cured, even promoting health equity and inhibiting inequality in society. What if I were to tell you that epidemiology could help with all of these goals and more?

'Epidemiology', taken from the Greek words '**epidemic**' (first used by Hippocrates, way back around 400 BC) and '-ology' (science or discipline) is traditionally defined as 'The study of the distribution and determinants of health-related states or events in specified populations, and the application of this study to the control of health problems' (1, p 42).

Although historically thought of as concerned primarily with disease and disease **risk factors**, in more recent times there has been far greater recognition of epidemiology's capacity to explore the social, political and health experience of populations (2). Yet epidemiologists tend to be thought of by many as 'disease detectives' – complete with metaphorical trenchcoats and deer hunter hats, sniffing out causes of disease and identifying the culprits and their associates. Although there is some truth in this stereotype, in fact there are multiple 'flavours' (or fields) of epidemiologists who work across the gamut of health-related scientific endeavour. These flavours include, but are not limited to: communicable and non-communicable disease **surveillance** and control; immunology and vaccine development; medical, clinical and pharmaceutical; veterinary science; environmental health; and the analysis of '**big data**'. In this book, we will be discussing examples of research in many of these fields of epidemiology and more.

Hugo: I was thinking epidemiology had something to do with skin disorders – I guess I got confused because the word 'epidermis' is about skin.

Rachael: You're not the only one. When she heard I was learning about epidemiology, my Aunt Mary started talking to me about her rash!

Big data: Very large population-level datasets that are analysed for epidemiological trends and patterns in health, risk and human behaviour.

Outcomes: The different health states a person might experience.

What all fields of epidemiology have in common is the application of critical thinking to understand and describe phenomena, identify causative or contributing factors to **outcomes**, provide and evaluate evidence from which to develop actions to modify health outcomes, and even evaluate the effect of those actions once they are taken. Of course, critical thinking is not just the preserve of epidemiology; it has wide and important application in just about every field of human endeavour. Developing your critical thinking skills can help you with all parts of your current studies and future work. In fact, the ability to question, analyse, interpret and reach an informed judgement could be seen as vital to making sense of just about everything that happens in the modern world (3).

As well as raising the quandary of the best place to put your chair, Example 1.1 describes a hypothetical case of everyday critical thinking: questioning the source of information, seeking opposing arguments and synthesising the evidence before reaching an informed judgement or conclusion. In this chapter, we will learn a bit more about critical thinking in epidemiology and how this is used to identify, prioritise and address health priorities in society.

EXAMPLE 1.1

You hear you could catch a cold from the draught of an open window. Your first instinct might be to move your chair as far away from the window as possible, but then you might start thinking about this a bit more:

- I wonder how many of the colds I have caught in the past might have happened after I sat next to an open window?
- What about those people having their lunch outside in the cold – will they get more or fewer colds if they eat their lunch indoors?
- What about the person who told me about the window thing – would I normally trust their advice?
- Do other people have different theories about the risk of sitting near open windows?

Based on these ruminations, you could either conclude that the original advice is likely to be correct or begin to wonder whether you should be looking into this further.

An approach to critical thinking

The concept of critical thinking is not new but, in what is starting to be a repeating theme here, goes back at least as far as ancient Greece. The idea of critical thinking was born from the work of Socrates, around 2500 years ago (4). His research indicated that the majority of people in his own society, even those who were supposed to be in charge, were prone to irrational and often contradictory beliefs that were usually based on little or no evidence. Socrates stressed the importance of gathering good evidence and developed a method of challenging underlying assumptions and beliefs, and their implications, through an approach known as 'Socratic questioning', a method that is still used in psychotherapy and teaching (5) – although, in true critical thinking style, there is some debate about the consistency of understandings and application of Socratic questioning in practice (6).

While Socrates' observations were made about the illogical thought processes prevailing at the time, it could be argued that the tendency to build irrational systems of beliefs (what I like to term '**feel-osophy**' – based on a mixture of emotional reaction, peer influence, resentment, misunderstandings and personal agenda), is ever present when it comes to human beings. Illogical and irrational assumptions arising from the absence of critical thinking can have devasting consequences on personal, societal and global levels. These consequences can range from the breakdown of personal relationships to the type of shared societal hysteria that brought about the cruel and deadly witch trials that occurred periodically across Europe and North America between the fourteenth and eighteenth centuries (7, 8). More recently, a lack of critical thinking in relation to COVID-19 vaccinations could well have had global health impacts. In one example, the owner of a multinational technology corporation stands accused of a plan to microchip the whole world population using vaccines – a surprisingly widespread belief that seriously impacted vaccination rates in the United States and elsewhere (9). You may have heard about this and other COVID-19 related 'feel-osophies' and the conspiracy theories they spawn (10). Reduced protective behaviour – such as decreased mask-wearing, social distancing and handwashing – combined with low vaccination coverage and high

Feel-osophy: A made-up term denoting systems of belief relying on inaccurate information selected on the basis of factors such as peer influence, resentment, misunderstandings and personal agenda.

infection rates generates the perfect environment not only for more virus transmission, but also for the development of new variants of the virus. As the continuing emergence of new COVID-19 variants also makes the task of developing specific vaccines more difficult (11), pandemics are probably not a great time to be forgoing critical thinking.

Recognition of the importance of critical thinking today is reflected in the explicit goals of most universities in striving to produce graduates with critical thinking skills as a core attribute. This is because critical thinking is strongly associated with academic success and employment opportunity (12). Critical thinkers have the capacity to be innovative, to solve problems, are often creative and reach evidence-based conclusions. In fact, one study found that critical thinking was a better predictor of positive life outcomes than intelligence (13).

Hugo: That might explain how really smart people can make some really silly decisions.

Rachael: Maybe it also explains how my big, dumb brother always wins at chess – actually, he always wins at everything …

Fortunately, unlike inherent traits such as intelligence, critical thinking is something people can learn and develop over time. As touched on, critical thinking is a cognitive process that involves questioning, analysing, evaluating and reaching a judgement about information you might hear or read. It can be applied to information coming from social media, television, news sources, family and friends, your teacher or lecturer, and all published works (even this book!). Transferability across contexts and tasks is in fact an important and useful hallmark of critical thinking skills (14). Critical thinking provides a way of sorting out, on a preponderance of the evidence, what is most likely to be the most accurate version of reality. Being able to reach reliable judgements and then apply this to problem-solving is important across all social, academic and professional activities in life, but has particular relevance to the health sciences. People working in the health sciences may be providing clinical services, developing clinical guidelines or health policy, or researching and providing the evidence to inform all of these activities. Without trying to sound melodramatic here, the well-being of the population or even people's lives might well depend on those judgements (15).

And how do we 'do' critical thinking? Well, there is much written on the topic (and you should check out the 'Further reading' section at the end of the chapter to find out more), but most methods include the following components: analysing, evaluating, reasoning, problem-solving and decision-making.

Analysing

Analysis may sound like something that could be complicated, involving numbers and possibly the wearing of lab coats, but you are probably doing it all time without thinking too much about it. When first presented with new information, unless you are the type to automatically let your eyes glaze over, you will make an assessment of how relevant those data are to you. As in the window-opening example (Example 1.1), you could think about how much you trust the source of the information and whether there are alternative facts to consider. This natural ability (not the eye glazing-over thing) can be harnessed and improved in a logical way.

At the core of analytical thought is questioning the argument being proposed. In this context, the argument is a proposition or claim. The claim may be in the form of a statement of belief or may be more extensive, such as a theory (a system of ideas aimed at explaining a phenomenon) or even a feel-osophy (just had to get that term in there one more time).

In epidemiology, a claim might be about what causes disease. In Example 1.1, the claim was that the draught coming in through the window could cause the body to become more susceptible to respiratory illnesses. This is actually a common belief with its roots in folklore, where illness is thought to emanate from body temperature changes caused by exposure to cold or damp in the environment (e.g. 'catching a chill') (16). This theory may have developed to explain the objective observation that most respiratory illnesses are associated with the colder months of the year. This is a kind of theory involving reasoning to connect conditions – it is colder outside than inside, and colds are associated with colder seasons. The competing argument, particularly reinforced by recent observations involving COVID-19, is that air movement from open windows might dilute virus particles that could be in the indoor environment, usually secreted from people huddling inside, therefore decreasing the likelihood of being infected (17). This is also based on a theory: when it is cold, people tend to congregate inside for longer, heightening the risk of virus transmission between people who may be infected. But how do we sort out which claim is likely to be the most accurate? The first claim comes along with years of tradition, handed down from trusted personal authority to trusted personal authority. The competing claim comes from people we have never met, who tend to use complicated methods and language that is barely comprehensible at times.

Well, let's break it all down ...

Collecting and synthesising data

To begin, we need to analyse these claims about windows in the context of the events to which they pertain. They are both about contracting a respiratory illness in cold weather and the risk associated with airflow (increased or decreased). The first task might be to find out how many respiratory viruses arise in a given population and when they occur. For that we will need to collect some reliable data on how many people are getting respiratory illnesses and when. Friends and family members would probably not make the best source of information, as there are several potential factors that would impact the quality (or reliability) of the data. Personally, I have increasing trouble remembering accurately all that transpires the further that time moves on from the event. Your friends and family might not always be able to give you accurate information about whether or when they contracted a respiratory virus last year, for instance. Relying on this information could introduce a type of unintentional systematic error in your data known by epidemiologists as **'recall bias'**.

A **bias** can occur due to the existence of any factor or trend in the collection or analysis of data that can lead people to arrive at erroneous conclusions. Epidemiologists know about many different types of bias, some of which could arise from asking your friends and family for information. Another type that springs to mind here is the potential for **selection bias** – the type of bias that can occur when we select people to provide data who may have characteristics that differ from those about whom we want our conclusions to make a claim (such as the population in general). Those closest to you might share many genetic and/or behavioural characteristics that are related in some way to infection transmission but may differ from other people in society. Further, respiratory infections are transmitted from person to person so we might not be able to tell whether the open window is implicated in transmission or the

Recall bias: Occurs when there is differential recall of exposures or experiences between comparison groups, which is most likely to occur in studies using self-reported data (a form of measurement bias).

Bias: Any unintentional systematic factor, or trend in the collection or analysis of data, that leads to erroneous conclusions.

Selection bias: Systematic error introduced by the selection of participants, or inclusion of their information, with characteristics that differ from those not included in the study.

Confounding: Occurs when understanding of the relationship between one potential cause and an outcome is distorted by one or more additional factors associated with both that potential cause and the outcome.

De-identified data: Information about characteristics of a population (or sample from a population) from which all identifying information has been removed; it is not possible to recognise particular people from whom the data have been collected.

virus spreads since friends and families tend to hang out together, regardless of proximity to windows. This last is an example of another potential source of error called **confounding**, when the true relationship between one potential cause and an outcome is distorted by the existence of another factor that is associated with both that potential cause (being near an open window) and the outcome (viral transmission). You will be hearing much more detail about bias and confounding and their various impacts in later chapters, but this is enough to be going on with.

So where do we get the required reliable information? Happily, we are now living in an era of unprecedented access to high-quality information about almost every part of human experience. This is a time I like to call 'paradise for nerds'. All this information is collected across the population, turned into **de-identified data** (all identifying information is removed) and regularly presented in downloadable number files (e.g. in Microsoft Excel and similar) or summarised in reports. Assuming one has access to the internet, in many countries it is now possible to access the latest population data on health, welfare, workforce, housing and more. International health data are available online from institutions such as the World Health Organization (18). I have included a link to this website in the 'Further reading' section near the end of this chapter for you to go and see what is there, but you could and should do some exploring online to see what is available from government and non-government agencies in your country.

Accessing data from one such public health organisation in my own country, I learnt that there were 12 083 cases of influenza reported in 2022 in the population of around 1.8 million people of South Australia (19, 20). This was quite a big year for influenza following some quiet years, which was thought to be due to international border restrictions in place in Australia during the earlier years of the COVID-19 pandemic (21). Influenza is not the only virus that causes respiratory infections like colds, but it does follow a similar pattern of occurrence to most other respiratory viruses and, handily for us, is subject to surveillance in many jurisdictions. Looking at the information available, and loosely estimated in Figure 1.1, it is clear that most of the cases of influenza in South Australia occurred in late autumn and winter – the same seasonal pattern that has been note around the world (22).

Rachael: I knew there would be graphs!

Hugo: Do you think you could explain it a bit, Emma?

Author (Emma): Reading graphs can be a bit daunting, but the best thing to do is to always take it step by step, as even seasoned graph readers are well advised to do. The title of this graph (Figure 1.1) indicates that it shows the number of cases of influenza reported each week over the seasons in the year 2022. Along the upright axis (known as the y-axis) is depicted the range of the potential number of cases from zero to 1400. Along the horizontal axis (known as the x-axis) are the seasons flowing from summer to summer – left to right. Because the graph concerns influenza in Australia, you can see that winter occurs in the middle of the year and the year starts and ends with summer seasons. The columns (or bars, as this type of graph is called a 'bar chart') across the x-axis represent the number of cases reported each week (refer back to the title). The height of the bars represents the number of cases reported in that week measured against the y-axis.

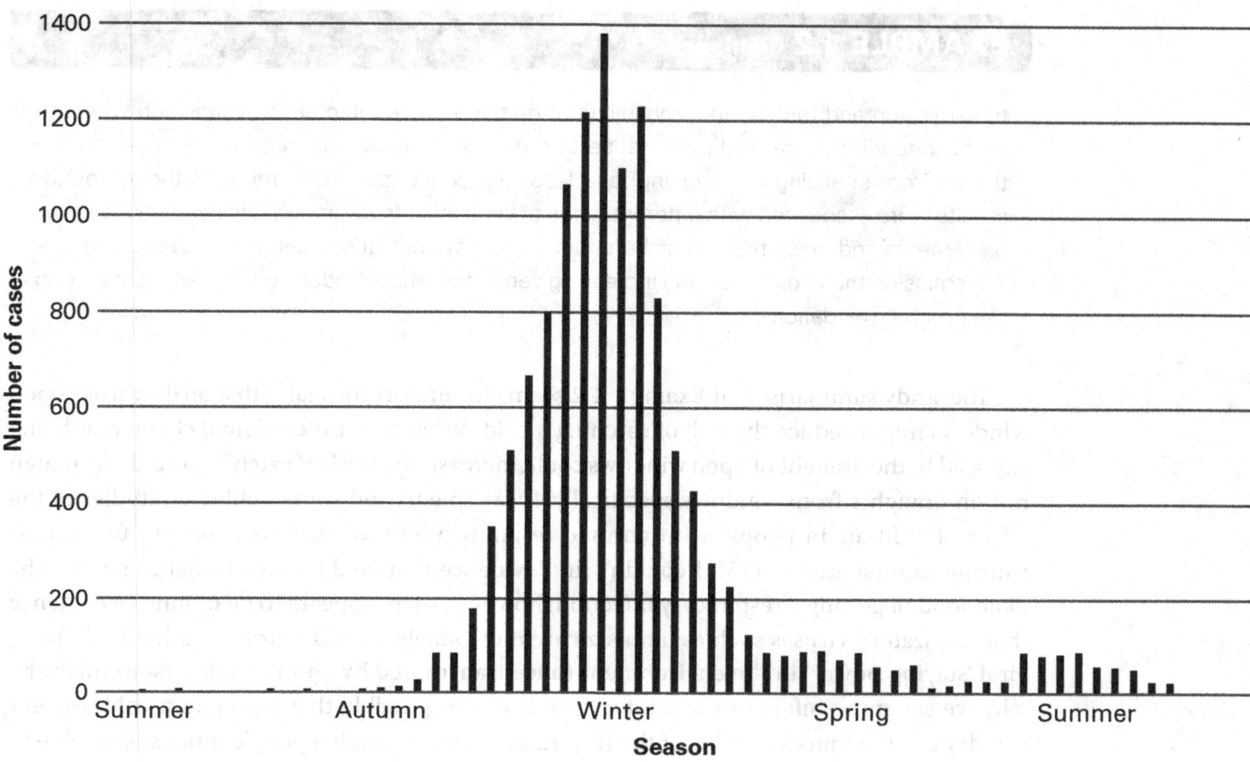

Figure 1.1 Laboratory-confirmed influenza cases per week by season in 2022 in South Australia. Adapted from (20).

We now begin to suspect there may be some truth in at least the first part of both claims: increases in respiratory infections are associated with colder weather. But what about the second part, the risks associated with cold air flow? Although there are unlikely to be handy population data sets to access on this issue, there may well be some other evidence in the form of published studies. A lot of research has been done in this area in recent times, particularly in relation to COVID-19, which is caused by a particular respiratory virus type known as a *coronavirus*, **SARS-CoV-2** (Severe Acute Respiratory Syndrome Coronavirus 2). Non COVID-19 type coronaviruses are thought to cause up to 15 per cent of cases of what most people call the 'common cold' (23). So, the real-life study summarised in the Example 1.2 could be highly relevant to our current critical thinking activity.

SARS-CoV-2: Severe Acute Respiratory Syndrome Coronavirus 2, the virus that causes COVID-19.

Systematic review: A review that aims to identify, evaluate and synthesise all available evidence from quality-assessed studies, using predetermined explicit and systematic methods to address specific research questions (may or may not involve a meta-analysis).

Rate: The occurrence of an event (e.g. counts of disease or death) divided by the number of a specified population at risk over a specified period of time.

EXAMPLE 1.2

In a special kind of study called a **systematic review**, in which the researchers locate and review as many quality published studies as they can find to fully understand a particular topic, Thornton and colleagues (24) synthesised the findings of 32 different studies that investigated the effectiveness of ventilation – for example, window opening and their placement in the building, exhaust systems, air conditioners – on the transmission of coronaviruses. They found that increasing of ventilation decreased both the **rate** of virus

EXAMPLE 1.2 Continued

transmission and the risk (or probability) of getting infected. Increased ventilation was also associated with decreased persistence of droplets (infected watery particles released into the air from sneezing or coughing) and less viral concentration in the air. Although better results were associated with different types of ventilation (such as exhaust systems, window placements and fans), the researchers found that any ventilation was better at reducing viral transmission than none at all and increasing ventilation and introducing fresh air were among their recommendations.

The study summarised in Example 1.2 seems to support the claim that airflow from open windows might reduce the risk of catching a cold. What about the original claim: that being exposed to the draught of open windows could increase your risk of catching a cold? Although not on draughts from windows specifically, I was able to find some published studies of the effect of cold air in people with chronic respiratory illness, such as exposure to cold air causing asthma attacks (25). I couldn't find evidence that cold air alone might increase the likelihood of getting a respiratory infection; however, there appears to be mounting evidence that respiratory viruses such as influenza are more stable in colder drier weather (26). Thus, viral 'staying power' in the environment (once transmitted by an infected person) might be why we see more infections in winter (27). It is also possible that sitting in a cold draught can dry out the mucosal lining of the respiratory system, making people more susceptible to infection should they be exposed to a virus (28).

Evaluating

It is here that we return to considering the quality of the information underlying the competing claims. This is part of the process of evaluation: assessing the strength, authority, credibility or value of the argument. The quality of information is greatly influenced by the authority and agenda of its source. First, I always like to ask: who is saying this and why they are saying it? The 'who' is the person, author or organisation presenting the information. Finding out the 'why' can be a relatively simple exercise, but sometimes can take a bit more investigation.

From time to time, you may hear about methods to preserve health and prevent illness as you navigate your way through cyberspace. Many theories of health and illness are espoused on social media by 'friends', or presented on the internet via 'influencers' (people who appeal to large online audiences, and who often are paid in money or goods to promote commercial products). Developing, or ascribing to, alternative (and sometimes irrational) explanations for health phenomena is extremely common and has been studied for many years (29). The emergence of social media has allowed for the rapid and unprecedented propagation of information and misinformation across the world (30). In the social media environment, it is not always easy to answer the 'who' question and can be even more difficult to uncover what the motivation for presenting any information might be. While some posters might genuinely wish to pass on what they believe is good health advice, misinformation may also be promoted deliberately. One study suggests that the intentional posting of misinformation may be due to people having a high degree of trust in the online environment and therefore being willing to take risks in passing on unverified information, the fear of missing out (FoMO) and a sort of indifference to caution arising from social media fatigue (31). Overall, the inability to assess the authenticity of the information and the authority of its source suggests that basing one's health beliefs on information solely obtained from social media might be a risky proposition.

Being well known is kind of the point when it comes to influencers, so we can be more confident about who is providing any particular fact. Although not always as transparent as they could be, the underlying motivations of many influencers are also more obvious, promoting the sale of commercial products. Companies form legitimate relationships with influencers to harness the trust they have built with their online followers to promote their products (32). Recognising the potential that this trust might be exploited to pressure their followers to purchase goods or services, government consumer regulators in countries such as Australia have recently reminded influencers that failure to disclose their commercial relationships or to deliberately manipulate consumers with misleading endorsements are crimes under Australian law (33). Whether such reminders will be sufficient to 'influence the influencers' (that has a nice ring!) around the globe remains to be seen. In the meantime, we can assume that the primary motivation of many influencers is to endorse services and products, and it is not necessarily easy to discern the quality of the evidence underlying their advice.

The internet is also heaving with direct marketing of goods and services. A simple search on health and well-being issues may produce long lists of websites advertising a range of commercial products purporting to address every known health issue. Such products might promise to protect your body from a range of **infectious diseases**, such as colds and influenza, stop allergic responses and improve heart health and circulation. The webpage authors might assert that their device uses 'scientifically proven' methods and may even offer the reassurance of a guarantee against faulty manufacture (but will probably not guarantee the actual performance of the device). Who is saying this and why are they saying it? The answer to both questions is clear: the information is presented by the very people who want to sell the product and their agenda is just as clearly commercial.

Infectious diseases: (synonym 'communicable diseases') A class of illnesses resulting from specific infectious agents or their toxic products.

Rachael: Does that mean we can't trust any information about products on the internet?

Hugo: What about product reviews?

Author (Emma): Well, it depends on what type of information you are seeking. If you have a serious question about a health issue (and maybe have to write a paper or other assignment on it), then relying on the information provided by commercial sites (or referencing them in a paper or other assessable task) is unlikely to be helpful (or to get you a good grade). Instead, search for objective information about the issue from reputable sources, such as published scientific studies or technical reports, or statistics published or posted by government health agencies. If you want to find information about a product to purchase, you would still be better applying critical thinking and seeking corroborative information from sources with less of an agenda than the people selling the product. And yes, Hugo, product reviews might help here!

Although they should always be asked, the 'who' and 'why' questions are generally easier to answer when it comes to information provided by government agencies (or those supported by or affiliated with government), non-government and community-based organisations that conduct their own research and the publications of reputable scientific journals. The names of the respective agencies, scientific journals, research teams and their institutional affiliations are always provided. The purpose of any reputable organisations is clearly stated on their webpages or in their reports, and any of their (equally reputable) associates are listed. Reputable scientific journals have clearly defined and strict standards for the authors they publish. Any funding bodies associated with published studies are listed, as are the institutional affiliations of each member of the research team that authored the paper. Conforming with explicit journal guidelines, the aims of published papers will be clearly described and any potential conflicts of interest (any financial, commercial or other relationship with organisations or people who could potentially influence the research) are disclosed. If you ever find that any of the above is not the case, this is your first clue that you are not dealing with a reputable information source.

Evaluating is not just about assessing the authority of the information source or claim, but also the quality of the evidence underlying the claim. You may very well trust the person who told you that sitting in a draught from an open window could cause a cold, but how did they come by the information in the first place? It is likely that they also heard this from someone they trust. Alternatively, they may have undertaken extensive research or even have gone through a careful process of critical thinking on this very issue. I guess you would need to ask them ...

Exposure: A behavioural or genetic characteristic, toxin or other substance in the environment, or a lifestyle factor that is associated with an increase/decrease in the risk of a defined outcome.

We have noted that things such as bias and confounding can affect how we understand relationships between an apparent **exposure** and an outcome. Luckily, scientific studies are usually designed to identify and minimise the impact of such factors on their conclusions, as we will discover further in later chapters. The quality of the information presented in reports of quantitative studies is largely measured by the methods used and how well these methods were implemented. In published studies, you will find a whole section detailing the methods used by the researchers, who participated in the study, and what was measured and how. When authors (usually the researchers involved in the study) submit a paper to a journal, the manuscript is reviewed by other researchers who have published papers or have expertise in a similar field, on whose critique the paper is either rejected, revised and possibly reviewed again and, ultimately, published if deemed appropriate. This process is known as 'peer review' and is the main method used by journals to ensure the research is valid and original prior to publication. Peer review is essentially intended to 'weed out' poor-quality studies. The whole review process can be quite slow, is perceived by some to be subject to editor and reviewer bias and has been accused of stifling innovation (34). Thus, peer review is not completely without its critics. Yet the process is currently considered the best way to support the integrity of science, at least as it is reported.

This is not to say that anything you see published must be of good quality, even if it is published in a reputable journal. As mentioned, the peer review process is good but not perfect, and peer reviewers are not infallible. Further, even very good studies come with an explicit statement of the probability that their findings might be wrong (more on this later). Consumers of the scientific literature should refrain from assuming certainty from a single study, but instead consider the balance of evidence from more than one publication.

Reasoning

Critical thinking is about following a logical pathway of collecting information, sorting it into categories, systematically comparing the evidence and its quality, and making links between ideas. In applying this process to our open window example, we have collected the relevant data and carefully analysed this information. Now we are at the point of applying reasoning to all we have learnt – the process of developing an argument or arriving at a position on the two claims.

We now have good evidence that respiratory infections chiefly occur in colder seasons of the year, supporting the idea that colder temperatures have something to do with increased transmission. We have also learnt that respiratory viruses tend to be more stable in colder environments, so it follows that they would hang around longer to represent a greater exposure risk to susceptible people. Further, while we were not able to find direct evidence of harm from sitting near windows, there is a possibility that cold air might damage the mucosal lining of the respiratory system, making it easier for viruses to be transmitted. The one constant linking all these facts is that there must be virus around in the first place – if there is no virus, there is no transmission. From here we might start to doubt that merely sitting in the draught of a cold window will cause a cold, as it is unlikely to do so without circulating viruses.

So, assuming we are operating under the condition that it is winter and respiratory viruses are in circulation, we now need to work out which of the competing claims is most likely to be accurate: that cold draughts caused by open windows can cause people to catch colds or that the open window would help to reduce the risk of people catching colds. If we want to address the problem (viral transmission), we need to be able to apply logical reasoning here to inform the development of a potential solution (the next stage in the process).

Let us return to our evaluation, in which we examined the quality of the information underpinning each claim. On the balance of probabilities, it is most likely that the person who first told you that sitting in cold draughts causes colds has not undertaken comprehensive research on the issue, although they may be very fond of the person who first advised them of this. Both points of view (amended to include the existence of circulating virus) can be supported by quality evidence coming from reputable sources, although it was a lot easier to find quality evidence supporting the case for opening the window due to the recent interest in ventilation and COVID-19 prevention. You might recall the studies looking at cold air-related damage to the lining of the respiratory system, and the systematic review of 32 studies that concluded any ventilation was better than none. We could go on researching but, on balance, do we have sufficient evidence to reach a judgement here?

We now think that the cold draught itself is unlikely to cause you to catch a respiratory illness. We have established that cold weather is associated with increased circulation of respiratory viruses but these are chiefly spread from person to person by droplet infection or by the persistence of the virus in the environment. We could even deduce that the risk of infection is likely to be increased due to the tendency of humans, including those who are infected, to congregate together indoors during cold weather. From our research, we might determine that opening the window can introduce outdoor air that has a lower viral concentration as well as helping to circulate the air inside, potentially diluting the concentration of viruses inside (24).

Problem-solving

Now we have reached a judgement on the claims, we can apply this information to the problem of catching winter colds. This is where we turn our attention from carefully examining the issue itself to focusing on potential solutions. We won't need to make any firm decisions yet, but we can use our new understanding of the issue to identify and evaluate potential alternatives.

From all our work, we have determined that the main factors contributing to the transmission of respiratory viruses are the cold weather, circulating viruses and (potentially) inadequate indoor airflow. We can apply the same steps of critical analysis to identifying and evaluating potential solutions. There is not much we can do about the seasons, but perhaps we could educate people on protective behaviour when infection risk is high. For instance, social distancing, handwashing and mask-wearing have all become very familiar strategies in COVID-19 prevention. There is evidence that these same behavioural measures can be employed to reduce the transmission of most types of respiratory and other infections (35). Increasing education about the benefits of engaging in personal protective behaviour might help to address the problems associated with more time spent indoors with others during winter. However, evidence shows that people have grown increasingly tired of following these practices – a phenomenon known as 'pandemic fatigue' (36).

Vaccinations have the potential to reduce the concentration of virus circulating around the population. Currently, vaccines are available for COVID-19 and seasonal influenza, and there is plenty of research showing that vaccinating the population leads to lower rates of infection with both viruses (37, 38). While these vaccines are great for preventing severe disease, neither vaccine stops all infection and there is still no vaccine available for the all the other viruses that cause what we refer to as the 'common cold' (39). As well, history shows there will be a whole lot of work to do if we want to increase the uptake of seasonal vaccines among those known as the 'vaccine hesitant' (40).

Various methods to improve ventilation have been found to be effective in decreasing the viral transmission indoors (40). There is a range of lower- and higher-tech ways to mechanically increase rates of ventilation, decrease the amount of recirculated and (potentially) contaminated air, regulate humidity, expel contaminated air (exhaust systems), control temperature and provide 'natural ventilation' (opening windows). Some of these measures might be more or less feasible in different locations, depending on funds and enthusiasm.

Decision-making

The various solutions put forward to address increased winter time transmission of respiratory viruses boil down to:

- personal protective behaviour (social distancing, handwashing and mask-wearing)
- vaccination (influenza and COVID-19)
- improving indoor ventilation (range of low- to high-tech solutions).

All these strategies were found to be effective at reducing viral transmissions, but they also had problems that might affect their feasibility. These issues included pandemic fatigue, vaccine hesitancy and funding. We could apply critical thinking to examine all of those issues and, over time, develop potential strategies to address them. For now, based on all our critical thinking to date, the best decision might be, when finding yourself inside in winter with other people, dress warmly, open the window and sit wherever you wish.

Hugo: Phew! I'm so glad we sorted all of that out!

Rachael: Yes, what a relief!

EXAMPLE 1.3

Across the nineteenth century, Europe was beset by waves of cholera – a diarrhoeal disease, now known to be caused by the bacterium *Vibrio cholerae*, that can result in death if left untreated. At the time, the prevailing theory of infectious diseases was that they were caused by bad air arising from dank water and rotting organic matter, evil gases known as 'miasma' (41). During the 1849 and 1854 London cholera epidemics, a distinguished physician and anaesthetist called John Snow decided to conduct some observational studies. He undertook a statistical mapping exercise to investigate the pattern of disease (who it affected and where), ultimately linking water quality to the **outbreaks** and recording cases that were associated with the Broad Street Pump (42). At that time in London, people obtained water from community pumps for drinking, cooking and washing. Because homes and businesses didn't have septic systems, much of the untreated sewage produced was dumped into the Thames River or into streets, where it could contaminate the town wells supplying communal water pumps, such as the Broad Street Pump (43). Once he was able to convince the local authorities about the findings of his rigorous investigation, the pump was disabled and was therefore implicated in no further outbreaks (although later analyses did show that this particular outbreak of cholera was receding anyway (44), not that this takes away from the illustration).

Snow did not believe in miasma theory and instead, based on his own years of research, had developed an alternative theory involving living particles in the diarrhoea of infected patients that then contaminated the drinking water and infected others (45). Strikingly, Snow's explanation anticipated germ theory, some 20 years prior to the first writings about germs and their role in disease. Often now referred to as the 'Father of Modern Epidemiology', although his methods and theories were strongly criticised by powerful medical authorities at the time (46), Snow demonstrated that rigorous observations of epidemiological associations could be used for the basis of public health intervention even before necessarily understanding the precise biological mechanism of disease.

Outbreak: (synonym 'epidemic') An increase in the number of cases, which is beyond that normally expected for a particular region during a particular period of time.

Example 1.3 describes the competing claims of miasma and 'germ' theory; the analysis of information from collecting observations; the evaluation of this information against prevailing belief; reasoning to arrive at a judgement on the cause of the outbreak; the application of this information to problem-solving; and then the action of advocating that the pump be disabled. The story of John Snow and the Broad Street Pump demonstrates how critical thinking has underpinned epidemiology since its birth.

How are health priorities determined?

We have spent quite a bit of time applying critical thinking to the pressing issue of window opening so far in this this chapter, and you might be wondering why I decided to choose this topic. Sadly, I can pretend to no rigorous thinking here, with the concept merely arising at whim. When it comes to priority-setting in health, however, I am happy to report that the approach tends to be rather less cavalier. In fact, strictly evidence-based health priorities are routinely established by authorities at local, national and global levels. The World Health Organization (WHO) is a global body working with nearly 200 member states, with the explicit aim of achieving better health for everyone in the world (47). Commitment to the cause is really important as the WHO priority programs are very expensive and donations by member states make up a large proportion of the budget. The WHO's program in 2020–21 alone, which admittedly did include extra COVID-19 program responsibilities, cost more than US$6 billion, with donations from member states providing 73 per cent of the funding (48). The WHO regularly establishes global health priorities that inform the national health priorities of wealthy countries and has specifically set goals and standards to improve the health of lower-income countries. For instance, for much of this century, member countries have been working towards achieving WHO's eight Millennium Development Goals (MDGs). These included targets for reducing poverty and hunger, improving maternal health, reducing child mortality (deaths) and addressing HIV/AIDS, malaria and a range of other diseases (49). The MDGs have now been superseded by the Sustainable Development Goals, which apply to all countries, not just lower income countries. They are made up of 17 interconnected goals (complete with 169 targets), all supporting the three WHO priorities (also committed to by all member states) of 'moving towards universal health coverage, better protecting people [in] health emergencies and ensuring [good health] and well-being' for people of all ages (50).

In addition to the WHO's global agenda, many countries set their own health priorities. In Australia, for instance, national health priorities have included specific health conditions such as cardiovascular disease, mental health, diabetes and obesity, and also the health of priority populations, such as Indigenous Australians, the aged and prisoners (51, 52). Similar nation-specific health priorities have been set just about everywhere across the globe (53–55).

Determining health priorities involves identifying the main health issues of concern in a given population, evaluating the best ways of addressing those issues, then selecting strategies that are likely to approach the solution in the most effective way at a reasonable cost. Talking about cost here might seem a bit harsh, but in fact this has long been recognised as the best way to ensure equity across populations (56). Governments need to decide how best to spend funds on health from the resources that are available, so taking economics into account when deciding on health programs and services is actually the most ethical way to fairly distribute scarce resources (57). Relative to low-income countries, wealthier countries with fully functioning clinical and public health systems tend to have an easier time addressing priorities. Yet, careful planning and sustained technical and financial support for lower income countries have led to real successes in addressing their particular priority health issues. These successes include controlling guinea worm in Asia and Africa; improved poverty and mortality rates **mortality rates** in Mexico; HIV/AIDS prevention in Thailand; and family planning in Bangladesh (58). Recognising economic reality here, it stands to reason that not everything health-related can be funded even in wealthier countries. Prioritising is a way to ensure that precious funds are spent on the most important issues in each setting.

Mortality rate: Any *rate* where the phenomenon of interest is death. A measure of *mortality*.

But how are these health priorities determined in the first place? Should they be determined on the basis of politics, the level of public outrage or because they are celebrity causes? Or should they be based on how common or serious the problem is and whether it is actually amenable to some sort of (affordable) intervention? All these considerations and more will play a part in deciding the final rankings. However, underpinning these deliberations will be some sort of epidemiological analysis, which requires good-quality data.

One of the earliest types of data collected by the state comprised mortality (death) data, cases of which were first tabulated by John Graunt in London in the seventeenth century (59). I have included a link to a scan of Graunt's original book in the 'Further reading' section at the end of this chapter; see whether you can guess the modern names for the fatal conditions Graunt has tabulated. Graunt has become known as the world's first demographer (although he was actually a successful haberdasher), due to his study of the patterns of deaths recorded in the parishes of London (60). As we heard earlier, data on almost all aspects of human and societal experience are now being collected and stored in surveillance databases and registries all over the world. As well as being extraordinarily useful to researchers (and a source of much entertainment to nerds like me), these data perform a vital function in protecting the health of populations and allowing the identification of emerging priorities in health.

Further enhancing the usefulness of all the information being collected is the introduction of data standards, which have made it possible to compare data from different countries and time periods. For instance, one important standard is known as the 'International Classification of Diseases'. This is an internationally agreed upon, legally mandated system for coding every type of human health issue and it is used around the word at all levels of healthcare (61). The coding system, which includes country-specific adjustments, allows for the surveillance of diseases and conditions and monitoring health service usage, and is linked to medical insurance and payment systems in some countries (62). Introduced for the first time in the nineteenth century, the International Classification of Diseases is now in its 11th revision (ICD-11), with emergency codes for COVID-19 (U07.1 and U07.2) available for both ICD-10 and ICD-11, depending on which revision is in use. Presumably, the ICD-12 revision will formally include new standards for reporting COVID-19.

The mandatory use of international classifications makes it possible for the identification of changes in the pattern of presentations to hospitals across various locations and can be the first sign of a new public health emergency. It is even possible that ICD codes played a part in Chinese authorities noticing the uptick in unspecified viral pneumonia cases (ICD code: J12) when these started turning up in hospitals across Wuhan City.

EXAMPLE 1.4

The WHO China County Office was informed on 31 December 2019 about several pneumonia cases of unknown cause that had been identified in Wuhan City, Hubei Province of China. As of two days ago [3 January 2020], the national authorities in China had reported 44 such cases to WHO, of whom 11 are severely ill. All of the patients are isolated and receiving treatment in hospitals in Wuhan. The main symptom is fever, some are exhibiting breathing difficulty and scans have revealed invasive lesions in both lungs.

Early investigations have suggested an association with a seafood market in Wuhan, where some of the patients were working. There is currently little evidence for person-to-person transmission as none of the healthcare workers involved in the care of patients are reported to be infected. The market has now been closed for sanitation and disinfection.

Public health responses to date:

- Authorities have identified 121 close contacts of the cases. These contacts are now under medical observation and follow-up of further close contacts continues.
- Investigations to identify the pathogen and other causal factors have been implemented.
- Closure and sanitation of the market was undertaken from 1 January and further hygiene investigations are being undertaken.
- The situation is being monitored closely by the WHO, in communication with Chinese authorities.

Source: WHO Disease Outbreak News, 5 January 2020 (63).

Disease surveillance

As well as healthcare settings, data on a large range of human conditions are collected and notified to population-specific surveillance systems in most countries, as well as reported to international bodies. Disease surveillance, the routine collection and evaluation of health data by states, plays a critical role in identifying new health issues and monitoring those already prioritised. Routine data collection and evaluation allow for the monitoring of changes in the occurrence of disease (or other health outcome), such as changes in disease frequency – whether sudden and requiring immediate action or occurring over a longer term, when they may guide future service need. Infectious disease surveillance also allows for the identification of outbreaks and new pathogens (64), such as SARS-CoV-2. Importantly, surveillance is used to inform public health action, evaluate prevention efforts and guide future resource planning (65).

Routine, and usually mandated, surveillance is conducted by states on a vast range of health issues, including (but not limited to):

- births, deaths and marriages
- communicable diseases
- cancer
- injuries
- birth and neonatal outcomes
- vaccination coverage
- hospital infection control
- zoonotic diseases (those that transmit from animals to humans)
- quality of life.

The 'routine' part of routine surveillance is its most important and useful aspect as continued scrutiny of the status quo is the only way to notice when changes occur. Crucially, surveillance must only be conducted on conditions for which some sort of prevention or remedial action is available. In addition to prevention opportunity, to make it on the surveillance hit list (or to be listed as 'notifiable'), the condition might affect a lot of people, be really serious or lead to deaths, have a large social or economic impact, be infectious and/or be associated with a high degree of public or political concern.

Hugo: Politics again?

Rachael: Yeah, that's a few times you have mentioned politics!

Author (Emma): Well, health and health policy doesn't happen in a vacuum. People working in health are always angling for funds for research and for health interventions, often requesting new laws and regulations to help them improve health. Politicians are more constrained by legislative agenda and budgetary concerns, as well as the need to respond to their constituents. Arriving at a consensus can be a tricky process of negotiating and balancing the scientific evidence against fiscal and political imperatives (66).

There are a few different approaches to undertaking surveillance, but the most common systems are either passive or active. Passive systems are the most common type of state surveillance systems that rely on health-related services, schools, councils and other agencies sending in notifications of particular disease. The notification usually comes with disease-specific and demographic data, and information about major disease risk factors. Once established, passive surveillance systems are inexpensive and simple to run compared with more active systems. However, relying on the ongoing cooperation of those reporting cases comes at a price. To keep the reporting burden as low as possible – which is essential to achieving ongoing effort from notifiers – only the smallest amount of accompanying information is usually requested, which means we get to know the bare minimum about each affected person. Sometimes not even the small amount of information requested is reported completely, and not reporting cases at all is common. This can all result in things like outbreaks and clusters being identified late or missed altogether.

Active surveillance, on the other hand, focuses on heath personnel periodically collecting data in defined populations. Surveillance staff might visit specific locations, either routinely or when several cases have emerged, to interview people and collect data on the condition of interest, environmental context, demographic details, social networks and family history. Relative to passive surveillance, active systems tend to produce the most complete data, and provide more capacity to detect outbreaks and the ability to identify potential contacts of the cases (in the case of communicable diseases). However, they can be far more expensive and labour-intensive than passive systems.

It is worth noting here that events such as of clusters of disease, outbreaks and new diseases identified via routine passive surveillance will usually trigger an investigation and/or period of enhanced surveillance. This combines the attributes and advantages of both approaches.

Disease surveillance provides the quantitative evidence required for determining health priorities that underpin equitable health policy. Yet, despite many improvements coming under WHO programs, not all countries have the same capacity to develop, implement and maintain surveillance systems that are appropriate to their regions (67). There are some examples of effective global surveillance efforts, which include surveillance programs focusing on antimicrobial resistance (a gonococcal-specific program and antimicrobial resistance in general) and influenza (68–70), but there is still a lot of work to do. Improving the capacity for identifying and responding to global health priorities, infectious and non-communicable, new and emerging will need the concerted effort and investment of all countries to improve surveillance globally.

Using epidemiology

We have heard a bit about the need for good-quality data and how they can be collected. The next chapters of this book will discuss methods of data collection in more detail and how this information can be analysed and used to describe health and social phenomena, identify associated risk factors and disease causes, and inform the development and evaluation of effective health interventions. For now, though, we will have a brief taste of some of the methods that epidemiology can bring to bear on issues of concern today.

First, we do need to get something clear – it might seem obvious, but surveillance is not the same as research. Surveillance is about using epidemiological information so appropriate monitoring and control measures can be used and (most importantly) it must be linked to a public health response. The purpose of research is to contribute to the scientific body of knowledge by identifying or synthesising epidemiological data, or evaluating new interventions – all of which can then inform the development of appropriate control measures. Both strengthen and inform each other and both are concerned with obtaining and analysing accurate, high-quality data. But in characterising these information sources, we really need to consider intents, motivations and objectives as these have implications for the conclusions that can be drawn from the data derived. For instance, with surveillance data we must be aware that only a fraction of cases are notified to the state (called the 'reporting fraction'), and with data emerging from research we have to be concerned with representativeness of samples selected for research. Essentially, there are overlapping agendas, but surveillance is governed by regulation and research by ethical responsibilities and expectations. One is almost always linked to public health action based on the data (which can lead to research questions); the other is almost always linked to discovering new information (which can inform the development of public health strategies). In practice, it is not always easy to define the borders!

Types of study epidemiological designs

From the enormous number of studies published in the scientific literature over the years, you might imagine there could be an almost infinite variety of research designs. In reality, there are just a handful of broad epidemiological approaches to collecting data, with all the fancy study types you might read about essentially representing variations to the theme as well as a bunch of synonyms (with which, I am afraid, epidemiology abounds). In Figure 1.2, you can see that I have boiled down the types of studies to two main categories: experimental designs that mainly involve doing things to people, and **non-experimental designs** that mainly involve observing what happens to people. The real complexity lies in posing a measurable scientific question, then selecting the most appropriate study type (or types) and data sources to answer it.

Non-experimental design: A type of epidemiological study that utilises data on exposures and outcomes without any intervention on behalf of those conducting the study, other than to analyse the data in some way. 'Observational study design' is another term used here.

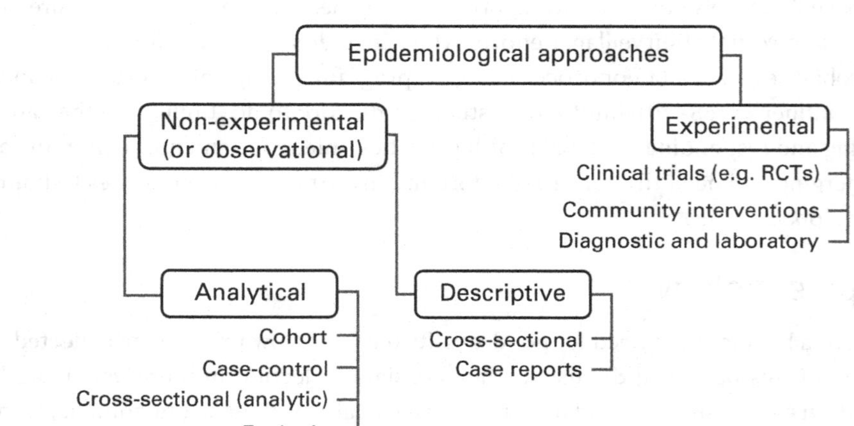

Figure 1.2 Epidemiological study designs

Study design: The way an epidemiological study has been executed.

In Figure 1.2, the non-experimental arm branches off into two basic types of **study design**. The descriptive branch list study types that can be designed to describe health states and events and/or their distribution in the population. The sorts of information that descriptive studies can determine are: what proportion of a specified population is affected by a particular phenomenon (epidemiologists call this **prevalence**), or how many people developed a particular health condition in a specified population over a specified period of time (epidemiologists calculate these as **incidence rates**).

Typically, descriptive studies can be considered as a type of 'snapshot' of what the story is in a given population at a particular point in time. You could say that descriptive studies address the 'what' and 'how much' question. The types of scientific questions that could be answered by descriptive designs are presented in Example 1.5.

Prevalence: The proportion of a specified population affected by a specified disease or health state at a specified point in time.

Incidence rate: The rate at which new cases of a specified disease or health state arise in the population at risk over a specified period of time.

Analytical study design: A type of epidemiological study in which the analytical intent is to explore causal relationships.

Relative risk: (synonym 'rate ratio') A ratio of the risk of an event in those exposed to a specified risk factor to the risk of the same event in those not exposed. In a cohort study, the observed incidence in the exposed group is divided by the observed incidence in the unexposed group to calculate the relative risk.

Odds ratio: (synonyms 'cross-product ratio' and 'relative odds') A ratio of the odds of exposure in cases (or an affected group) relative to the odds of the same exposure in cases (or an unaffected group).

Cohort study: (synonyms 'concurrent', 'prospective', 'follow-up', 'incidence' studies) An observational study in which defined populations are identified on the basis of whether they have been exposed to specific health-related factors; health outcomes for exposed and unexposed groups are compared over time. Data collection may be prospective or retrospective.

EXAMPLE 1.5

What proportion of people in my country were vaccinated against COVID-19 in 2022?

- *A cross-sectional study.* This could involve accessing data from a vaccine surveillance system (or administering a survey if no data were available), and calculating the proportion (or prevalence) using data on the size of the population of interest in 2022.

What's up with that guy that turned up at the hospital with the strange rash?

- *A case report.* This could involve producing a detailed description of the appearance of the patient's strange rash and any other symptoms they might have. The report could include patient accounts of any known risk factors, the treatment applied and any resolution to the issue.

The second branch of the non-experimental arm in Figure 1.2 depicts **analytical study designs.** These studies use a range of sophisticated methods for investigating the determinants of health and illness. The sorts of information that analytical studies can provide include whether potential exposures and outcomes are related to each other (epidemiologists call these 'associations') and what the strength of those relationships is (epidemiologists often measure this with ratios such as **relative risk** and **odds ratios** – much more on this later). These analytical studies are still observational, in that nobody is intervening or doing things to people, but they build on purely descriptive studies to address the 'how' and 'why' questions. The types of scientific questions that could be answered by analytic observational designs are presented in Example 1.6.

EXAMPLE 1.6

Over 2022, how did COVID-19 outcomes differ between people who got vaccinated in January and those who didn't get vaccinated?

- *A **cohort study**.* This could involve collecting information from people at the beginning of the year (the **cohort**), sorting them into vaccinated ('exposed') and unvaccinated ('unexposed') groups, then following them up to learn what happened to them by the end of the year. A range of outcomes could be compared between the two groups, which might include contracting COVID-19, **severity** of illness, hospitalisations and deaths.

Cohort: A group of people who share certain characteristics, such as being in the same work environment or being born in the same year. Also refers to the participants in a study being followed up over time.

Severity: The impact of a health phenomenon.

Case-control study: (synonyms 'case-referent' and 'retrospective' studies) An observational study that starts by identifying people with a condition of interest and a comparable group of people without the condition and retrospectively comparing their exposure histories to determine which exposures might be associated with case status.

Ecological studies: These are also known as correlational studies. Building upon our understanding of 'longitudinal' cross-sectional surveys, ecological studies analyse existing data at the group or population level. The quantitative measure used to determine a relationship between exposure and outcome in these studies is correlation.

Incidence: Synonymous with 'incident case' or 'incidence rate', depending on context.

Randomised controlled trial (RCT): an experimental study design in which participants are randomly allocated to intervention (or study) groups or control group to receive a treatment or therapy or not. The outcomes are rigorously compared (performance, cure or improvement, deaths, safety, side-effects, etc.).

EXAMPLE 1.6 Continued

What sorts of things might have been involved in the development of the strange rash that guy at the hospital had?

- *A **case-control study**.* This could involve finding people who had developed the same type of rash at some stage ('cases'), and another group that didn't develop a rash but were otherwise pretty much the same sorts of people ('controls') and asking them about things that may have been exposed to in the past that could be associated with the rash. History of a range of potential exposures could then be compared between the two groups, which might include dietary factors, travel history, environmental factors and pet ownership.

Is there something different about students who benefit from meditation compared with those who remain stressed?

- *An analytic cross-sectional study.* This might involve surveying a group of students who have completed a session of meditation therapy and comparing those with stress levels (the outcome) against a range of things that might be affect treatment outcome, such as age and sex, educational achievement, financial status and housing situation, and previous history of stress.

What is the relationship between COVID-19 cases and vaccination in different countries?

- *An **ecological study**.* This could involve finding estimates of COVID-19 vaccine coverage (the proportion of the population who had been vaccinated) from multiple countries and then comparing that information with COVID-19 country-specific **incidence** over the same time period to see whether the relationship between vaccine coverage and infection rates follows a similar pattern across countries.

The other broad category of study designs (according to Figure 1.2) includes the experimental types. In very general terms, these are studies that are designed to evaluate interventions such as treatments and therapies, vaccinations and diagnostic tests. The sorts of information that experimental studies can provide include how effective and safe interventions are, how well they are tolerated by people and what outcomes they are associated with. Some experimental studies are conducted entirely in laboratories and don't really involve doing things to people in themselves, but instead provide evidence to inform the development of new tests, treatments and procedures. Experimental studies address the 'how good' questions. The types of scientific questions that could be answered by experimental designs are presented in Example 1.7.

EXAMPLE 1.7

Can worm treatment help people with a touch of COVID-19 get better more quickly?

- A ***randomised controlled trial (RCT)***: This real-life study (71) involved randomly allocating people with mild COVID-19 infection into two groups. One group took three days of the worm treatment (the intervention group) and the other took an identical-looking but inactive treatment (**placebo**) for the same amount of time (the control group).

Neither the participants nor the researchers knew which group they were in during the study. Information about symptoms were collected before and during treatment (worm treatment and placebo) and follow-up continued after all symptoms had resolved. Various outcomes were compared between the two groups, such as length of time experiencing COVID-19 symptoms, side-effects, hospitalisations and deaths. In this study, worm treatment didn't make a difference to the length of COVID-19 symptoms.

Placebo: An inactive or inert medication or procedure that simulates an experimental medication or procedure being evaluated in a trial.

How can we reduce stress in the community?

- *A community intervention.* This could involve surveying the stress levels and related factors in the residents of two geographically separate communities (or local government areas) with similar demographic and economic profiles. The intervention community could be provided with free access to new health and well-being programs, while the control community could be directed to existing services in their area. After the study period, all residents could be surveyed again and a range of outcomes compared between the two communities, such as change in stress levels, health program access and satisfaction with services provided.

Are self-administered rapid tests for COVID-19 as accurate as PCR tests administered by health professionals?

- *A diagnostic study.* Another real-life study (72) compared the accuracy of a number of rapid antigen tests (RATs) with a 'gold standard' test (the PCR test that only health professionals can administer). On average, it was found that the RATs were only able to detect the virus in known PCR positive samples 30 per cent of the time (epidemiologists call this **sensitivity**), although they were 100 per cent accurate in testing negative from samples that were known to have no virus (epidemiologists call this **specificity**). I guess a test that mostly tests negative is not that useful, although if you got a positive RAT result you could be pretty sure you have COVID!

Sensitivity: The ability of a test to identify a particular disease (or disease marker) in people who truly have the disease. Measured as a proportion against a 'gold standard' test.

Specificity: The ability of a test to identify the absence of disease in those who truly don't have the disease (or disease marker). Measured as a proportion against a 'gold standard' test.

It is important to note that not all questions can be answered using epidemiological techniques. If we wanted to understand the phenomenon of homelessness, for instance, we might use epidemiological methods to determine how many people are currently homeless, identify risk factors for homelessness and quantify the strength of relationship between those risk factors and homelessness. But if we wanted to understand the actual experience of homelessness – how it makes individuals feel and what meaning homelessness has for them – only qualitative methods would do. Qualitative methods use non-numerical methods including in-depth interviewing of people experiencing phenomena of interest to explore things such as people's attitudes and beliefs, social context and cultural realities. Increasingly, researchers employ both quantitative and qualitative approaches in a single study (known as 'mixed methods') to ensure a more complete understanding of health issues. Deciding which approach and which study design to use really depends on what you want to know – the scientific question.

Rachael: That was a lot of information!

Hugo: Is this going to be in the test?

Author (Emma): Those examples were intended to demonstrate how important the scientific question is to determining the type of approach required to address it. In the coming chapters, a lot more detail will be provided about all these types of epidemiological concepts and approaches.

Role of epidemiology

Commonly referred to as the 'epidemiological transition', the world has shifted from an environment where infectious diseases were overwhelmingly the main health threats to an environment in which non-infectious and chronic disease predominate, at least in industrialised countries. The changing environment has been linked to widespread population changes and public health advances that have included the end of waves of cholera and plague, improved sanitation and food availability, and the introduction of antibiotics and vaccinations (73). The focus of epidemiology is also thought to have transitioned from its early days, from being mostly preoccupied with clean air, clean water and infectious disease to concentrating on non-communicable diseases, the ageing population and so-called 'lifestyle' diseases and their risk factors. In reality, this shift is probably as illusionary as the concept of the single 'epidemiological transition' itself, which has now turned out to be neither as linear nor as unidirectional as was once assumed (74).

As well as strictly physiological factors, it is now understood that health is influenced by a number of social, economic, political and cultural influences, collectively known as the 'social determinants of health' (75). These social determinants can determine the health of individuals, societal groups and whole populations. The world hasn't so much transitioned to a new health reality as splintered into different health realities everywhere all at the same time. We have actually transitioned to a state of greater inequity in health, within and between countries. It is now also clear that epidemiology has not changed focus but spread its attention wider and transitioned to a role that recognises the social determinants of health and understands social and economic inequity and the health outcomes associated with them.

At the start of this chapter, I mentioned that multiple 'flavours' (or fields) of epidemiologists work across the gamut of health-related scientific endeavour. Every one of these flavours is currently responding to the multiple issues arising in a world that is defined by economic and health inequity. The patchy 'epidemiology transition' has ushered in the emergence of new communicable diseases and the re-emergence of diseases thought to have long disappeared. Diseases of the aged have increased in some places, while infants and young children continue to die from preventable diseases elsewhere (76). Nutritional deficiency and over-nutrition are occurring side by side (77); even access to clean water is no longer a sure bet and in some countries it never has been (78).

Thinking about the COVID-19 pandemic, it is easy to see the footprint of epidemiology everywhere, from the identification of the first cases arising, to characterisation of the new virus and its genomic analysis, to describing transmission modes and identifying protective behaviours, to new vaccinations and treatments and their evaluation. Epidemiologists are involved in surveillance of COVID-19 in populations, as well as the surveillance and evaluation of new strains of the coronavirus. They continue to investigate new COVID-19 outbreaks, predict new waves of infection in the population and investigate behavioural trends in protective behaviours and vaccination uptake and 'hesitancy'.

Rachael: I never thought about being an epidemiologist, but it sounds cool!

Hugo: Yeah, seems like there's lots of cool stuff to do, but let's see what else in this book …

Conclusion

In this chapter, we have learnt about epidemiology, the importance of good-quality data and how they can be collected. We also had a whirlwind tour of a variety of different ways to collect data in examining surveillance and epidemiological research designs. Hopefully, we have now managed to achieve all the learning objectives of the chapter, as summarised below.

Learning objective 1: Appreciate the importance of critical thinking and understand how it underpins epidemiology

In this chapter, we learnt how the process of critical thinking could be applied to everyday and epidemiological problems to arrive at informed decisions. Together, we employed the stages of analysing, evaluating, reasoning, problem-solving and decision-making to a hypothetical claim (that you could catch a cold from the draught of an open window), and along the way learnt a good deal about what constitutes quality data and how to evaluate information.

Learning objective 2: Describe the role of epidemiology in identifying and responding to health priorities

We heard how evidence-based health priorities are routinely established by authorities at local, national and global levels on the basis of epidemiologically identified health issues, and the selection of the most effective and affordable solution to address those issues. We explored different types of disease surveillance and how surveillance data could be used to identify emerging health issues and monitor health issues that are already prioritised.

Learning objective 3: Understand the relationship between the scientific question and epidemiological research methods

The various types of epidemiological studies were introduced. Hypothetical scientific questions were posed to demonstrate how each type of study could feasibly answer those questions. In doing so, we touched on the types of measurements and outcome measures associated with each type of study design, which will be explored in much detail in the coming chapters.

Further reading

Graunt J. *Natural and Political Observations Mentioned in a Following Index, and Made upon the Bills of Mortality*. John Graunt; 1665. https://echo.mpiwg-berlin.mpg.de/ECHOdocuView?url=/permanent/echo/mpi_rostock/Graunt_1665/index.meta&pn=1

Murray J, Cohen AL. Infectious disease surveillance. In *International Encyclopedia of Public Health*. Elsevier, 2017:222–9. https://doi.org/10.1016/B978-0-12-803678-5.00517-8

The Foundation for Critical Thinking. A brief history of the idea of critical thinking. 2019. www.criticalthinking.org/pages/a-brief-history-of-the-idea-of-critical-thinking/408

World Health Organization. *The Global Health Observatory.* 2023. www.who.int/data/gho/publications/world-health-statistics

World Health Organization. *International Statistical Classification of Diseases and Related Health Problems (ICD).* 2023. www.who.int/standards/classifications/classification-of-diseases

Questions

Answers are available at the end of the book.

Multiple-choice questions

1. Which of the following is true about critical thinking?
   A – Describes a largely negative outlook on life
   B – Critical thinkers are born, not made
   C – Provides a way to come to evidence-based conclusions
   D – Applies only to limited fields

2. What are some important ways to critically evaluate information?
   A – Assess the authority and agenda of the information source
   B – Consider the level of trust in the person providing the information
   C – Measure the amount number followers that person has on social media
   D – All of the above

3. Which of the following would you say best describes the chief purpose of health-related surveillance?
   A – Prevent disease occurrence and maintain good health and well-being across populations
   B – Provide quality data to undertake research on specific health issues and contribute to the knowledge base
   C – Monitor changes in disease occurrence and identify emerging health issues in populations that are linked to public health responses
   D – Track disease progression, evaluate treatments and contribute to evidence-based clinical decision-making

4. What are the main considerations for global and national bodies in determining health priorities?
   A – The prevalence and/or severity of health issues of concern in a given population
   B – The availably of cost-effective strategies for addressing particular health concerns
   C – Technical and financial capacity to implement appropriate health programs
   D – All of the above

5. Which of the following questions could be answered by using an observational epidemiological design?
   A – What was the lived experience of being locked down during the COVID-19 pandemic?
   B – Does the use of antiviral medications decrease the duration of illness in people infected with SARS-CoV-2?
   C – How many vaccinated people were diagnosed with COVID-19 during 2022 relative to unvaccinated people
   D – How accurate are later generation rapid antigen tests (RATs) for COVID-19?

Short-answer questions

1. During the COVID-19 pandemic, many governments and organisations mandated COVID-19 vaccines in health settings, workplaces, sporting venues and even for entry into some countries by travellers. Undertake a quick search of the internet (don't spend too long on this!) and outline the competing claims of proponents and opponents of mandating vaccinations for healthcare workers.
2. Evaluating the authority of information was an important part of critical thinking. Visit the site of the open-access journal *BMC Public Health* (https://bmcpublichealth.biomedcentral.com) and search for a paper on any topic, then report the affiliations of the authors, the funding sources for the research they reported and whether they reported any competing interests (which is usually found at the end and/or under the 'ethics declarations' section).
3. In your own words, describe how you think epidemiology applies critical thinking to health problems.
4. International Classification of Diseases (ICD) (now in its 11th revision) is the internationally agreed upon coding system for every type of human health issue requiring care, which is used all around the word at all levels of healthcare. Think of a specific health condition of interest to you, access the ICD-11 browser hosted by the World Health Organization (https://icd.who.int/browse11/l-m/en) or search for 'ICD' at the World Health Organization website (www.who.int). Locate the ICD-10 code that best describes your selected disease.
5. Visit the World Health Organization and review the Sustainable Development Goals (SDG) (www.who.int/europe/about-us/our-work/sustainable-development-goals). The three interconnected SDG goals are to end poverty, protect the planet and promote health for all. See whether you can find and name the broad areas of the nine targets associated with Goal 3.
6. At a communicable disease control branch, notification data are discussed by the public health team every week. They report patterns of specific diseases occurring up to that week and compare these with notifications up to the same date on previous years. They notice that one particular disease, commonly caused by bacteria contamination, has a larger number of cases reported relative to normal (from past patterns), which have been notified from roughly the same geographical area. They suspect there may be an outbreak of some kind and send out a public health team to collect further information and investigate epidemiological links between the cases. What sort of surveillance system (passive or active) do you think helped to identify this potential outbreak, and why do you think so?
7. In your own words, how would you describe the role of epidemiology in determining health priorities?
8. Look at Figure 1.3. Can you describe and interpret the chart?
9. You work in a city office and have noticed that a lot of people are taking time off on Mondays. What sort of scientific question would you pose, and what general epidemiological approach would you select to answer this question?
10. What are some of the key changes that have occurred during the period often referred to as the 'epidemiological transition'?

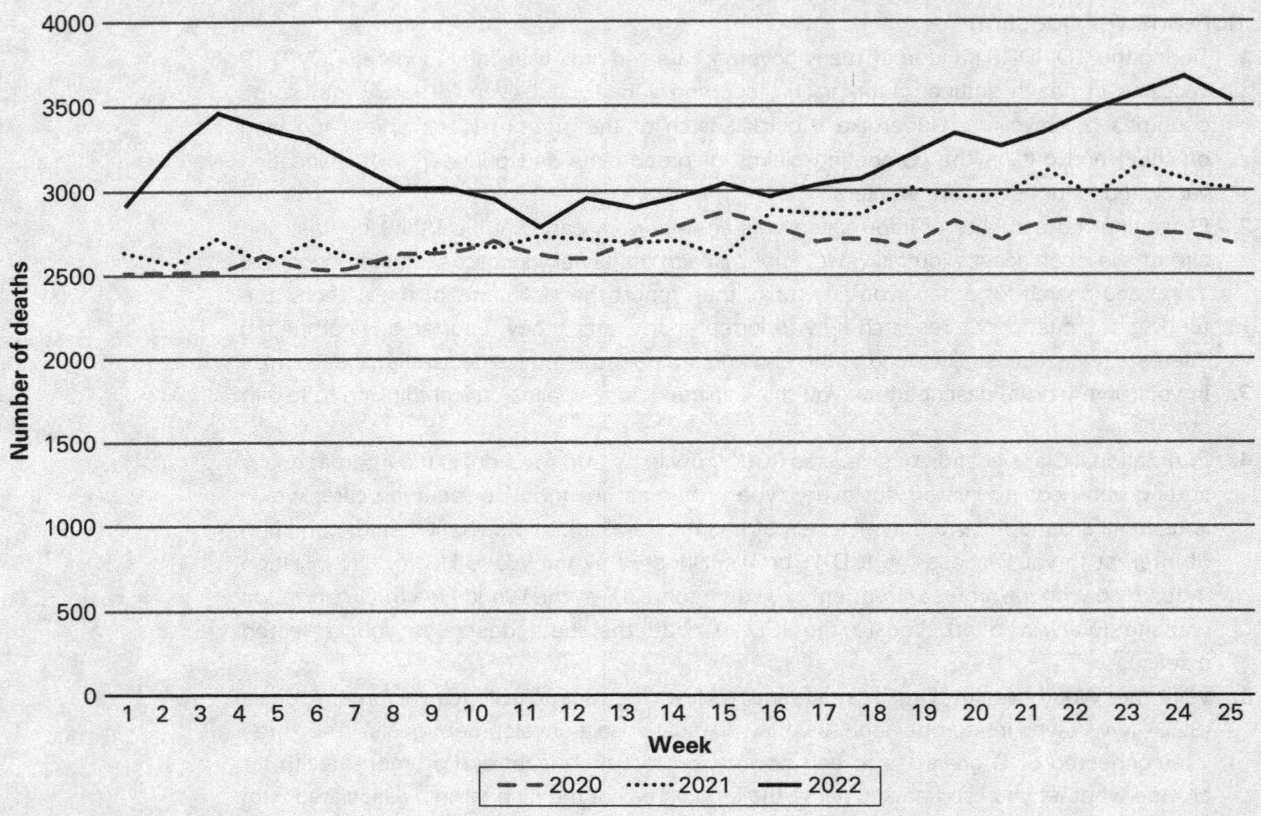

Figure 1.3 Medically certified deaths per week in Australia, January to June, 2020– 22. Data from (19).

References

1. Last J. *A Dictionary of Epidemiology*. 2nd ed. Oxford University Press; 1988.
2. Krieger N. *Epidemiology and the People's Health: Theory and Context*: Oxford University Press; 2011.
3. Bassham G, Irwin W, Nardone H, Wallace JM. *Critical Thinking: A Student's Introduction*. 4th ed. McGraw-Hill; 2011.
4. The Foundation for Critical Thinking. *A Brief History of the Idea of Critical Thinking*. Foundation for Critical Thinking; 2019.
5. Paul R, Elder L. Critical thinking: The art of Socratic questioning. *Journal of Developmental Education*. 2007;31(1):36–7.
6. Carey TA, Mullan RJ. What is Socratic questioning? *Psychotherapy: Theory, Research, Practice, Training*. 2004;41:217–26.
7. Decarlo J, Eliason G. Salem Witch Trials. In: Bernat FP, Frailing K, eds. *The Encyclopedia of Women and Crime*. Wiley; 2023:1–6.
8. Goodare J. *The European Witch-Hunt*. Routledge; 2016.
9. Khubchandani J, Sharma S, Price JH, Wiblishauser MJ, Sharma M, Webb FJ. COVID-19 Vaccination hesitancy in the United States: A rapid national assessment. *Journal of Community Health*. 2021;46(2):270–7.
10. Goodman J, Carmichael F. Coronavirus: Bill Gates 'microchip' conspiracy theory and other vaccine claims fact-checked. *BBC News*; 2020. www.bbc.com/news/52847648
11. Callaway E. Fast-evolving COVID variants complicate vaccine updates. *Nature*. 2022;607:18–19.

12. Stupple EJN, Maratos FA, Elander J, Hunt TE, Cheung KYF, Aubeeluck AV. Development of the Critical Thinking Toolkit (CriTT): A measure of student attitudes and beliefs about critical thinking. *Thinking Skills and Creativity*. 2017;23:91–100.

13. Butler HA, Pentoney C, Bong MP. Predicting real-world outcomes: Critical thinking ability is a better predictor of life decisions than intelligence. *Thinking Skills and Creativity*. 2017;25:38–46.

14. Butterworth J, Thwaites G. *Thinking Skills: Critical Thinking and Problem Solving*. 2nd ed. Cambridge University Press; 2013.

15. Facione NC, Facione PA. Critical thinking and clinical judgment. In: Facione NC, Facione PA, eds. *Critical Thinking and Clinical Reasoning in the Health Sciences: An International Multidisciplinary Teaching Anthology*. California Academic Press LLC; 2007. p.1–13.

16. Helman CG. 'Feed a cold, starve a fever': Folk models of infection in an English suburban community, and their relation to medical treatment. *Culture, Medicine and Psychiatry*. 1978;2(2):107–37.

17. Kohanski MA, Lo LJ, Waring MS. Review of indoor aerosol generation, transport, and control in the context of COVID-19. *International Forum of Allergy & Rhinology*. 2020;10(10):1173–9.

18. World Health Organization. *The Global Health Observatory 2023*. www.who.int/data/gho/publications/world-health-statistics

19. Australian Bureau of Statistics. National, state and territory population. ABS; 2022. www.abs.gov.au/statistics/people/population/national-state-and-territory-population/latest-release

20. SA Health. Disease notification: 5 year & YTD comparisons as at 11-Feb-2023. SA Health, Communicable Disease Control Branch; 2023. www.sahealth.sa.gov.au/wps/wcm/connect/public+content/sa+health+internet/about+us/health+statistics/surveillance+of+notifiable+conditions/surveillance+of+notifiable+conditions

21. Sullivan SG, Carlson S, Cheng AC, Chilver MB, Dwyer DE, Irwin M et al. Where has all the influenza gone? The impact of COVID-19 on the circulation of influenza and other respiratory viruses, Australia, March to September 2020. *Eurosurveillance*. 2020;25(47):2001847.

22. Chowell G, Miller MA, Viboud C. Seasonal influenza in the United States, France, and Australia: Transmission and prospects for control. *Epidemiology & Infection*. 2008;136(6):852–64.

23. Heikkinen T, Järvinen A. The common cold. *The Lancet*. 2003;361(9351):51–9.

24. Thornton GM, Fleck BA, Kroeker E, Dandnayak D, Fleck N, Zhong L et al. The impact of heating, ventilation, and air conditioning design features on the transmission of viruses, including the 2019 novel coronavirus: A systematic review of ventilation and coronavirus. *PLOS Global Public Health*. 2022;2(7):e0000552.

25. Koskela HO. Cold air-provoked respiratory symptoms: The mechanisms and management. *International Journal of Circumpolar Health*. 2007;66(2):91–100.

26. Lowen AC, Steel J. Roles of humidity and temperature in shaping influenza seasonality. *Journal of Virology*. 2014;88(14):7692–5.

27. Leung NHL. Transmissibility and transmission of respirator viruses. *Nature Reviews Microbiology*. 2021;19:528–45.

28. Mourtzoukou EG, Falagas ME. Exposure to cold and respiratory tract infections. *The International Journal of Tuberculosis and Lung Disease*. 2007;11(9):938–43.

29. Furnham A. Explaining health and illness: Lay perceptions on current and future health, the causes of illness, and the nature of recovery. *Social Science & Medicine*. 1994;39(5):715–25.

30. Wang Y, McKee M, Torbica A, Stuckler D. Systematic literature review on the spread of health-related misinformation on social media. *Social Science & Medicine*. 2019;240:112552.

31. Talwar S, Dhir A, Kaur P, Zafar N, Alrasheedy M. Why do people share fake news? Associations between the dark side of social media use and fake news sharing behavior. *Journal of Retailing and Consumer Services*. 2019;51:72–82.

32. Farivar S, Wang F, Turel O. Followers' problematic engagement with influencers on social media: An attachment theory perspective. *Computers in Human Behavior*. 2022;133:107288.

33. Taylor J. ACCC to crack down on misleading influencer endorsements across social media. *The Guardian*. 27 January 2023.

34. Kelly J, Sadeghieh T, Adeli K. Peer review in scientific publications: Benefits, critiques, & a survival guide. *EJIFCC*. 2014;25(3):227–43.

35. Chiu N-C, Chi H, Tai Y-L, Peng C-C, Tseng C-Y, Chen C-C et al. Impact of wearing masks, hand hygiene, and social distancing on influenza, enterovirus, and all-cause pneumonia during the coronavirus pandemic: Retrospective national epidemiological surveillance study. *Journal of Medical Internet Research*. 2020;22(8):e21257.

36. Haktanir A, Can N, Seki T, Kurnaz MF, Dilmaç B. Do we experience pandemic fatigue? Current state, predictors, and prevention. *Current Psychology*. 2022;41(10):7314–25.

37. Dawood FS, Chung JR, Kim SS, Zimmerman RK, Nowalk MP, Jackson ML et al. Interim estimates of 2019–20 seasonal influenza vaccine effectiveness – United States, February 2020. *Morbidity and Mortality Weekly Report*. 2020;69(7):177–82.

38. Tregoning JS, Flight KE, Higham SL, Wang Z, Pierce BF. Progress of the COVID-19 vaccine effort: Viruses, vaccines and variants versus efficacy, effectiveness and escape. *Nature Reviews Immunology*. 2021;21(10):626–36.

39. Morens DM, Taubenberger JK, Fauci AS. Rethinking next-generation vaccines for coronaviruses, influenzaviruses, and other respiratory viruses. *Cell Host & Microbe*. 2023;31(1):146–57.

40. Nair AN, Anand P, George A, Mondal N. A review of strategies and their effectiveness in reducing indoor airborne transmission and improving indoor air quality. *Environmental Research*. 2022;213:113579.

41. Karamanou M, Panayiotakopoulos G, Tsoucalas G, Kousoulis AA, Androutsos G. From miasmas to germs: A historical approach to theories of infectious disease transmission. *Le Infezioni in Medicina*. 2012;20(1):58–62.

42. Newsom SWB. The history of infection control: Cholera – John Snow and the beginnings of epidemiology. *British Journal of Infection Control*. 2005;6(6):12–15.

43. Newsom SWB. Pioneers in infection control: John Snow, Henry Whitehead, the Broad Street Pump, and the beginnings of geographical epidemiology. *Journal of Hospital Infection*. 2006;64(3):210–16.

44. McLeod KS. Our sense of Snow: The myth of John Snow in medical geography. *Social Science & Medicine*. 2000;50(7):923–35.

45. Tulodziecki D. A case study in explanatory power: John Snow's conclusions about the pathology and transmission of cholera. *Studies in History and Philosophy of Biological and Biomedical Sciences*. 2011;42(3):306–16.

46. Cameron D, Jones IG. John Snow, the Broad Street Pump and modern epidemiology. *International Journal of Epidemiology*. 1983;12(4):393–6.

47. World Health Organization. *Working for Better Health for Everyone, Everywhere*. www.who.int/about/what-we-do/who-brochure

48. World Health Organization. *For a Safer, Healthier, and Fairer World: Results Report – Programme budget 2020–2021*. www.who.int/about/accountability/results/who-results-report-2020-2021

49. World Health Organization. *Millennium Development Goals (MDGs)*. www.who.int/news-room/fact-sheets/detail/millennium-development-goals-(mdgs)

50. World Health Organization. *Sustainable Development Goals*. www.who.int/europe/about-us/our-work/sustainable-development-goals

51. Australian Government Department of Health and Aged Care. *National Preventive Health Strategy 2021–2030*. Commonwealth of Australia; 2021.

52. Australian Institute of Health and Welfare and Commonwealth Department of Health and Family Services. *First Report on National Health Priority Areas 1996*. AIHW and DHFS; 1997.

53. Ministry of Health. *New Zealand Health Strategy: Future Direction*. NZ Government; 2016.

54. Public Health England. *PHE Strategy 2020–25*. UK Government; 2019.

55. National Prevention Council. *National Prevention Strategy: America's Plan for Better Health and Wellness*. US Department of Health and Human Services; 2011.

56. World Bank. *World Development Report: Investing in Health*. Oxford University Press, World Bank; 1993.

57. Tragakes E, Vienonen M. *Key Issues in Rationing and Priority Setting for Health Care Services*. World Health Organization; 1998.
58. Jamison DT, Breman JG, Measham AR, Alleyne G, Claeson M, Evans DB et al. *Priorities in Health*. International Bank for Reconstruction and Development; 2006.
59. Graunt J. *Natural and Political Observations Mentioned in a Following Index, and Made upon the Bills of Mortality*. John Graunt; 1665.
60. Encylopaedia Britannica. John Graunt. 2022. www.britannica.com/biography/John-Graunt
61. World Health Organization. *International Statistical Classification of Diseases and Related Health Problems (ICD)*. WHO; 2023. www.who.int/standards/classifications/classification-of-diseases
62. National Center for Health Statistics. *International Classification of Diseases (ICD-10-CM/PCS) Transition – Background Atlanta, USA*. Centers for Disease Control and Prevention; 2015. https://archive.cdc.gov/#/details?url=https://www.cdc.gov/nchs/icd/icd10cm_pcs_background.html
63. World Health Organization. Pneumonia of unknown cause. Media release; 5 January 2020. www.who.int/emergencies/disease-outbreak-news/item/2020-DON229
64. Murray J, Cohen AL. Infectious disease surveillance. In: *International Encyclopedia of Public Health*. 2017:222–9. https://doi.org/10.1016/B978-0-12-803678-5.00517-8
65. Bonita R, Beaglehole R, Kjellström T. *Basic Epidemiology*. 2nd ed. World Health Organization; 2006.
66. Hunter EL. Politics and public health: Engaging the third rail. *Journal of Public Health Management and Practice*. 2016;22(5):436–41.
67. Worsley-Tonks KEL, Bender JB, Deem SL, Ferguson AW, Fèvre EM, Martins DJ et al. Strengthening global health security by improving disease surveillance in remote rural areas of low-income and middle-income countries. *The Lancet Global Health*. 2022;10(4):e579–e84.
68. World Health Organization. *Global Influenza Surveillance and Response System (GISRS)*. WHO; 2023. www.who.int/initiatives/global-influenza-surveillance-and-response-system
69. World Health Organization. *Gonococcal Antimicrobial Surveillance Programme (GASP)*. WHO; 2023. www.who.int/initiatives/gonococcal-antimicrobial-surveillance-programme
70. World Health Organization. *Global Antimicrobial Resistance and Use Surveillance System (GLASS)*. WHO; 2023. www.who.int/initiatives/glass
71. Naggie S, Boulware DR, Lindsell CJ, Stewart TG, Gentile N, Collins S et al. Effect of Ivermectin vs placebo on time to sustained recovery in outpatients with mild to moderate COVID-19: A randomized clinical trial. *JAMA*. 2022;328(16):1595–1603.
72. Scohy A, Anantharajah A, Bodéus M, Kabamba-Mukadi B, Verroken A, Rodriguez-Villalobos H. Low performance of rapid antigen detection test as frontline testing for COVID-19 diagnosis. *Journal of Clinical Virology*. 2020;129:104455.
73. Wahdan MH. The epidemiological transition. *Eastern Mediterranean Health Journal*. 1996;2:8-20.
74. McKeown RE. The epidemiologic transition: Changing patterns of mortality and population dynamics. *American Journal of Lifestyle Medicine*. 2009;3(1 Suppl):19s–26s.
75. Baum F. The New Public Health. 4th ed. Oxford University Press; 2022.
76. Karlsson O, Kim R, Hasman A, Subramanian SV. Age distribution of all-cause mortality among children younger than 5 years in low- and middle-income countries. *JAMA Network Open*. 2022;5(5):e2212692.
77. Peng W, Berry EM. Global nutrition 1990–2015: A shrinking hungry, and expanding fat world. *PLOS ONE*. 2018;13(3):e0194821.
78. United Nations. *Sustainable Development Goals Report*. United Nations; 2022.
79. Australian Bureau of Statistics (ABS). *Provisional Mortality Statistics, Australia – Jan to Nov 2022*. ABS; 2023. www.abs.gov.au/statistics/health/causes-death/provisional-mortality-statistics/latest-release#data-downloads

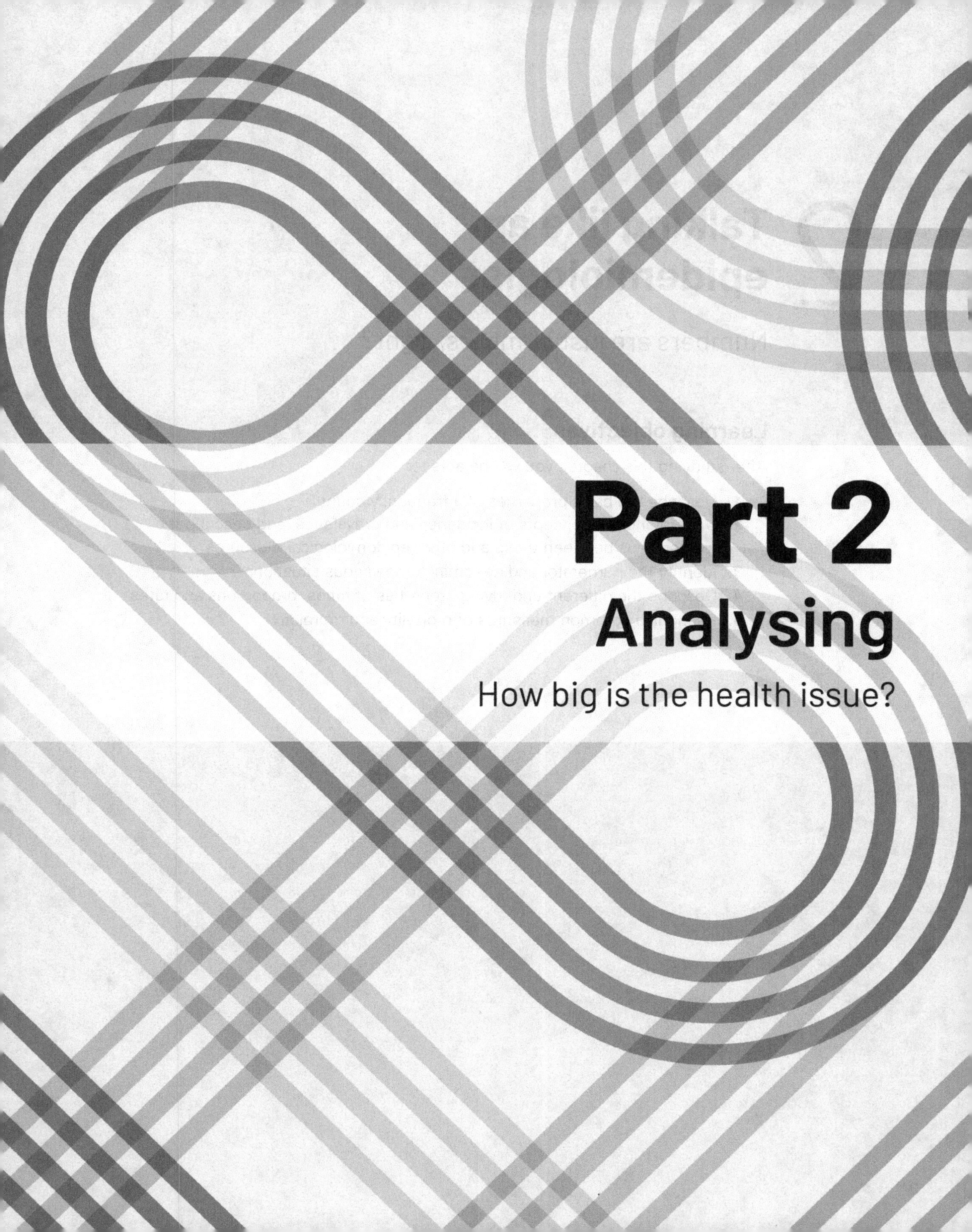

Part 2
Analysing
How big is the health issue?

2 Talking like an epidemiologist

Numbers are just numbers, right?

Learning objectives

After studying this chapter, you will be able to:

1. Describe the basic properties of a frequency count
2. Understand the concepts of incidence and prevalence, and describe the relationships between these and other epidemiological measures
3. Identify the numerator and denominator in various situations
4. Describe the different underlying properties of ratios, proportions and rates
5. Recognise common measures of mortality and morbidity

Introduction

Congratulations, you've made it this far. Now is probably a good time to recap what we learned about epidemiology in Chapter 1. It is not the study of skin (although it may include studies about skin); it involves the application of critical thinking (a valuable skill that can be learned and that involves questioning, analysing, evaluating and reaching a judgement about information you might hear or read); it is useful if you want to pursue a career in the health sciences (you're reading this book so you don't have to just have to take our word for this!); and numbers are involved. So what's the big deal? At this stage, it is worth letting you in on a secret. When students are asked about the difficulties they experience in their epidemiology classes, one of the biggest barriers they report is the language their teachers use to describe the concepts being explained (note, it is the *language* rather than the concepts themselves). And here's the thing: it is epidemiologists who are largely to blame, not the teachers! Being a relatively young discipline, it is not unusual to come across different words being used to describe the same concept, or the same word being used to describe different concepts – sometimes fundamentally different. Confusing, right?

Hugo: Confusing is not the word for it.
Rachael: Yes, try bewildering!
Author (Stephen): Well, yes. But to be fair, it has been a bit like building the plane as we learn how to fly.

Sometimes imprecision and lack of consistency are the price we pay for progress, and progress we have! By the end of this book, we hope that you too may share the view that epidemiology has a great deal to celebrate. For now, however, we trust there is at least some comfort in knowing that the discipline has matured to the point where epidemiologists can agree on a core group of numerical concepts, even if not necessarily the labels we might attach to them. Which brings us to the overarching question of this chapter: numbers are just numbers, right?

Well, no – not to an epidemiologist. Different numbers have different underlying properties, and it is worth understanding these differences if we are to talk about epidemiological concepts with any degree of precision. So, let's take a look at these differences and start talking like an epidemiologist!

Frequency counts

The most basic number in epidemiology is the **frequency count**, used to answer the question 'How many?' as in 'How many cases of influenza were there in South Australia in 2022?' You saw this type of number in the previous chapter and there is nothing complicated about it, except to note three points. First, while the information presented in Figure 1.1 comes from a reputable source and paints a compelling picture about the seasonality of influenza, it is not unreasonable to ask how much faith we should be placing in the figures being presented.

Frequency count: Number of cases of the phenomenon of interest within a specified period.

Do they reflect the actual number of influenza infections in the community or are they more or less than this number? It is easy to think of reasons why they might be less – for example, not every case was included in the counting process because not everyone with influenza seeks treatment and these other people are never tested for the virus. But there are also plausible reasons why they might be more – for example, some people may have been counted twice due to administrative errors. Maybe these two factors cancel each other out. Maybe not. We don't know without knowing a lot more about influenza and how it is counted and reported in South Australia.

The second point is more subtle and goes to the heart of epidemiological inquiry. If you look again at Figure 1.1, you will see not only that it tells us influenza is more common in winter than at other times (at least in South Australia); it also tells us how many new cases were recorded in that population week by week *for every week in the year 2022.* The point, in case you missed it, is that the graph represents a snapshot in time and that every frequency count should include a time dimension (in this example, a year); if it doesn't, we should be asking why. To put this another way, it is meaningless to say there were so many new cases of a particular illness without also stating the period over which these cases were observed. It can be a year, but this is more by convention than necessity and any unit of time is acceptable; the choice really depends on the situation. The essential point is that the unit is expressed unambiguously together with the frequency count. So, for example, the statement '23 083 South Australians were reported as contracting influenza in 2022' contains everything we need to know for it to be complete, as does the statement '2022 was quite a big year for influenza following some quiet years', but the statement 'There were X cases of influenza in the summer of 2022' would be less helpful because it is not clear over which period these cases were observed (just the sequential months of January and February 2022 or December 2022 as well?) and the statement 'There were 12 083 cases of influenza in South Australia' is incomplete because it lacks a time dimension altogether (don't laugh, we see this in student assignments quite frequently).

Rachael: So, is this why, during the COVID-19 pandemic in Australia, we were getting daily updates from health officials on the number of new cases reported to authorities in the last 24 hours compared with previous days?
Author (Stephen): Exactly!

In an emerging crisis such as the early days of the COVID-19 pandemic, a period as short as 24 hours might well be the unit of time that makes the most sense for health officials to be reporting new cases because everyone would want to know, in as close to real time as possible, whether the measures being put in place to slow the spread of the disease were having the desired effect. But you would not expect these same officials to be providing daily updates on the number of cases of heart disease, despite heart attacks causing almost twice as many deaths each year than COVID-19. We will have more to say about this later when we return to other types of frequency counts.

Hugo: They wouldn't be able to say exactly how many new cases of COVID-19 there were in the last 24 hours anymore would they?

Author (Stephen): No, they wouldn't, which gets back to the first point about frequency counts.

As the situation unfolds and the crisis passes, official responses change, which can affect the type and quality of the information there is to work with. Polymerase chain reaction (PCR) testing is the gold standard for diagnosing COVID-19. At the height of the pandemic, PCR testing was widespread and even a requirement in many countries if you had COVID symptoms. So, you would expect official daily reports to be a pretty accurate reflection of the actual number of new symptomatic COVID-19 cases at that time, at least in these countries, give or take a few because of delays in reporting and the rarer instances of misdiagnosis (no test is 100 per cent accurate and PCR testing for COVID-19 is no exception). But now PCR testing has been wound back in most places, official counts of new COVID-19 diagnoses will under-represent the true number in the population by a large margin. And while officials may still be able to say how many cases of COVID-19 were *reported* to them in the last 24 hours, there is no longer a need for such frequent reports of this information and, in any event, the value of this information is greatly diminished by the much lower use of PCR testing and the biases introduced by changes in eligibility for this service.

The final point to note about frequency counts is probably the most obvious. Certain attributes about the population that gives rise to the phenomenon being counted matter, principally its size. Put simply, the larger the population, the more chance (usually) of observing the phenomenon of interest. So, is 12 083 reported cases of influenza in South Australia in 2022 a lot or a little? It certainly seems a lot and we have been told that it was more than in previous years – but how would we really know?

Incidence and prevalence

Before turning to this question, we need to distinguish between the *frequency* of a phenomenon and other attributes about it that epidemiologists might be interested in counting. In both the above examples, you will notice that the word 'new' was used or implied when referring to the cases being counted. This stems from the fact that these examples involve a disease for which it is relatively easy to say when someone became a *new* case – that is, when they became infected with the influenza or COVID-19 virus. The explicit nature of this transition from not being a case to being a one is a characteristic of *infectious diseases* and is in contrast to many **chronic conditions** – for example, diabetes or dementia – for which a formal diagnosis can lag the onset of pathology by quite some period. Epidemiologists refer to this type of case (a new one) as an **incident case** and use the term 'incidence' to refer to the number of new cases in a defined population within a specified period. So, the statement 'there were 23 083 incident cases of influenza in South Australia in 2022' simply means there were 23 083 new cases of influenza in that population and year; it is the same as saying 'the incidence of influenza in South Australians in 2022 was 23 083'. Remember, of course, that the period over which the cases were observed does not have to be one year, but it does have to be specified for the statement to be complete.

Chronic conditions: A class of health conditions that last a long time (typically one year or more).

Incident case: A new case of the phenomenon of interest in a defined population within a specified period. A measure of *morbidity*.

If incidence refers to new cases in a defined population within a specified period, you might be wondering what is left to tally up. Well, there are other ways epidemiologists count things, one of which involves considering existing cases rather than new ones. If you look again at the influenza example, you will see that at any point during the year 2022, it is possible to classify people into two groups: those who have influenza and those who don't. Epidemiologists agree on labelling the former group **prevalent cases**. (Unfortunately, they are less united when it comes to the term *prevalence*, so we will put that to one side for moment and focus on where there is agreement.) The key difference between a count of incident cases and of prevalent ones defined in this way is that the latter does not require a period of time to pass for the cases to occur *because they already exist*; all that is required is to count them. This is called **point prevalence** to remind us that it is undertaken with reference to a point in time rather than a period and is the main way of counting prevalent cases. The other way is to count them over a period of time. This tally combines new and existing cases between two time points into a single measure and is called **period prevalence** to remind us that it is undertaken with reference to a period of time rather than a point in time. Twelve months is a commonly used period, but you will sometimes see 'lifetime prevalence' being reported as well. Explanation 2.1 illustrates these different ways of counting incident and prevalent cases using influenza as an example.

Prevalent case: An existing case of the phenomenon of interest in a defined population at a specified point in time (*point prevalence*) or over a period of time (*period prevalence*). A measure of *morbidity*.

Point prevalence: Existing cases of the phenomenon of interest in a defined population at a specified point in time.

Period prevalence: Existing cases of the phenomenon of interest in a defined population over a period of time.

EXPLANATION 2.1: Incidence, point prevalence and period prevalence – what's the difference?

Imagine you had access to the South Australian Infectious Diseases Register presented in Figure 1.1 and this allowed you to plot the day every reported case of influenza was diagnosed as having this illness and the day they reported feeling better. Such a plot would look something like those presented in Figure 2.1.

Each of the plots in Figure 2.1 illustrates a different way of representing the same data, with sad faces indicating the start of a period of illness and smiley faces indicating recovery from this period of illness. In the first (Figure 2.1a), the nine new cases that occurred between the start of week 26 and the end of week 27 are represented by black sad faces. This is an example of incidence. In the second, (Figure 2.1b), the five existing cases at the start of week 27 are represented by black horizontal lines. This is an example of point prevalence. In the third (Figure 2.1c), the 14 cases represented by black horizontal lines can be broken down into the five existing cases at the start of week 26 and the nine new cases that occurred between the start of week 26 and the end of week 27. This is an example of period prevalence.

Each of these measures provides a different insight into the burden of disease or condition within a population. Counting incident cases helps to capture the speed of new occurrences or onset of the disease or condition, providing insights into its **temporal** trends and patterns. Incident cases are useful for studying risk factors, identifying potential causes and evaluating the effectiveness of prevention and intervention strategies. Counting prevalent cases, on the other hand, provides a snapshot of the total burden of the disease or condition within the population, regardless of when the cases initially occurred. Prevalent cases are useful for understanding the overall prevalence and distribution of the disease or condition within the population, assessing the need for healthcare resources and estimating the impact of a disease on society.

Temporal: Synonymous with time.

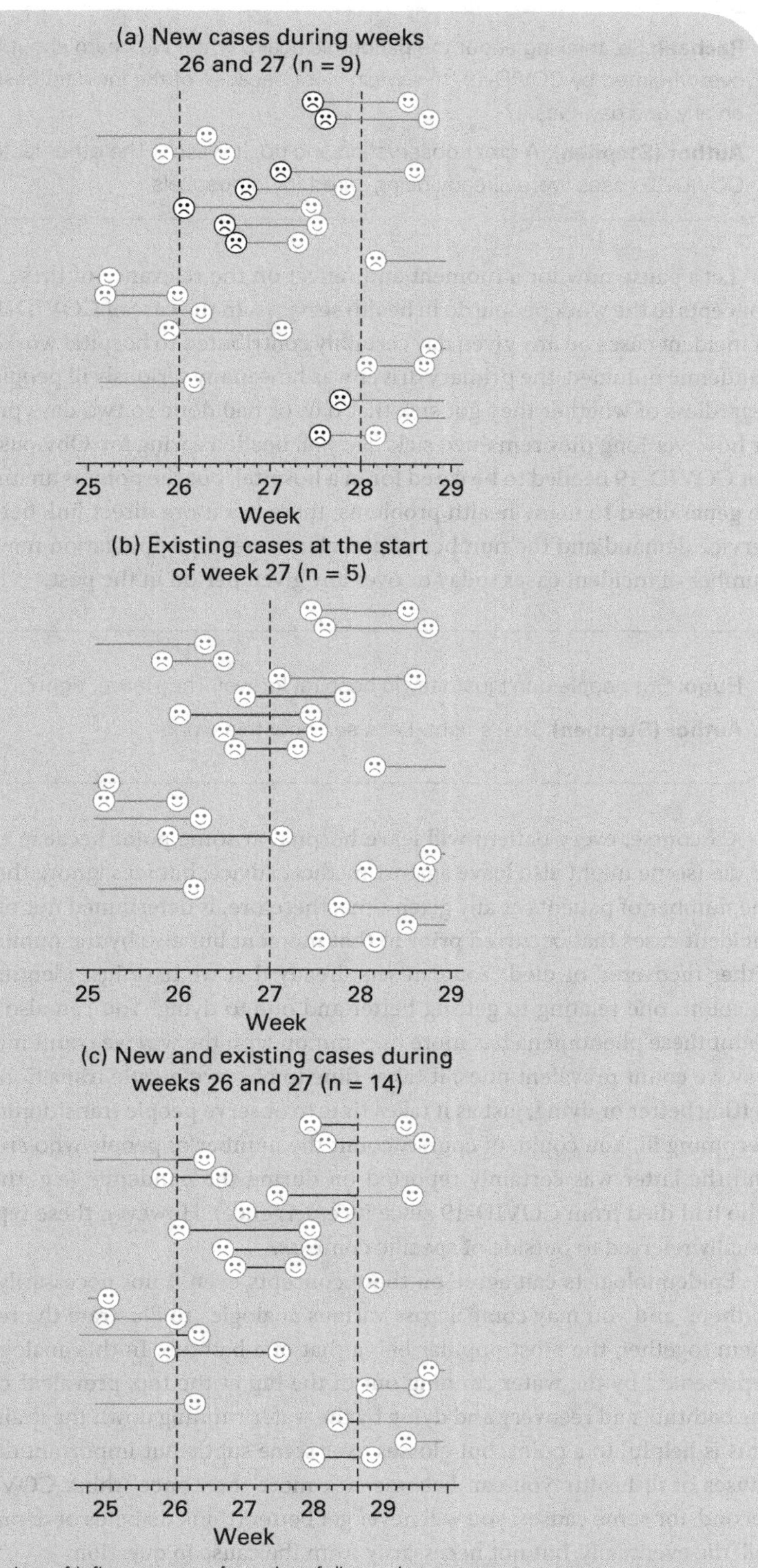

Figure 2.1 Imaginary plots of influenza cases from day of diagnosis to recovery

Rachael: So, thinking about the pandemic again, when we heard about hospitals being overwhelmed by COVID-19, this wasn't just because of the incident cases being reported on any one day, was it?

Author (Stephen): A great observation and no, it wasn't! The other factor was how many COVID-19 cases were already being cared for in hospitals.

Let's pause now for a moment and reflect on the relevance of these two epidemiological concepts to the work people do in health services. In the case of COVID-19, while the number of incident cases on any given day certainly contributed to hospital workload pressures as the pandemic unfolded, the primary driver was how many seriously ill people there were to treat, regardless of whether they got sick that day, or had done so two days prior, two weeks prior or however long they remained sick. They all needed caring for. Obviously not everyone who got COVID-19 needed to be cared for in a hospital, but the point is an important one and can be generalised to many health problems; there is a more direct link between current health service demand and the number of prevalent cases in a population now than there is to the number of incident cases today or over any given period in the past.

Hugo: But people don't just stay in hospital forever. They leave, right?

Author (Stephen): That's right. Let's see how this works.

Of course, every patient will leave hospital at some point because either they get better or die (some might also leave against medical advice, but let's ignore them for the moment); the number of patients at any given time, therefore, is determined not only by the number of incident cases that occurred prior to that moment but also by the number who, before then, either recovered or died. You can see already that we have just identified two other things to count: one relating to getting better and one to dying! You can also see that the way we count these phenomena has more in common with the way we count incident cases than the way we count prevalent ones; it takes time to observe people transitioning from being ill to getting better or dying, just as it takes time to observe people transitioning from being well to becoming ill. You could, of course, count the number of people who *ever* got better or died, and the latter was certainly reported on during the pandemic (e.g. the number of people who had died from COVID-19 since its emergence). However, these types of counts are not usually referred to outside of specific contexts.

Epidemiologists can agree on these concepts even if not necessarily the labels to attach to them, and you may come across various analogies to illustrate the relationships that link them together, the most popular being that of a bathtub. In this analogy, incident cases are represented by the water running out of the tap at the top, prevalent cases by the water in the bathtub, and recovery and dying by the water running down the drain hole at the bottom. This is helpful to a point, but glosses over some subtle but important details: first, for many causes of ill-health, you can become sick more than once (think COVID-19 or influenza); second, for some causes, you will never get better (think diabetes or dementia); and third, you will die eventually, but not necessarily from the cause in question.

Hugo: In other words, some of the water is recycled, but the bathtub never overflows because it's got more than one hole in it.

Author (Stephen): That all depends on whether the outflows match the inflows! And this is exactly what we were worried about with COVID-19 and our hospitals.

Figure 2.2 seeks to address these shortcomings with the bathtub analogy using the language we have discussed so far but with a few modifications to the plumbing. First, we have added being born to indicate the ultimate source of water in the system. Second, we have split 'dying' into dying from the cause in question and dying from other causes. Finally, for each of the counts that can only be observed over time – that is, the frequency counts – we have included a noun equivalent of the verb in parentheses for ease of reference later. These are represented by arrows in the diagram and are sometimes referred to as 'flow variables' (think of water flowing through a pipe). The buckets, on the other hand, represent the point-in-time concepts we have discussed thus far and are sometimes referred to as 'stock variables' (think of how much water there is in each of the buckets).

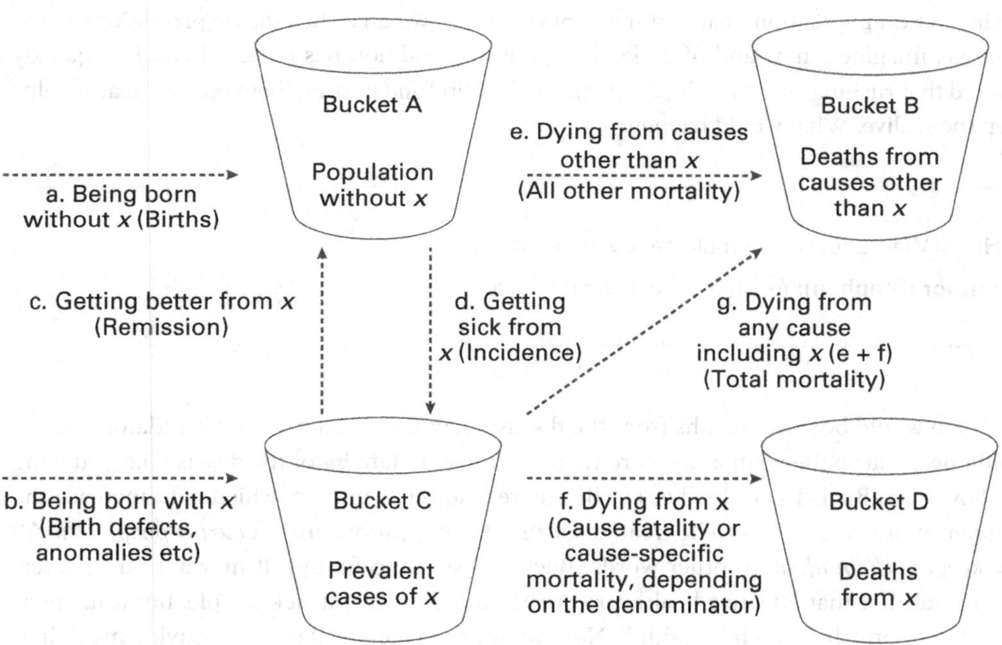

Figure 2.2 Putting it all together: a more complete depiction than the bathtub analogy.

Figure 2.2 has several interesting implications. First, it shows that both the size of the group of prevalent cases (Bucket C) and how long one spends in this group (i.e. the average **duration** of the phenomenon of interest) are determined by the flow variables leading into and away from that part of the system. In fact, the dependency of these variables on the others is such that it is possible to paint a complete picture of the epidemiology of a phenomenon even when you have only partial information. This can occur with chronic conditions such

Duration: The average length of time someone spends as a prevalent case before leaving this group either due to getting better or dying.

as diabetes and dementia where, as we have already noted, the transition from being disease-free to becoming an incident case can be gradual and therefore difficult to observe. So, for example, if all you knew about diabetes was how many people had this condition and their risk of mortality compared with non-diabetics, then assuming the **remission** from diabetes is zero (i.e. once you are a diabetic, you stay that way for life), you could work out values for the other variables (i.e. their incidence and average duration).

Remission: A measure of *morbidity* concerned with the speed with which people recover from the phenomenon of interest.

While these relationships can be expressed precisely, this is straying into a more advanced area of descriptive epidemiology and the calculations themselves are best undertaken using specialist software such as Dismod (1). A simplified version is therefore often used instead. This is typically expressed as:

$$p \approx i \times d \qquad \text{(Equation 2.1)}$$

Where p is the number of prevalent cases, i is the number of incident cases and d is duration expressed in the same unit of time over which i was observed.

Equation 2.1 is useful in situations where you have only two of the three named parameters and want to know the third. However, it only works for conditions of relatively short duration (e.g. less than a year), whereas the precise approach has no such limitation and accommodates all the variables identified in Figure 2.2 (rather than just p, i and d).

The second implication of Figure 2.2 is that it provides a visual framework for understanding the impact on population health of many of the things we do as healthcare professionals. For example, imagine a new and often fatal respiratory condition has emerged and it is quickly realised that rushing severely affected people to hospital and putting them on a ventilator helps keep them alive. What would happen?

Hugo: Well, a few lives would be saved, obviously.

Author (Stephen): Yes, that would be one outcome ...

There would be fewer deaths from the disease than if they hadn't used ventilators, which would be because the ventilators were reducing the **case fatality** of the disease (i.e. reducing the flow from Bucket C to Bucket D). But there is another impact, which is to increase the number of prevalent cases to be treated *because the ventilators are not curing people, they're just keeping them alive* (in other words, Bucket C starts to fill up). It may appear counter-intuitive at first that effective healthcare creates more prevalent sick people, but it happens more frequently than you might think. Now, what would happen if certain antiviral medicines were found, when given early in the infection, to help those who were hospitalised fight the disease?

Case fatality: A measure of *mortality* and a *frequency count* that includes the number of deaths from the phenomenon of interest over a specified period.

Rachael: The number of prevalent cases would start to decrease.

Author (Stephen): True again!

The effect of the antiviral medicines would be to increase the speed with which people get better (i.e. increasing the flow from Bucket C to Bucket A) so the number of severely affected cases would begin to decrease (Bucket C would start to subside again) as the average duration of illness declines. It may also result in fewer deaths by reducing case fatality, but both these observations rely on the assumption that incidence is not changing. Now let's assume that this is not the case and that incidence is rapidly increasing (i.e. the flow from Bucket A to Bucket C is getting faster). In other words, it turns out that the new disease is highly contagious. Unless the antiviral medicines provide an instant cure and are given to everyone presenting to hospital, then the number of severely affected cases needing hospital care is going to rapidly increase as well, as will both the number of people being put on ventilators and the number who die. So, what is our best hope of stopping this situation from spiralling out of control (i.e. everyone in Bucket A ending up in Buckets C or D)?

Rachael: Reducing incidence?

Author (Stephen): Spot on!

Our best hope in this situation is to decrease incidence and, because this is a new and highly infectious disease, one of the quickest ways to do that is to limit transmission between people through public health measures such as limiting the frequency and duration of public gatherings. By getting incidence under control in this way (i.e. by slowing down the flow from Bucket A to Bucket C), severely affected cases and deaths from the disease will reduce, even if there are no further breakthroughs with respect to increasing remission or reducing case fatality (i.e. the flows from Bucket C to Buckets A and D remain constant). Over the longer term, of course, the development of a vaccine to increase immunity to this disease is the pathway back to normality.

Sound familiar? It should because this is pretty much what we went through with the COVID-19 pandemic. But the broader point is this: Figure 2.2 neatly captures the different levels of prevention that you might encounter in your work as a healthcare professional. In ascending order, primary prevention is concerned with preventing the onset of disease altogether; reducing incidence is the focus here. Secondary prevention is concerned with early intervention to limit disease progression, and remission or recovery is the focus here. And tertiary prevention is concerned with improving survival or quality of life once a disease has occurred; reducing case fatality is often the focus here. Of course, not every level is relevant in every situation (primary prevention, for example, is much more effective for infectious diseases than it is for dementia), but every prevention activity will be aimed at having an impact on at least one of these levels. Figure 2.3 summarises these relationships with examples.

Having established the relevance to healthcare of the aspects of disease and disease progression that epidemiologists are interested in counting and the relationships that bind them, let's now return to the question of whether 12 083 reported cases of influenza in South Australia in 2022 was a lot or a little.

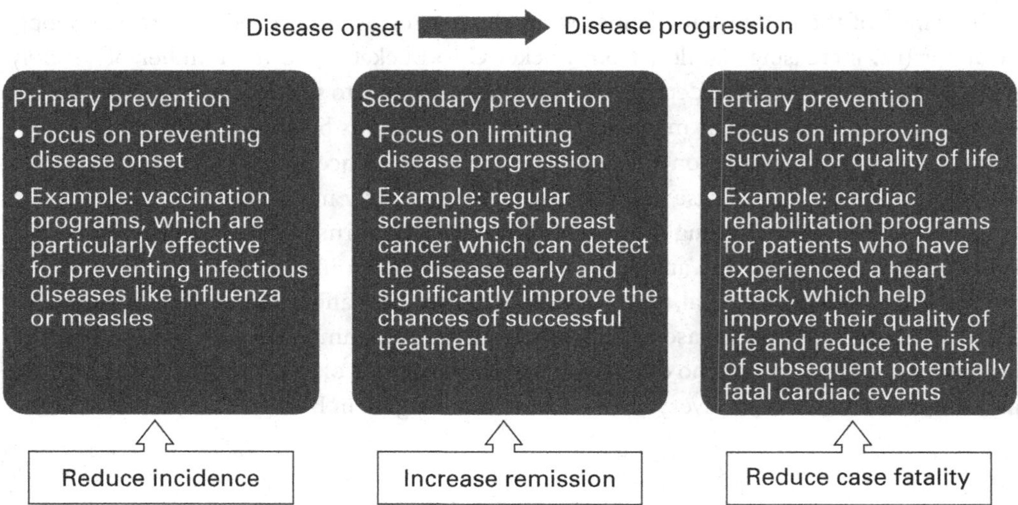

Figure 2.3 Relationship between epidemiological parameters and different levels of prevention activities.

Numerator and denominator

To answer this question, we need to transform this simple frequency count (which we now know is related to incidence) into something else. The actual transformation will vary depending on the situation, but the objective is the same: to express the count on a different scale numerically and, by so doing, to make it more interpretable or comparable with other similarly transformed counts. We will explore making comparisons in greater detail in the next chapter. For now, it is worth observing only that comparing raw counts side by side is rarely useful, except under very specific circumstances.

At its most basic, the types of transformations we are talking about involve dividing one number by another number, as in

$$\frac{x}{y}$$

Numerator: The number above the fraction bar.

Denominator: The number below the fraction bar.

You would have first come across this transformation in primary school in the context of learning fractions and the maths is simple enough. You may also recall that the number above the fraction bar is called the **numerator** and the number below is known as the **denominator**. Epidemiologists use these same labels quite a bit and, as we shall see, apply them not just to fractions but to other transformations as well.

Ratios, proportions and rates

The types of transformations that epidemiologists routinely perform can be classified into one of three broad groups: *ratios*, *proportions* and *rates*. It is worth exploring the properties of each in turn.

Ratios

Ratios are the most generalised transformation of the three and simply involve dividing one quantity (the 'numerator') by another like quantity (the 'denominator'); the result has no dimensions and can take any value, where a ratio of 1 simply means equality between the two quantities being compared. Unlike a proportion, therefore, there is no requirement when calculating a ratio for the numerator to be a subset of the denominator for the result to be meaningful. An example of a ratio is the number of nurses to allied health professionals on a hospital ward. If the answer is 5 it simply means there are five nurses for every allied health professional on the ward. The reverse of this also makes sense; there are 0.2 allied health professionals for every nurse on the ward. The ratio of nurses to allied health professionals is 5:1 (five to one) is another way saying the same thing.

We will have a lot to say about certain types of ratios in coming chapters. For now, it is worth returning to Equation 2.1 and noting how, with some basic algebra, this formula can be rearranged as follows:

$$d \approx \frac{p}{i}$$

Thus, the duration of a phenomenon of interest can be thought of as the ratio of its prevalence to its incidence. If the answer is less than a year, then this a reasonable approximation of the true value.

Proportions

Proportions are a special type of ratio in which every entity counted in the numerator is also included in the denominator. The most common example you will encounter in epidemiology relates to prevalent cases, as in 'the proportion of people with this disease is X'. The calculation underlying such a statement is simple enough and includes the raw count of prevalent cases in the numerator (Bucket C in Figure 2.2) and the total number of people in the population in the denominator (Buckets A plus C in Figure 2.2). In other words, the number of prevalent cases is expressed as a proportion of the whole population, with a range of between 0 and 1 or, just as typically, between 0 per cent and 100 per cent (if the result is multiplied by 100). The obvious advantage of transforming a raw count in this way is that it converts it into a scale that is immediately familiar (everyone knows that 0.2 or 20 per cent is a fifth, 0.25 or 25 per cent is a quarter, 0.333 or 33.3 per cent is a third, and so on). It also allows you to compare the result with a proportion from another population and see which population has more of the attribute in question in proportion to its size.

So far, so good. A problem arises, however, when trying to attach a label to a proportional transformation involving prevalent cases, as in the above example. **Prevalence proportion** might seem appropriate enough and would be strictly correct. It is, however, rarely used. Instead, you will see *prevalence* or even *prevalence rate*. The former would be acceptable but for the fact that it is also sometimes used to refer to the simple frequency count of prevalent cases and thus is ambiguous. The latter is problematic because the word 'rate' implies there is some sort of time dimension to the measure when we have already learnt that a count of prevalent cases typically refers to a moment in time. Another consideration is the fact that in the case of rare diseases, multipliers other than 100 (e.g. 1000, 10 000, etc.) are sometimes used to reduce the number of decimal places that need to be reported.

Prevalence proportion: The number of *prevalent cases* divided by the whole population. Cannot be less than 0 or greater than 1. A measure of *morbidity*.

Hugo: Here we go!

Rachael: Right, so epidemiologists can't even agree on this thing called prevalence.

Author (Stephen): Well, not exactly. They agree on the underlying idea readily enough; it's just that sometimes the labels get a little muddled.

While the labels epidemiologists use for prevalence can be a bit inconsistent at times, this is not actually as big a deal as it might sound because, as with all communication, context matters and it is usually quite easy to work out what is meant, even if the labels are not quite as you might expect. The important point is to try to be as precise as you can when your turn comes to use or explain the concept.

There are several additional points worth noting about proportions before we move on. First, they are not, of course, limited to transformations involving prevalent cases. Another context in which you will see them being used is in discussions about causes of death, as in 'Heart disease causes X per cent of deaths every year, making it the leading cause of death globally'. There are only so many deaths in the world each year, and these can be allocated proportionally to specific causes such that, in total, they add up to 100 per cent. Second, you will sometimes see ratios dressed up as proportions, as in 'The prevalence of diabetes changed by X per cent from last year to this'. If you look closely at this statement, you will see that what is being expressed here is not a proportion, but in fact the *ratio* of the change in prevalence between the two years. When calculated as the difference in prevalence between this year and the last divided by prevalence in the last and then multiplied by 100, the answer could be –15 per cent, 15 per cent or 150 per cent, and each of these would make sense, whereas a proportion of less than 0 or greater than 1 does not (there cannot be *negative* sick people just as there cannot be more sick people at any one time than there are people). Thus, while it is true that all proportions are also ratios and can be expressed as percentages (or any other unit that is convenient), it is *not* the case that all ratios and percentages are necessarily proportions.

Rates

In many ways, rates are the preoccupation of epidemiology and are defined as a transformation in which the numerator must contain a frequency count that is measured over a period (e.g. any of the 'flow' variables depicted as arrows in Figure 2.2). This rules out prevalent cases as candidates – even though, as we have already mentioned, you may sometimes encounter the term 'prevalence rate' in the literature. The defining characteristic of a rate, therefore, is that it is a time-based measure that tells us how *quickly* cases are occurring. A useful starting point is to think about the speed of a car. For example, if I were to tell you that I drove 60 kilometres in one trip last week, I would in effect be telling you the total number of kilometres my odometer recorded, but not how quickly it recorded them. If I were then to add that it took an hour to complete the trip, you would have all the information you need to calculate my speed in kilometres per hour (km/h) (you would not, of course, be able to say how fast I was travelling at any point along the journey, just my average speed across the entire trip). If I then mentioned that the day after I travelled 40 kilometres in a 30-minute trip, you would be able to say without much difficulty in which trip my average speed was the fastest. The correct answer is, of course, the second because I travelled an average of 60 km/h in the first but 80 km/h in the second. What makes these numbers comparable is that they are expressed with respect to the same unit of time (i.e. one hour), even though the second trip lasted only half as long as the first.

Rates are like kilometres per hour in that they are a measure of the speed of a phenomenon, and we must express them with respect to the same unit of time if we want to make them comparable. What makes them different, however, is that there is an additional consideration – as we have already noted in the previous section, when comparing frequency counts from different populations, the size of each of these populations also matters. The larger it is, the greater its chance of giving rise to a case (all other things being equal). What we want to know is whether the speed with which cases are arising is the same (or different) after accounting for any such size differences. This additional consideration can be thought of in terms of the speed of water flowing through pipes with different diameters. Two pipes can have water flowing through them at the same speed (think rate), but the one with the larger diameter (think population size) will have more litres of water passing through it over any given period (think cases recorded). If all you measured was how much water had passed through each pipe at the end of the period, you could still prove that the speed was the same in both if you knew the diameter of each (Figure 2.4).

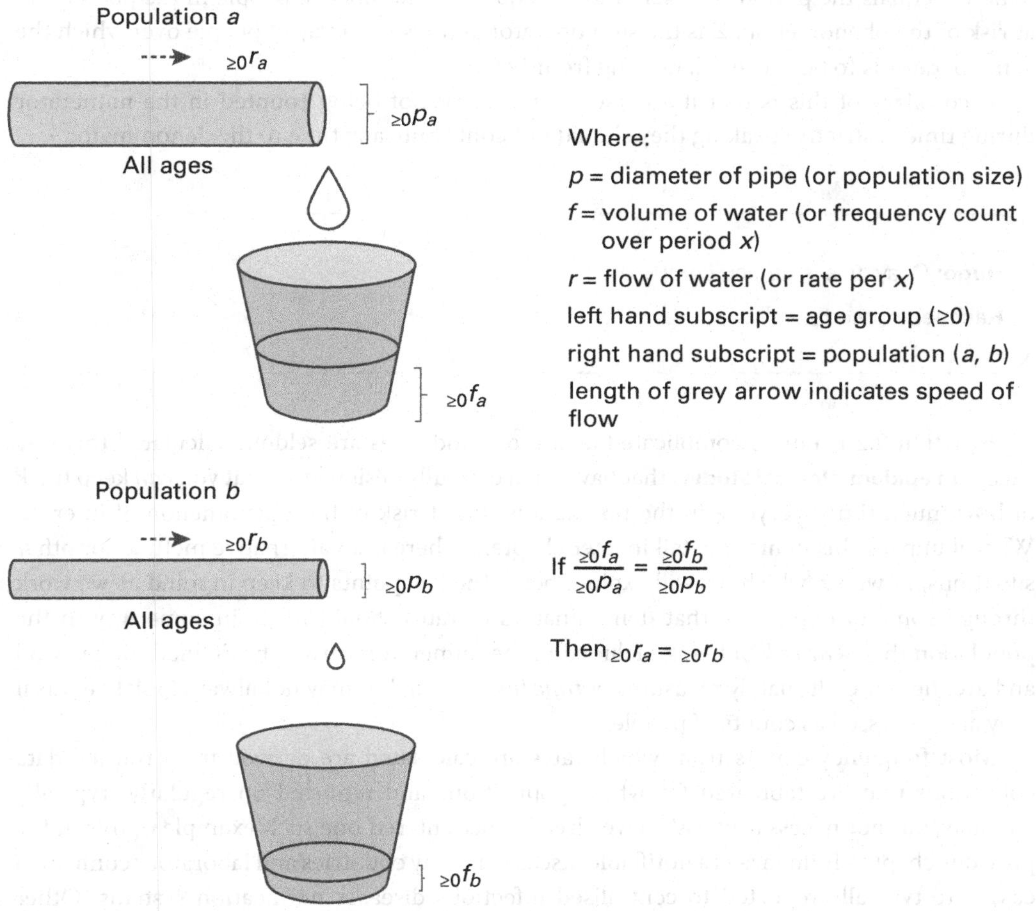

Figure 2.4 Relationship between population size, frequency counts and rates.

Frequency counts need to be similarly 're-scaled' in some way if we are to express their speed such that meaningful comparisons can be made. So, the obvious question is ...

Rachael: Well, you defined the numerator of a rate at the outset so ... what's in its denominator?!

Author (Stephen): Exactly (nicely put, by the way). And the short answer is, it depends.

Hugo: Ahh, I knew it!

... how do we know what to include in the denominator of a rate? Well, the long answer to this question is that, in an ideal world where you knew exactly how much time everyone in the population was *at risk* of the phenomenon of interest (i.e. the time spent in Bucket A of Figure 2.2) and you could add this up, then this would be your denominator. A rate can therefore be expressed most precisely thus:

$$\text{Rate} = \frac{\text{Number of cases of the phenomenon of interest during } x}{\sum_{i=1}^{n} \text{Time spent at risk of phenomenon during } x_i} \quad \text{(Equation 2.2)}$$

Where x equals the period of observation, n equals the number of people in the population at risk of the phenomenon, Σ is the sum operator and i is the array of people over which the sum operator is to be executed, ranging from 1 to n.

A corollary of this is that if a person is not at risk of being counted in the numerator during time x, strictly speaking they should not contribute any time to the denominator.

Hugo: Okay, this is getting complicated.

Rachael: Agreed ...

Epidemiological studies: Discrete attempts to pursue an epidemiological question, many of which get written up and published in scientific literature or elsewhere.

Equation 2.2 is not as complicated as it looks and rates are seldom calculated this way except in **epidemiological studies** that have been carefully designed so that you *can* keep track of how much time everyone in the population was at risk of the phenomenon of interest. We will unpack this in more detail in later chapters. There is an alternative method for other situations, however, which we will explore here. The key points to keep in mind as we work through some examples are that denominators of rates should relate in some way to the population that is *at risk* of being included in the numerator during the defined time period and are therefore ultimately measures of *time* (even though it may not always look like this if they are expressed as counts of people).

Most frequency counts from which rates are calculated are derived from routine data collections that are tabulated for whole populations and reported on regularly (typically annually, but not necessarily). We have already encountered one such example of this in the previous chapter. Influenza is a notifiable disease in many countries and laboratory confirmed cases are typically reported to centralised infectious diseases notification systems. Other examples of these types of collections include births and deaths registries, cancer registries and health service utilisation systems. For most of these, it is easy to think about who might be at risk of the phenomenon being counted and reported on. For example, anyone could die at any moment from something; it is therefore reasonable to consider everyone in a population as being at risk of ending up as a record in a deaths registry in countries with complete vital records (i.e. Buckets B and D in Figure 2.2). If we were then to restrict our timeframe to just the number of deaths recorded in a particular year (i.e. the number of new records that appear in Buckets B or D in that year), then we can say that everyone was at risk of being in included in this number for approximately *a one-year period.* The denominator in this case would therefore be the whole population (i.e. Buckets A and B) multiplied by one year. If the numerator were observed over a two-year period, the denominator would be the whole population multiplied by two years. If the observation period were three and a half years, the whole population would be multiplied by 3.5 years, and so on.

In each of these cases, the denominator represents an *approximation* of the total amount of time (in years in this example, but again not by necessity) the population was at risk of being included in the numerator, not the *exact* amount. The most obvious reason for this imprecision is that you are no longer at risk of dying once you are dead, but this is not accounted for by the method. Other reasons include babies being born and movements in and out of the population due to migration. The approximation is near enough, however, and a tell-tale sign that a rate has been calculated in this way is that it is expressed as *per X people per year* or even just *per X people* as in 'the global mortality was 8 *per 1000 people* in 2022'. The alternative expression is 'the global mortality was 8 *per 1000 person-years* in 2022' and might imply that every person in the world had been followed individually to determine the amount of time they were at risk of dying. This is sometimes referred to as **person-time**, but the distinction in usage is by no means guaranteed, so once again context is everything. Obviously, it is not feasible to follow every individual at a national level, let alone globally, so the chances are that a rate of global mortality will be calculated using the approximation rather than the exact method, regardless of how it might be expressed. This will be true for most of the population-wide rates you encounter.

Person-time: The combined time study participants are observed to be at risk of a particular outcome from the beginning of the observation period to developing the outcome, leaving the study (e.g. loss to follow-up, death) or the end of the study. Each person contributes only the time they spent under observation. May be defined as any period (days, weeks, years) and is used in the denominator of calculations of person-time incidence or *mortality rates*.

Several other points are worth noting before we move on. First, the contraction of 'per X people per year' to 'per X people' suggests that a rate is denominated by people, not time. This would be to misrepresent the nature of a rate, which – as we have already noted – is more accurately thought of as being denominated by the total amount of time these people were at risk of being included in the numerator. It just so happens that when the observation period is one year and the rate is being expressed as 'per year', the number of people and amount of time they are assumed to be at risk using the approximation method is the same. This is important to remember when you see the denominator in formulae for annual rates reduced to simply the number of people in the population. The person-time construction typically reserved for the exact method does not lead so readily to this type of misrepresentation. Second, just as with proportions, rates can be expressed in terms of any multiple of 10 (e.g. 1, 10, 100, 1000, 10 000, 100 000) without affecting the underlying information being conveyed. This extra step after the division of the numerator by the denominator is done simply to reduce the number of decimal places that need to be reported without losing precision.

What we have been discussing here is a type of *mortality rate* that goes by various names (depending on the situation) but is one of the most basic pieces of information epidemiologists might want to know about a population together with its birth rate (epidemiologists are a bit like demographers in this respect). We will return to these and other types of rates epidemiologist like calculating shortly. For now, however, it is worth distilling what we have learnt about the approximation method thus far to:

$$\text{Rate per } y \text{ people per } x \approx \frac{\text{Number of cases of the phenomenon of interest during } x}{(\text{Number of people assumed to be at risk of phenomenon during } x) \times x} \times y$$

(Equation 2.3)

Where x equals the period of observation and y equals some multiple of 10 (e.g. 1, 10, 100, 1000). If x is one year, don't be surprised to see the expression to the left of the approximation symbol reduced to simply 'Rate per y people'. Multiples of 10 are used for y rather than some other unit because they represent a familiar scale.

Rachael: Okay, so if the numerator in Equation 2.3 comes from routine data, where does the denominator come from?

Author (Stephen): That is a good question.

Determining an appropriate source of information from which to derive the denominator for population-wide rate calculations (i.e. rates calculated using Equation 2.3) is just as important as knowing what is included in the numerator. For any given geographic area, such as a country or region, it is quite difficult to say with any degree of precision exactly how many people there are at any one time that might be giving rise to the phenomenon of interest without reference to multiple sources of information such as population-wide censuses, births and deaths registries, and migration records. The gold standard would be for every person to have a unique identifying number that allowed data to be linked across these datasets; even then, various sources of error could affect the integrity of such a system. In practice, therefore, we tend to rely on estimates produced on a regular basis by national statistics agencies and sometimes referred to as **estimated resident population** tables. These seek to describe how many people *resided* in a geographic area at a point in time after accounting for any population movements captured by official records. The most basic level at which this type of information can be disaggregated is typically age and sex, but other levels, such as sub-regions and/or ethnic groupings, are sometimes possible. These tables are usually the best source of information from which to derive the denominator when using Equation 2.3. Standard practice is to use tables estimated for the mid-point of the period over which the numerator has been collated (or to impute such figures if a table for the required timepoint is unavailable) on the assumption that this most accurately reflects the composition of the population at risk of being counted in the numerator. The tables are only estimates though (by definition), so this additional consideration implies a greater degree of precision than, in all likelihood, is realistically achievable given that the method is only ever going to approximate the underlying rate of interest anyway.

Estimated resident population: Official estimates of how many people resided in a geographic area at a point in time.

Hugo: What about dying from childbirth? Only women are 'at risk' here, aren't they?

Author (Stephen): Another good question! And the answer is yes indeed, only women can give birth or die from this experience. And more precisely still, only women of child-bearing age are at risk of these phenomena.

A more important consideration is to not cast the net too wide when thinking about the population at risk of being included in the numerator. There are some illnesses, for example, that only affect one sex (e.g. prostate cancer, testicular cancer, cervical cancer), although the number of these conditions is smaller than you might think (both sexes can get breast cancer, for example). In these situations, those at risk are quite clearly a subset of the whole population. More common, however, is that one sex is more *susceptible* than the other (e.g. breast cancer is more common in women) or that susceptibility is **age-dependent**, such that certain age groups (typically older people) are more likely to become ill than others. To explore these differences, a common approach is to *stratify* the population into separate groups (e.g. males and females, young and old people) and compare the rates in each. When the population is stratified in this way, it is useful to distinguish between **crude rates** – that is, rates for the whole population, without stratification – and those for the separate strata. An **age-specific rate** is an example of this type of stratification and is any rate for a specific age group where the numerator and denominator refer to the same age group (2). The other terms you will come across in relation to rates are *standardised* and *adjusted*. These indicate that specific techniques have been used to reduce the influence of certain aspects of the population (most typically its **age structure**, but not exclusively) on the crude rate to reveal any underlying differences. We will explore these concepts in more detail in Chapter 3. For now, it is worth pausing to reflect on what we have just learnt about the different transformations epidemiologists perform on raw frequency counts and how these might be useful in addressing the question of whether 12 083 reported cases of influenza in South Australia in 2022 was a lot or a little.

Age-dependent: The risk of health-related phenomena changes with age.

Crude rate: A rate that is calculated for all ages combined.

Age-specific rates: Rates that are calculated after stratifying the population into specific age groups that define both the *numerator* and *denominator*.

Age structure: The total number of people alive at different ages at a point in time.

We have already determined that the 12 083 cases are *incident* cases – that is, they are the people who transitioned from the influenza-free bucket to the influenza bucket in 2022 – so we can now consider which of the three transformations from incident cases to something else might be appropriate, or even informative, and why. First, we could calculate the *ratio* of the 12 083 cases in 2022 to the number in a previous year. This would be one of the few situations where comparing raw frequency counts side by side might be useful. The reason for this is that the counts are derived from a single population that is unlikely to have changed much in terms of its size over such a short period. A ratio calculated in this way could be used to convey the percentage change in influenza case numbers from one year to another, as in the following equation:

$$\text{Percentage change in } n \text{ from } t_1 \text{ to } t_2 = \left(\left(\frac{n_{t=2}}{n_{t=1}}\right) - 1\right) \times 100 \qquad \text{(Equation 2.4)}$$

where n equals the number of cases (incident cases in this example, but any frequency count could be used here) and t_1 and t_2 are the two time points. At the heart of this is a ratio. It may look complicated, but this is just because of the bracketing, which tells you the order in which to do the calculations (ratio first, then subtract 1, then multiply by 100).

Say the South Australian Notifiable Diseases Surveillance System indicated that were 40 influenza cases reported to it in 2021. Using Equation 2.4, the calculations would look like this:

$$\begin{aligned}\text{Percentage change in } n \text{ from } t_1 \text{ to } t_2 &= \left(\left(\frac{12\,083}{40}\right) - 1\right) \times 100 \\ &= (302.1 - 1) \times 100 \\ &= 30\,107\%\end{aligned}$$

In other words, the incidence of reported influenza increased by a massive 30 107 per cent between the two years, suggesting that 2022 was indeed a very big year for influenza in South Australia, at least compared with the previous year!

Of course, 2021 was an exceptional year globally due to the mobility restrictions imposed during the COVID-19 pandemic so it is perhaps not surprising to see such a large increase in influenza numbers when these restrictions started to ease the following year. To be sure that changes in population size alone did not account for this increase, however, we could perform a different sort of transformation involving one of the rate formulae (Equations 2.2 or 2.3). Because we know that the data we have on influenza cases are derived from a routine collection rather than an epidemiological study, Equation 2.3 is the only feasible way to perform this transformation, so we would also need an estimate of the number of people we could reasonably assume to be at risk of influenza in South Australia at the relevant time. We have already been told that the population of South Australia was about 1.8 million in 2022 but we can be more precise than this by referring to the estimated resident population tables for South Australia, which the Australian Bureau of Statistics produces on a regular basis (3). These indicate that 1 821 537 people were estimated to be residing in South Australia at the end of June 2022 (i.e. at the middle of that year). If we assume that all these people were at risk of contracting the virus (this is not strictly true because many will have received Fluvax and will therefore be at a reduced risk of infection, but we will make the assumption anyway), then the calculations using Equation 2.3 would look like this:

$$\begin{aligned}\text{Rate per 1000 population per year} &= \left(\frac{12\,083}{1\,821\,537 \times 1}\right) \times 1000 \\ &= 0.00663 \times 1000 \\ &= 6.6\end{aligned}$$

In other words, the incidence rate of reported influenza in South Australia was 6.6 per 1000 population per year in 2022. This could be contracted to '6.6 per 1000 population in 2022' without any loss of meaning (the one-year timeframe is implied by saying 'in 2022'). You might even see it contracted to '6.6 per 1000 in 2022' and it would still be interpretable. We chose a multiplier of 1000 in these calculations because this was the smallest unit that allowed the result to be presented with sufficient precision at one decimal place (we could have used 10 000 but 66.3 per 10 000 does not add a lot to the accuracy of the information being conveyed). If we were then to perform the same calculations for each of the four years preceding 2022 and plot the results, we would get the information depicted in Figure 2.5.

This suggests that while 2022 was indeed a big year for influenza in South Australia, at least compared with the previous two years, it was a relatively mild year compared with 2019, the year just before the COVID pandemic, even accounting for changes in population size over this period.

One important point to note about incidence rates before we move on is that they are unlike proportions and mortality rates in that they have no upper limit. An incidence rate of 2000 per 1000 people per year simply means that, on average, everyone gets sick twice a year. In other words, incidence rates do not share all the properties of either proportions or mortality rates; while they can't be less than 0, they can be greater than 1.

There is one other type of transformation we could perform with the information we have from South Australia, and it does not rely on any additional data, just some assumptions.

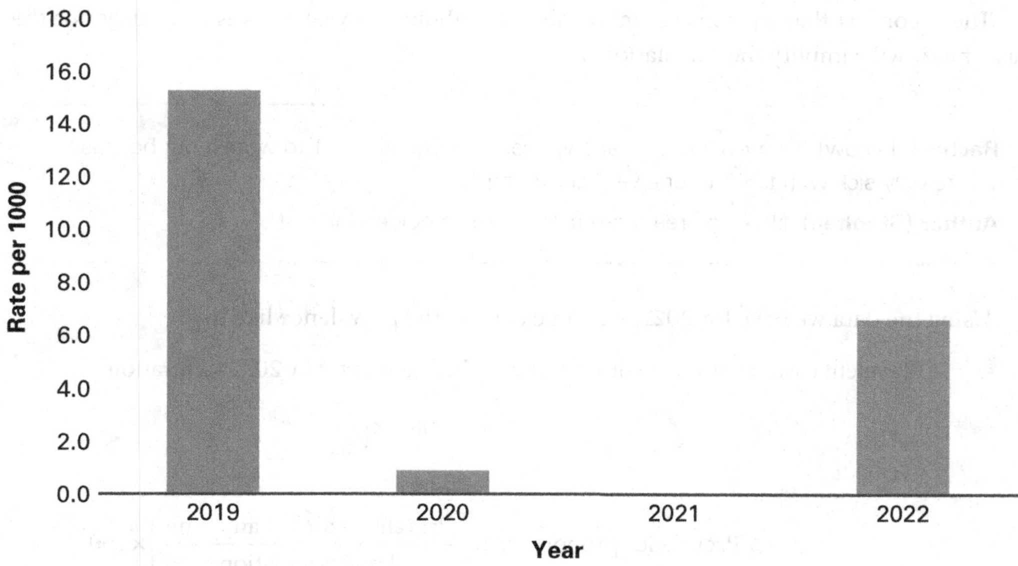

Figure 2.5 Incidence of reported influenza cases in South Australia, 2019–22. Adapted from (2).

Hugo: Well, we haven't calculated a proportion yet, so I guess it involves a proportion.

Rachael: But hang on, incidence is a flow variable, and you can't calculate proportions with flow variables.

Author (Stephen): These are great observations. Actually, there is no law that says you can't calculate proportions from counts of incident cases, and in fact there are situations where what you want to know about them is in this form. It's just that we haven't covered these yet since they sit better with our discussions on epidemiological studies in coming chapters.

The transformation we have in mind is a proportion and relies only on a formula we have learnt so far (not those we will learn about) plus two assumptions.

Hugo: Give us a clue.

The first assumption is that an influenza infection lasts, on average, one week.

Hugo: Give us another clue.

The second is that they occur uniformly throughout the year (this is obviously not the case, but it will simplify the calculations).

Rachael: I know! It's prevalence ... and we can use Equation 2.1 to work it out because you're only sick with the 'flu for a very short time!

Author (Stephen): Now you really are talking like an epidemiologist!

Using the data we have for 2022, we can calculate the prevalence like this:

$$\begin{aligned}
\text{Prevalent cases at any time during } 2022 &= \text{Incident cases in } 2022 \times \text{Duration} \\
&= 12\ 083 \times \left(\frac{1}{52}\right) \\
&= 232.4 \\
\text{Prevalence proportion } &= \left(\frac{\text{Prevalent cases at any time}}{\text{Total population}}\right) \times 100 \\
&= \left(\frac{232.4}{1\ 821\ 537}\right) \times 100 \\
&= 0.0001275 \times 100 \\
&= 0.013\%
\end{aligned}$$

In other words, assuming that influenza lasts, on average, one week, and that infections occur evenly throughout the year, then at any time during 2022, 0.013 per cent of the South Australian population was infected with the virus. This could be expressed as 1.3 per 10 000 and it would still make sense. Either way, the answer is a proportion in the strict sense of the definitions discussed thus far (i.e. it is bounded by 0 and 1) and has been worked out using the data we have on incidence cases and what we now know about the relationship between incidence, prevalence and duration. Note that if the answer were to have not conformed to the properties of a proportion, something would have been wrong with either our data on incidence or our assumption regarding duration. Of course, the real prevalence proportion would have been higher in colder months and lower in warmer months, but when averaged over 2022, this figure is about right.

Hugo: That's pretty neat.

Morbidity and mortality

There is only one more topic we need to address before finishing up this chapter on language and this relates to how epidemiologists like to differentiate between different types of measures. Broadly speaking, these can be divided into two categories: those relating to

morbidity and those relating to **mortality**. The latter is the easier term to define because death is unequivocal. Thus, any ratio, proportion or rate that involves this outcome can be regarded as a measure of mortality. We have already discussed mortality rates in these terms and case fatality is another example. Because of the unambiguous nature of death and the fact that authorities tend to put effort into counting this phenomenon (with varying degrees of rigour, as we will explore in coming chapters), it is not surprising that measures of mortality have become *the* most basic way to track changes in the overall health of a population over time, or to compare the relative health of different populations at a single point in time. The most ubiquitous of these is **life expectancy**, but there are others as well. Life expectancy tells you the average number of years an individual of a given age can be expected to live and is calculated using age-specific mortality rates (2). We will learn more about how to make comparisons using life expectancy and other common measures of mortality in Chapter 3.

Morbidity: Any measure that does not include death as an outcome. Includes measures such as *incidence, prevalence, remission, duration* and *severity*.

Mortality: Death, often expressed as the rate of death occurring in a given population over a specified period of time.

Life expectancy: The average number of years an individual of a given age can be expected to live. A measure of *mortality*.

Of course, epidemiologists are interested in much more than just how many people are dying (and what they are dying from), and measures that involve outcomes other than death are grouped under the morbidity heading. While morbidity may therefore initially appear to be an all-encompassing concept without clear boundaries (other than it excludes mortality), in fact epidemiologists tend to focus on specific attributes when talking about this concept. As far back as 1959, the World Health Organization characterised these in terms of three measurable 'units': '(1) persons who are ill; (2) the illnesses (periods or spells of illnesses) that these persons experienced; and (3) the duration (days, weeks, etc.) of these illnesses' (in 2). Thus, the claim that incidence, prevalence and duration are all measures of morbidity is consistent with this definition. In addition, you will see people's interaction with health services discussed as a measure of morbidity, although this is only true to the extent that their illness results in them seeking treatment. None of these measures, however, fully captures the differential impact of different health conditions on a population. For example, two illnesses may be highly prevalent and long-lasting, but the illness with severe symptoms will have more impact than the illness with only mild symptoms, all other things being equal. This observation has given rise to a new generation of epidemiologists who see *severity* as the missing link and very much an attribute to be considered when talking about morbidity (e.g. 4). We will explore examples of composite measures that seek to incorporate this dimension in our discussion about life expectancy in the following chapter.

Just a few comments about *remission* and *case fatality* before we finish up. You will notice that we have italicised these terms in the discussion about responses to the COVID-19 pandemic above but have not defined them further, except with reference to two of the three outflows from Bucket C in Figure 2.2. In other words, we have identified them as flow variables, the frequency of which – like incidence – is counted over time. Unlike incidence, however, we have not talked about possible transformations to make them more interpretable or comparable with similarly transformed remission or case fatality frequency counts. There are reasons for this. In the case of *remission*, it is because, as a whole, epidemiology has not engaged with the idea, as evidenced by the fact that it does not feature in even the most recent version of *A Dictionary of Epidemiology*, now in its sixth edition (2). Synonyms (e.g. recovery) are similarly absent; thus, the term tends to be overlooked outside of specific areas such as cancer and infectious disease epidemiology. Nevertheless, it can be considered relevant

Cause-specific mortality rate: A measure of *mortality* and a *mortality rate* that includes in the *numerator* the number of deaths from the phenomenon of interest over a specified period and in the *denominator* the product of the number of people in the population and the period over which the numerator was observed. Shares a numerator with *case fatality risk.*

Case fatality risk: (synonyms 'case fatality rate', 'case fatality ratio') A measure of *mortality* that includes in the *numerator* the number of deaths from the phenomenon of interest over a specified period and in the *denominator* the incident cases of this phenomenon over the same period. Shares a numerator with *cause-specific mortality rate.*

to morbidity because, as we learnt in Figure 2.2, the speed with which people get better is central to describing the complete epidemiology of any health condition (but particularly those where people can recover and become sick again).

In the case of *case fatality*, we have left the term undefined until now because there is debate over how this measure, once transformed, is to be classified. The above-mentioned dictionary classifies it as a rate (2), a respected textbook on epidemiology, now its fourth edition, maintains it is a ratio (5), while a scholarly review of the concept concludes that both understandings are outdated and that the emerging trend is to consider it a risk (6). Interestingly, this review is prefaced with the following quote from Lewis Carroll's *Alice Through the Looking Glass*:

> 'When I use a word,' Humpty Dumpty said, in a rather scornful tone, 'it means just what I choose it to mean – neither more nor less.'

What we can say about the outflow from Bucket C to D in Figure 2.2 (i.e. 'f. Dying from x') is that the label we attach to it depends on which denominator we chose for the transformation. If we choose a time-based denominator such as those defined in Equation 2.2 or Equation 2.3, we are calculating a rate. You will often see such a rate referred to in the literature as a **cause-specific mortality rate.** If, instead, we choose a case-based denominator such as the number of incidence cases (i.e. 'd. Getting sick from x') over a given period, we are calculating a proportion. You will see such a proportion variously referred to in the literature as a *case fatality rate, case fatality ratio* or **case fatality risk.**

Conclusion

In this chapter, we learnt that epidemiology is a relatively young discipline and that it is therefore not unusual to come across different words being used to describe the same concept or, even more confusingly, the same word being used to describe different concepts. However, we also heard that the discipline has matured to the point where there is agreement on a core group of numerical concepts, and therefore understanding the underlying properties of these concepts is critical if we are to talk about them with any degree of precision.

Learning objective 1: Describe the basic properties of a frequency count

First, we were introduced to the frequency count as being concerned with how quickly a health phenomenon is observed to have occurred in a given population. Points to consider in relation to this type of number include:

- how closely it reflects the actual number of cases in the population
- the unit of time over which the counting took place
- any attributes about the population, such as its size and age structure, that might influence the likelihood of the phenomenon occurring.

Learning objective 2: Understand the concepts of incidence and prevalence, and describe the relationships between these and other epidemiological measures

Next, we distinguished between the frequency of a health-related phenomenon and other attributes about it that epidemiologists might be interested in counting. In the first group we included the concept of *incidence*, which we learnt refers to new cases in a defined population within a specified period. In the second, we included the concept of *prevalence*, which we learnt refers to existing cases in a defined population at a point in time. To complete the picture, we introduced the concepts of getting better and dying, both of which we classified as frequency counts and included in the first group. We then learnt that these measures are mathematically related, such that it is possible to work out the complete epidemiology of a phenomenon even if you have information about only some of the variables.

Learning objective 3: Identify the numerator and denominator in various situations

Third, we noted that comparing raw counts side by side is rarely useful, except under specific circumstances, and that this limitation can be overcome by transforming them to a different scale numerically, thereby making them more interpretable or comparable with other similarly transformed counts. The transformations typically involve dividing one number by another, which we call the numerator and the denominator, respectively.

Learning objective 4: Describe the different underlying properties of ratios, proportions and rates

Fourth, we learnt that the types of transformations epidemiologists routinely perform can be classified into one of three broad groups: ratios, proportions and rates. Ratios are calculated by dividing one quantity (the 'numerator') by another like quantity (the 'denominator'). Proportions are a special type of ratio in which every entity counted in the numerator is also included in the denominator. Rates are another type of ratio in which the numerator is the number of cases of the phenomenon of interest in a specified population over a specified period and the denominator is the amount of time (whether measured exactly, or by an approximation method) for which everyone in that population was at risk of the phenomenon. Both proportions and rates can be expressed in terms of any multiple of 10 (e.g. 1, 10, 100, 1000, 10 000, 100 000) without affecting the underlying information being conveyed. Incidence rates do not share all the properties of either proportions or mortality rates; while they can't be less than 0, they can be greater than 1.

Learning objective 5: Recognise common measures of mortality and morbidity

Finally, we noted that epidemiologists like to differentiate between two broad categories of measures, those relating to *morbidity* and those relating to *mortality*. The latter is often easier to define and includes any measure where death is the outcome. Examples include mortality rates, case fatality and life expectancy. The former is made up of measures that involve outcomes other than death and includes traditional measures such as incidence, prevalence and duration, but also newer concepts such as severity.

Further reading

Bonita R, Beaglehole R, Kjellström T & World Health Organization. *Basic Epidemiology*. 2nd ed. World Health Organization; 2006. https://iris.who.int/handle/10665/43541

Questions

Answers are available at the end of the book.

Multiple-choice questions

1. Counts of prevalent cases are typically transformed into what kind of measure to make them more comparable and easier to interpret?

A – A ratio

B – A proportion

C – A rate

D – None of the above

2. Time is an essential component of what kind of measure?

A – A ratio

B – A proportion

C – A rate

D – None of the above

3. Health service demand is most influenced by what kind of epidemiological variable?

A – Incidence

B – Case fatality

C – Prevalence

D – None of the above

4. Which of the following statements is false?

A – All proportions are also ratios and can be expressed as percentages.

B – Proportions and rates can be expressed in terms of any multiple of 10 (e.g. 1, 10, 100, 1000, 10 000, 100 000) without affecting the underlying information being conveyed.

C – All ratios and percentages are necessarily proportions.

D – Incidence rates are unlike proportions and mortality rates in that they have no upper limit.

5. Which of the following is not a measure of morbidity?

A – Incidence

B – Health service usage

C – Case fatality

D – Disease severity

Short-answer questions

1. Explain the difference between counting incident cases and prevalent cases in epidemiology. What insights does each of these measures provide about the burden of a disease or condition within a population?

2. You are calculating the incidence rate of a relatively rare disease in a small population and have decided to use reported incident cases over a three-year timeframe to increase the robustness of your estimate. How does this influence your choice of denominator?

3. What is a ratio in epidemiological terms, and how does it differ from a proportion? Provide an example to illustrate your explanation.

4. How does the choice of denominator affect the interpretation of an epidemiological transformation in which the numerator is deaths from a cause?

5. Describe the different levels of prevention and their relevance in healthcare practice.

6. What is a proportion and how does this type of number relate to prevalence?

7. Explain the distinction between morbidity and mortality in epidemiology.

8. Discuss the bathtub analogy used by epidemiologists to explain the concepts of incident cases, prevalent cases, recovery and mortality.
9. Explain the use of the equation $p \approx i \times d$ in descriptive epidemiology and its limitations.
10. Describe the three levels of prevention that healthcare professionals may encounter. For each level, explain its primary focus in terms of an epidemiological parameter and provide an example of a disease where this level of prevention is particularly relevant.

References

1. Barendregt JJ, Van Oortmarssen GJ, Vos T, Murray CJ. A generic model for the assessment of disease epidemiology: The computational basis of DisMod II. *Population Health Metrics*. 2003;1(1):4.
2. Porta M. *A Dictionary of Epidemiology*. 6th ed. Oxford University Press; 2014.
3. Australian Bureau of Statistics. *National, State and Territory Population 2022*. ABS; 2022. www.abs.gov.au/statistics/people/population/national-state-and-territory-population/latest-release
4. Murray CJ. Quantifying the burden of disease: The technical basis for disability-adjusted life years. *Bulletin of the World Health Organization*. 1994;72(3):429–45.
5. Webb P, Bain C, Page A. *Essential Epidemiology*. 4th ed. Cambridge University Press; 2020.
6. Kelly H, Cowling BJ. Case fatality: Rate, ratio, or risk? *Epidemiology*. 2013;24(4):622–3.

3 Making comparisons

You can't compare apples with oranges – or can you?

Learning objectives

After studying this chapter, you will be able to:

1. Understand how to calculate crude, age-specific and age-standardised rates and when to use these measures for comparing the mortality or morbidity experience of populations
2. Describe life expectancy and potential years of life lost as two measures other than rates that are commonly used for comparing the mortality experience of populations
3. Identify the common links that allow mortality and morbidity data to be integrated and describe Health-Adjusted Life Expectancy (HALE) and Disability-Adjusted Life Years (DALY) as two popular measures that achieve this, thereby allowing us to compare the overall health of populations

Introduction

A fundamental problem in descriptive epidemiology is how to make meaningful and robust comparisons between different populations or within the same population over different periods. The problem has several dimensions. First, the data we have to work with (e.g. incident and prevalent cases, and deaths) are rarely usable in their raw form. We must therefore transform the data in some way before undertaking the comparison. Second, our data usually tell us about fundamentally different attributes of the populations we are seeking to compare. If we are only ever interested in comparing any one of these attributes at a time (mortality, for example), then one of several simple and well-established transformations is all that is typically required. Increasingly, however, epidemiologists are being asked to bring these attributes together into more integrated and meaningful comparisons. While simple transformations may well be necessary in these situations, they are by no means sufficient; additional, more elaborate techniques are therefore required. And finally, in developing these techniques, epidemiologists can find themselves making value judgements about how the world should be, rather than how they find it, or straying into territory that is beyond their training or unfamiliar to them in other ways. This can sit uncomfortably with some, leading to concerns about comparing apples with oranges. You can't do that, you might think. Or can you? Let's find out.

Crude, age-specific and age-standardised rates

In Chapter 2, we learnt that the key population characteristic that makes comparing raw frequency counts from different populations rarely very informative is size. Put simply, the larger the population the more chance (usually) of observing the phenomenon of interest. So, if we were interested in comparing the underlying force of, say, COVID-19 in two populations, the very least we would need to do would be to rescale the frequency count of infections by the amount of time everyone was at risk of getting the disease (or an approximation thereof). The analogy of two pipes of different sizes was used to illustrate the point that the pipe with the larger diameter (think population size) will have more water passing through it over any given period (think event frequency), even if the two pipes have water flowing through them at the same speed (think underlying force). Frequency counts rescaled in this way are called *rates*.

We say 'the very least' because there is another characteristic about a population in addition to its size that has a major bearing on the frequency of a phenomenon occurring, and this is its *age structure*. This is simply the total number of people alive at different ages at a point in time and is an important attribute of a population to both epidemiologists and demographers alike. It is best visualised using a type of graph called a **population pyramid**, where the x-axis (the horizontal axis) represents the size of the population, and the y-axis (the vertical axis) indicates the different age groups, starting with the youngest at the bottom. Males are typically represented on the left, females on the right. Represented in this way, the age structure of populations with high mortality rates resembles a pyramid, which is how this type of graph got its name. Figure 3.1 illustrates this by comparing the population age structure of sub-Saharan countries (high mortality) with Europe and North American countries (low mortality) in 2022.

Population pyramid: A type of graph that depicts the age structure of a population where the x-axis (the horizontal axis) represents the size of the population, and the y-axis (the vertical axis) indicates the different age groups, starting with the youngest at the bottom. Males are typically represented on the left, females on the right.

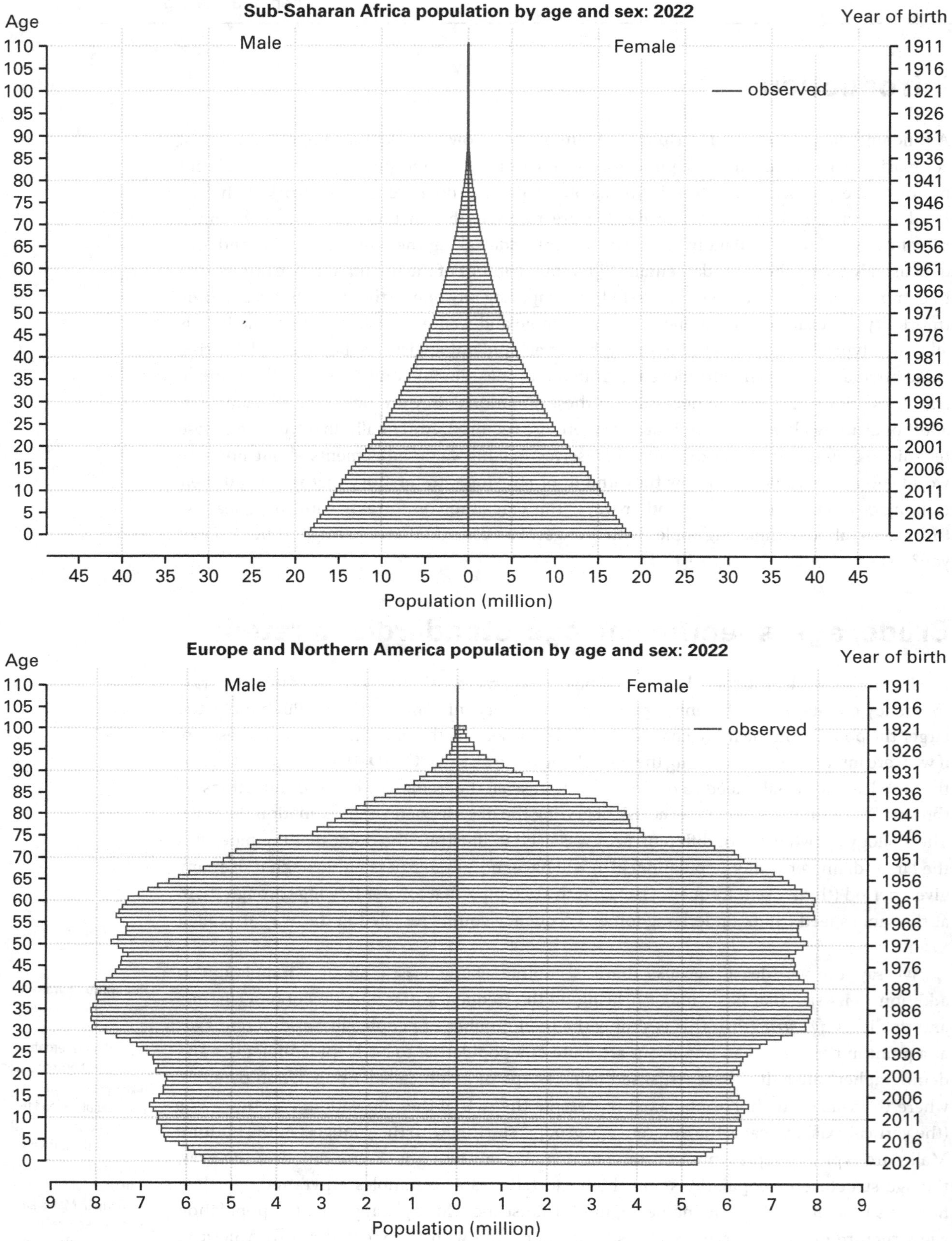

Sub-Saharan Africa population by age and sex: 2022

Age | Male | Female | Year of birth

— observed

Population (million)

Europe and Northern America population by age and sex: 2022

Age | Male | Female | Year of birth

— observed

Population (million)

Figure 3.1 Population by age and sex, sub-Saharan countries (top) and European and North American countries (bottom), 2022 (1)

The age structure of a population influences the frequency with which many health-related phenomena occur when the risk of these phenomena is *age-dependent* – in other words, when risk changes with age. For most chronic diseases – that is, those that last a long time – risk *increases* with age such that older people are much more likely to become ill than younger people. Dementia is a good example. People can get dementia at any age, but the chance of being affected is much greater in the very old than at any other age. For other diseases, however, risk is concentrated in age groups other than the very old. Figure 3.2 illustrates this point by comparing the incidence of Alzheimer's disease and other dementias, depressive disorders and transport injuries across the lifespan.

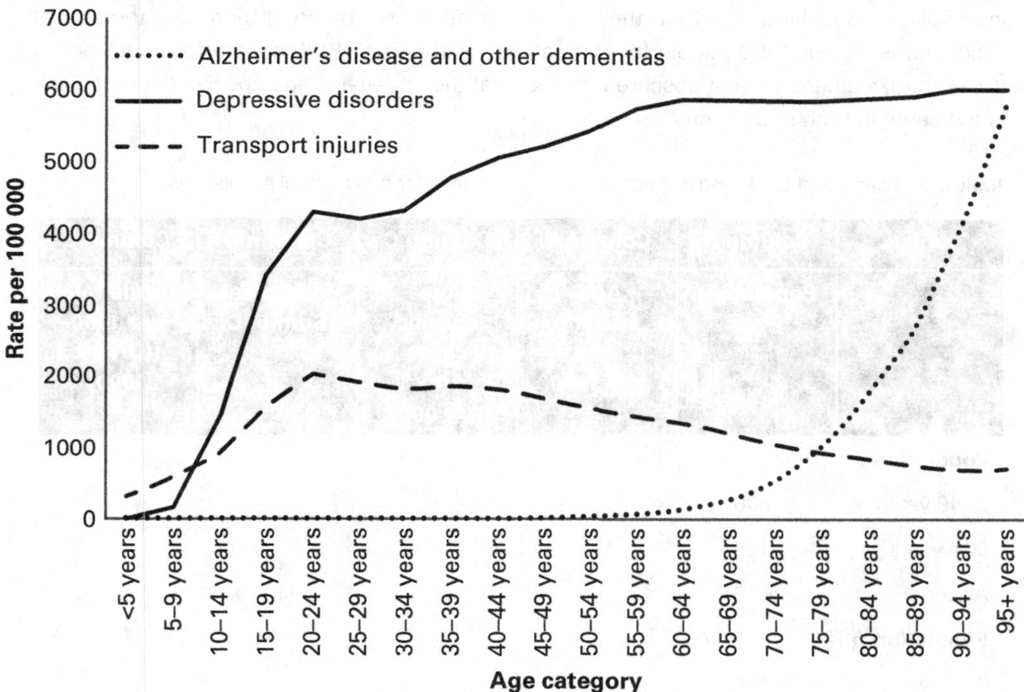

Figure 3.2 Global incidence per 100 000 by age, Alzheimer's disease and other dementias, depressive disorders and transport injuries, 2019 (2)

For any given phenomenon of interest, therefore, both the *size* of the population and its underlying *age structure* can influence the raw frequency count of that phenomenon, all other things being equal. Again in the case of dementia (which we now know has an age-dependent risk profile), the population with the older age structure – that is, the one with more older people in it – will experience both more new cases of this disease (incidence) and more cases living with this disease at any point in time (prevalence) than the population with the younger age structure – that is, the one with fewer older people in it – even when overall size and dementia risk are the same in both populations. Rescaling the frequency counts by population size alone will not help to reveal this underlying similarity in dementia risk.

Rachael: I don't get it. How can things be different but the same at the same time?

Author (Stephen): Okay, let's go through it step by step.

EXAMPLE 3.1

Imagine, for example, that there are two populations each with a total of 1000 people, but that the first (Population *a*) has 600 people in the 0–49 years age category whereas the second (Population *b*) only has 400. Now let's assume that, for both populations, the annual incidence of dementia is 10 per 1000 in the 0–49 years age category, but that this increases tenfold to 100 per 1000 in the 50+ years age category. In other words, the risk of getting dementia is age-dependent, but identical in both populations. Table 3.1 demonstrates that there will be a total of 46 incident cases in Population *a* in any one year compared with 64 in Population *b* (column D). If we then rescale these figures by population size, the annual incidence is 46 per 1000 people for Population *a* and 64 per 1000 people for Population *b* (Column E), a difference that obscures the fact that the underlying age-specific dementia risk is the same in both populations.

Table 3.1 Example of crude and age-specific rate calculations for two artificial populations

	Column A	Column B	Column C	Column D	Column E
	Population	Age-specific rate per 1000	Age-specific cases [A x (B/1 000)]	Total cases [Sum of C]	Crude rate per 1000 [(D/A) x 1000]
Population *a*					
0–49 years	600	10	6		
50+ years	400	100	40		
All ages	1000			46	46
Population *b*					
0–49 years	400	10	4		
50+ years	600	100	60		
All ages	1000			64	64

The difference in rates observed for all ages combined in Example 3.1 is due to differences in population structure alone, not differences in age-specific risk or overall population size. If we think back to our pipe analogy, the final section of pipe for all ages in both populations is the same diameter but Population *b*'s pipe is flowing faster because, even there is no difference in flow between the two population in any of the upstream pipes, Population *b* has a smaller pipe for younger ages where the flow is slower but a larger one for older ages where the flow is faster (Figure 3.3). For this reason, epidemiologists like to talk about rates calculated for all ages combined as *crude* rates. This is to remind us that no attempt has been made to account for the affect that age structure might have on the speed of the underlying force being calculated and compared. We came across these types of rates in the previous chapter when we compared the incidence of influenza in the South Australian population over time. In that example, any changes in age structure over the years for which we had data were likely to have such a small influence on the crude rates that we could safely ignore them. We did, however, account for changes in population size. This is what we can think of as the capability limit of crude rate transformations; they account for differences in population size, but not age structure.

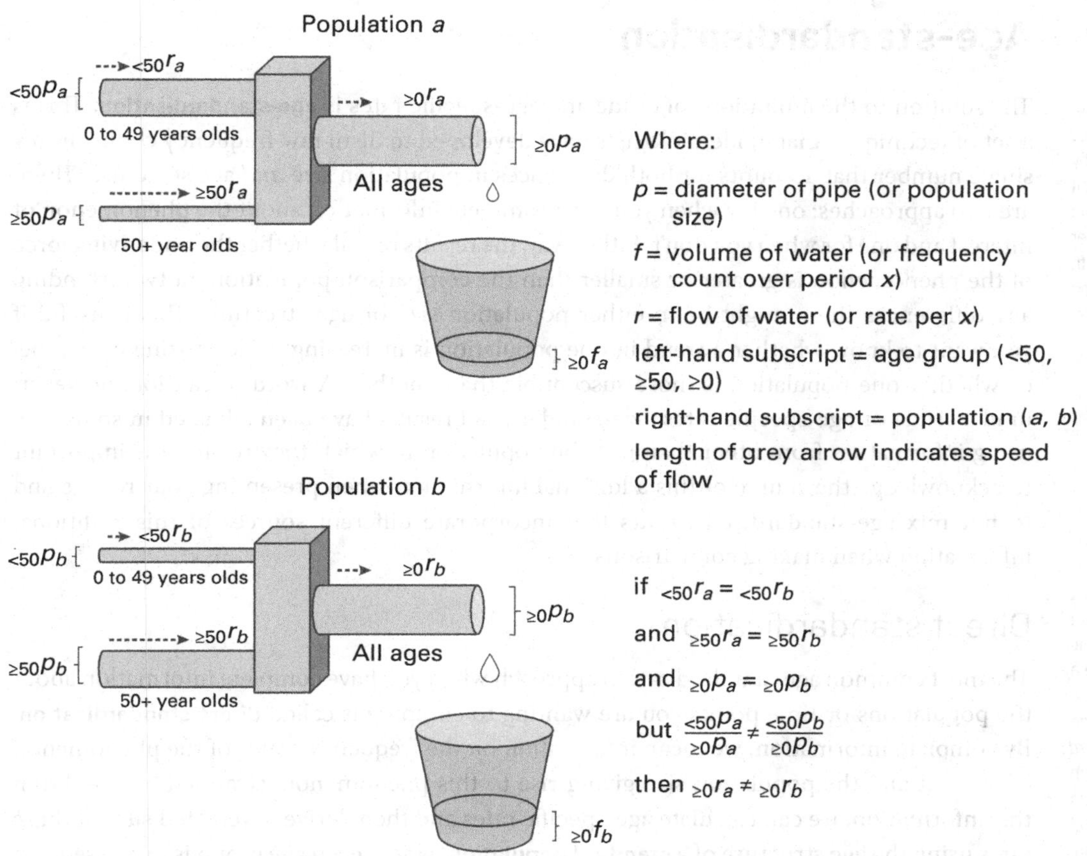

Figure 3.3 Relationship between population size, frequency counts and rates in populations with different age structures

If rates calculated for all ages combined are referred to as crude rates, then it follows that *age-specific* rates are those calculated after we have *stratified* the population into specific age groups. **Stratification** is simply the separation of a population into different groups on the basis of one or more attributes. In many ways, rates stratified by age are more useful for making comparisons with or between populations because they are, by definition, more specific. How specific really depends on the context, but five-year age groupings are as granular as you are likely to see in most situations. The age-specific rates presented in Column B of Table 3.1 are relatively coarse by comparison, but this is to simplify the example. And therein lies the problem with age-specific rates: the more specific they are, the greater the number of figures there are to compare, and this can quickly become unwieldy, making it difficult to synthesise the information into an overall picture.

Stratification: The separation of a population into different groups on the basis of one or more attributes.

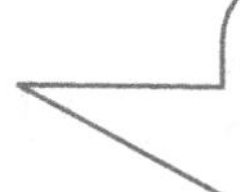

Rachael: So, if crude rates are too crude and age-specific rates are too specific, then I guess age-standardised rates are somewhere in between, right?

Author (Stephen): Not quite. We'll get to that next.

Age-standardisation

Age-standardisation: A set of techniques developed by epidemiologists to distil raw frequency counts into a single number that accounts for both differences in population size and age structure.

The solution to the limitations of crude and age-specific rates is **age-standardisation**. This is a set of techniques that epidemiologists have developed to distil raw frequency counts into a single number that accounts for both differences in population size *and* age structure. There are two approaches: one for when you have complete information about the phenomenon of interest and one for when you don't. Either way, the results reveal whether the underlying force of the phenomenon is greater or smaller than the comparison population, notwithstanding any differences there might be in either population size or age structure. This is useful if you want to know whether a trend in one population is increasing or decreasing over time, or whether one population is more susceptible than another. A word of caution, however: unlike crude or age-specific rates, age-standardised results have been adjusted in some way using information from other than just the population to which they relate. It is important to acknowledge the source of this additional information when presenting your results and to not mix age-standardised results that incorporate different sources of this additional information when making comparisons.

Direct standardisation: Where you calculate age-specific rates and then derive a weighted sum of these rates using the age structure of a *standard population*, where each age group is expressed as a proportion of the total in that population.

Standard population: The reference population used in age-standardisation procedures.

Direct standardisation

The most common age-standardisation approach when you have complete information about the populations or time points you are wanting to compare is called **direct standardisation**. By complete information, we mean information on the frequency count of the phenomenon of interest and the population size giving rise to this phenomenon, stratified by age. From this information, we can calculate age-specific rates and then derive a weighted sum of these rates using the age structure of a **standard population**, where each age group is expressed as a proportion of the total in that population. The standard population must be made explicit for the result to be replicable, but the choice about which standard to use is up to you. An age-standardised rate using this technique is therefore simply the weighted sum of age-specific rates using an agreed set of weights that add up to 1, as illustrated in Example 3.2.

EXAMPLE 3.2

In Table 3.2, we have reproduced the incidence of dementia in populations *a* and *b* from Table 3.1. The age-specific rates are the same in both populations (10 per 1000 in the 0–49 years age category and 100 per 1000 in the 50+ years age category) but the crude rates are different (46 per 1000 people for Population *a* and 64 per 1000 people for Population *b*) because, as we now know, the age structures are different (600 people in the 0–49 years age category in Population *a* compared with only 400 in Population *b*). The first step is to choose a standard population. In this example, we will standardise to the age structure of a hypothetical population that has equal proportions in both the 0–49 years and the 50+ years age categories (Column D). The next step is to multiply each of the age-specific rates from the populations being compared by the corresponding proportion from the standard population (Column E). The final step is to sum the weighted age-specific rates for each population (Column F).

Table 3.2 Example of direct age-standardisation rate calculations for two artificial populations using an alternative standard

	Column A	Column B	Column C	Column D	Column E	Column F
	Population	Cases	Rate per 1000 [(B/A) x 1000]	Standard population	Weighted age-specific rate per 1000 [C x D]	Age-standardised rate per 1000 [Sum of E]
Population *a*						
0–49 years	600	6	10	0.5	5	
50+ years	400	40	100	0.5	50	
All ages	1000	46	46	1		55
Population *b*						
0–49 years	400	4	10	0.5	5	
50+ years	600	60	100	0.5	50	
All ages	1000	64	64	1		55

In Example 3.2, the age-standardised rate is 55 per 1000 per year in both populations. In other words, by adjusting for the different age structures of the two populations, we can see that the underlying force of dementia is the same in both. We already knew this, since the age-specific rates are also the same, but the age-standardisation technique allows us to make the point by providing just two figures to compare rather than four (or potentially more if finer age groups are used). A comparison of crudes rates, on the other hand, might tempt us to reach a different conclusion.

The age-standardised rate itself is an artificial figure because it incorporates information from a standard population. A literal interpretation would be something like this: an age-standardised rate is what the crude rate would have been in a population had it had the same age structure as an arbitrarily chosen standard population. Or, in terms of our pipe analogy, what the speed of water in the final section of pipe for all ages would have been had the diameters of the upstream pipes been the same as in the standard population (Figure 3.4). However, you are unlikely to see words like this because the magnitude of an age-standardised rate in isolation is of little interest over and above what the crude rate already tells us; it is only when two or more standardised rates are compared that meaningful interpretations are possible. The power of the above analysis, therefore, is not that the age-standardised rates have a particular value but that it is possible to demonstrate that the underlying force of dementia is the same in both populations. We could have chosen another population with a different age structure to standardise to and the values of the standardised rates being compared would have been different, but the conclusion would have been the same.

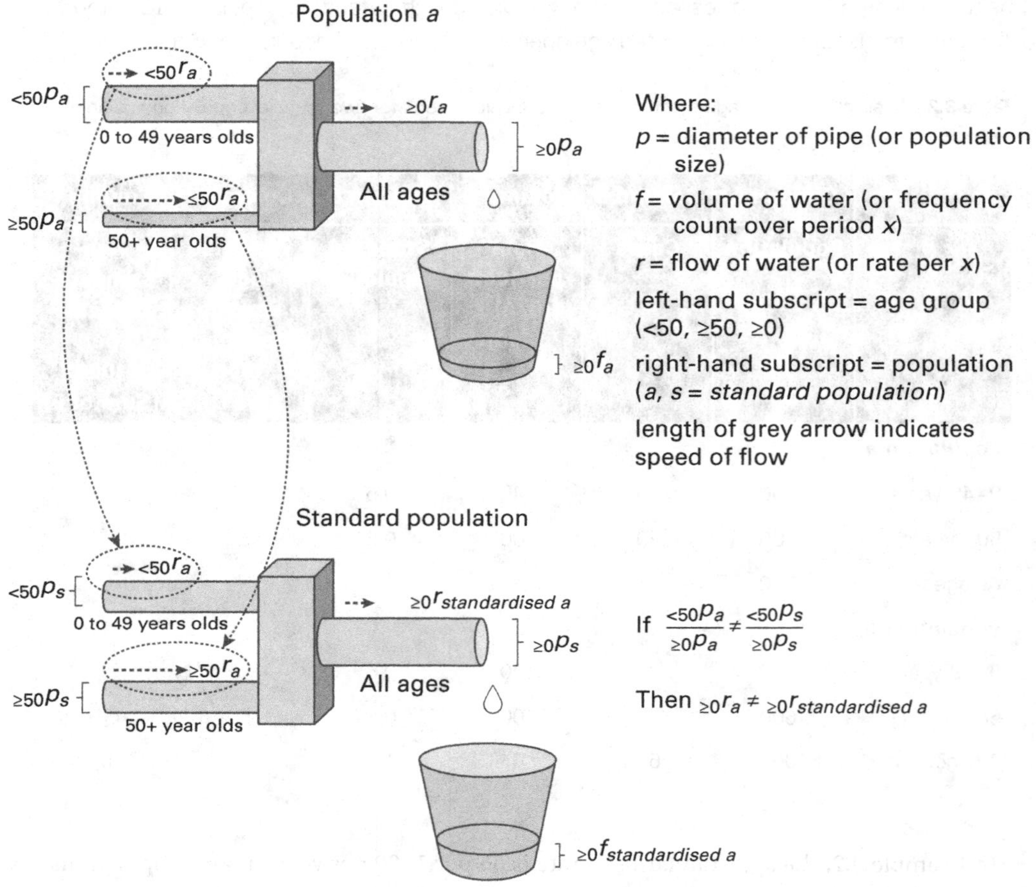

Figure 3.4 Direct standardisation

> **Hugo:** What about comparing crude rates and standardised rates? Is this a thing?
> **Author (Stephen):** A very good question, and there's a simple answer.

The magnitude of the difference between a crude rate and an age-standardised rate reflects the degree to which the age structure of the population in question differs from the chosen standard population. In the above example, the crude rate for Population *a* is slightly less than the age-standardised rate (46 compared with 55) because dementia is a disease of old age and Population *a*'s age structure is slightly younger than our standard population (60 per cent in the 0–49 years age category compared with 50 per cent). Conversely, the crude rate for Population *b* is slightly more than the age-standardised rate (64 per cent compared with 55 per cent) because its age structure is slightly older than our standard population (40 per cent in the 0–49 years age category compared with 50 per cent). When comparing rates between different populations, you would typically choose a standard population whose age structure is an average of the populations being compared, as we have done here. Authorities such as the World Health Organization, Eurostat and the US National Cancer Institute publish standard populations to use in various situations if ever you are in doubt.

When comparing rates from the same population over time, as in a trend analysis, it is not uncommon to choose one year of data from that population as your standard and use this to adjust all other years in the analysis. For example, assume that the data presented in Table 3.1 represents two different times (Year 1 and Year 1 + x) for one population rather than for two populations at the same time, and that you decide to choose population data for Year 1 as the standard. The calculations would look like those presented in Example 3.3.

EXAMPLE 3.3

Table 3.3 Example of direct age-standardisation rate calculations for one artificial population at two different times

	Column A	Column B	Column C	Column D	Column E	Column F
	Population	Cases	Rate per 1000 (B/A) x 1000	Standard population	Weighted age-specific rate per 1000 C x D	Age-standardised rate per 1000 Sum of E
Year 1						
0–49 years	600	6	10	0.6	6	
50+ years	400	40	100	0.4	40	
All ages	1000	46	46	1		46
Year 1 + x						
0–49 years	400	4	10	0.6	6	
50+ years	600	60	100	0.4	40	
All ages	1000	64	64	1		46

The first point to notice about the results in Example 3.3 is that the crude and standardised rates for Year 1 are the same. This is because the age structure at Year 1 is (by design) the same as the standard population in this analysis; hence the standardisation procedure has no effect. The next point is that the standardised rate for Year 1 + x is the same as for Time 1, reflecting the fact that the underlying force of dementia is the same at both time points; all that has changed over the period is that the population has aged. The final point is both an observation and a warning: the standardised rates in Table 3.3 are less than those in Table 3.2 for one reason alone: the age structure of the standard populations is different (the one in Table 3.3 is younger than in the one in Table 3.2). There is no difference in the underlying frequency data. This points to the danger of comparing standardised rates that have been adjusted using different standards; the results could suggest one conclusion when the underlying data support another.

Indirect standardisation

Indirect standardisation: Where you compare the raw frequency count of the phenomenon of interest in a population against the number you would expect to have observed had that population experienced the same age-specific rates as a standard population.

The other main approach to age-standardisation is called **indirect standardisation**. It is usually reserved for when you have incomplete information about the populations you are wanting to compare, or the numbers are too unstable to support the direct standardisation approach. Indirect standardisation is where you compare the raw frequency count of the phenomenon of interest in a population against the number you would expect to have observed had that population experienced the same age-specific rates as a standard population. The key difference with this approach compared with the direct standardisation approach is that it does not require you to stratify the frequency count in the population of interest by age. This means it can be used in situations where direct standardisation would not be possible. For example, official tabulations may record the number of incident cases of a health condition across different sub-populations, but not by the age at which they occurred. Even though you would be unable to apply the direct standardisation technique to these data, you would still be able undertake calculations using the indirect technique, provided you had more detailed information about the standard population.

EXAMPLE 3.4

Imagine a country is divided into three regions (A, B and C) and that official tabulations show over a one-year period 33, 77 and 55 new cases of tuberculosis in Regions A, B and C, respectively, but not the age at which they occurred. From other sources, we also know the population size of each region by age and have a recent epidemiological study for the entire country showing that the crude incidence of tuberculosis is 55 per 1000 person-years and that the age-specific rates are 10 and 100 per 1000 person-years in the 0 to 49 years and 50+ years age categories, respectively. We would not be able to calculate age-standardised rates using the direct method from these data because we are unable to calculate age-specific rates for each region. We can, however, proceed with the indirect method because we have raw frequency counts at the regional level.

Table 3.4 shows how to achieve indirect standardisation using the above information, which has been included in Columns A and B. The remaining steps are as follows:

1. Obtain age-specific rates of tuberculosis for a relevant standard population (Column C). We have been told that the epidemiological study is representative of the entire country so we will use data from this study.
2. Derive the expected number of cases in each region by age (Column D) by multiplying the age-specific rates from the standard population (Column C) by the population numbers for each region (Column A).
3. Derive the total number of expected cases for each region (Column E) by adding the figures in Column D.
4. Derive the ratio of observed to expected cases (Column F) by dividing Column B by Column E.
5. Optional: derive standardised rate (Column G) by multiplying Column F by the crude rate from the standard population (55 per 1000 person-years).

Table 3.4 Example of indirect age-standardisation calculations for three artificial populations

	Column A	Column B	Column C	Column D	Column E	Column F	Column G
	Population	Observed cases	Age-specific rate per 1000 from standard population	Age-specific number of expected cases [A x (C/1000)]	Total number of expected cases [Sum of D]	Ratio of observed cases over expected cases [B/D]	Standardised rate per 1000 [F x crude rate from std pop]
Region A							
0–49 years	600		10	6			
50+ years	400		100	40			
All ages	1000	33			46	0.7	39.5
Region B							
0–49 years	400		10	4			
50+ years	600		100	60			
All ages	1000	77			64	1.2	66.2
Region C							
0–49 years	500		10	5			
50+ years	500		100	50			
All ages	1000	55			55	1.0	55.0
Standard population							
0–49 years	1500	15	10				
50+ years	1500	150	100				
All ages	3000	165	55				

Several points are worth noting about Example 3.4. First, because it is based on incidence data, the figures in Column F are typically called Standardised Incidence Ratios (SIRs). When mortality data are used instead, they are typically called Standardised Mortality Ratios (SMRs). Ratios are the preferred way of expressing the results of indirect standardisation calculations, although the alternative rate expression (Column G) is also valid. Second, the SIR for Region A indicates that the incidence of tuberculosis in this region is 0.7 times less than would have been expected had it had the same age-specific rates as the standard population. For Region B, it indicates that it is 1.2 times more than would have been expected had it had the same age-specific rates as the standard population. For Region C, it indicates that it is the same as would have been expected had it had the same age-specific rates as the standard population. Taken together, these results indicate that, after accounting for age structure, Region B had the highest incidence of tuberculosis. Third, as with direct standardisation, comparing SIRs and SMRs based on different standard populations should be avoided.

Mortality-based measures

So far, we have looked at some basic transformations that epidemiologists have developed for comparing frequency counts from different populations or points in time. We have learned that the crude rate transformation rescales frequency counts according to population size alone whereas the standardisation transformation rescales them according to age structure as well. Although the examples we have explored have been based around incident cases, they apply equally to deaths because, as we learnt in the previous chapter, both incidence and mortality are time-based measures. They can even be used with prevalence data despite prevalence not being a time-based measure. There are several useful and popular transformations that can only be used on mortality data; however, the most ubiquitous of these is life expectancy. We will explore this and a related mortality-based measure in the following sections.

Life expectancy

The concept of life expectancy is something most people easily understand. For instance, if you are told that your current life expectancy is 75 years and that it could increase by eight years if you stop smoking, improve your diet and start exercising regularly, the message is clear. Your lifestyle choices are directly affecting how long you can expect to live, and you may want to think about changing your habits. This practical understanding is likely to have a greater impact than being told that your mortality risk is 10 per 100 000 person-years and could drop to five per 100 000 person-years if you were to adopt these healthier behaviours. So, what is the relevance to the goals of this chapter? It turns out that life expectancy isn't just a tool for predicting individual lifespans; it is also a valuable way to summarise and compare the mortality patterns of entire populations. It shares this feature with crude and age-standardised rates but can have a greater impact because it is easier to comprehend. Expressing mortality risk as a lifespan or parts of it is much more intuitive than presenting rates per some unit of the population.

For example, imagine you would like to make a simple comparison of the mortality experience of different populations around the world. One way to do this would be to look at age-specific or age-standardised mortality rates for each country. Another would be to compare life expectancy, as the Organisation of Economic Cooperation and Development (OECD) does on a regular basis. The latest data from this organisation reveals considerable differences in **life expectancy at birth** between OECD member countries in 2021, with Japan having the longest life expectancy (84.5 years) and Latvia having the shortest (73.1 years) (Figure 3.5). This is a gap of 11.4 years and a paints a sharper picture about the potential for health gain across these countries than would have been achieved using the other measures discussed thus far.

Life expectancy at birth: The average number of years a hypothetical newborn child could be expected to live if they were to experience the observed age-specific mortality rates of a population or group for the rest of their life.

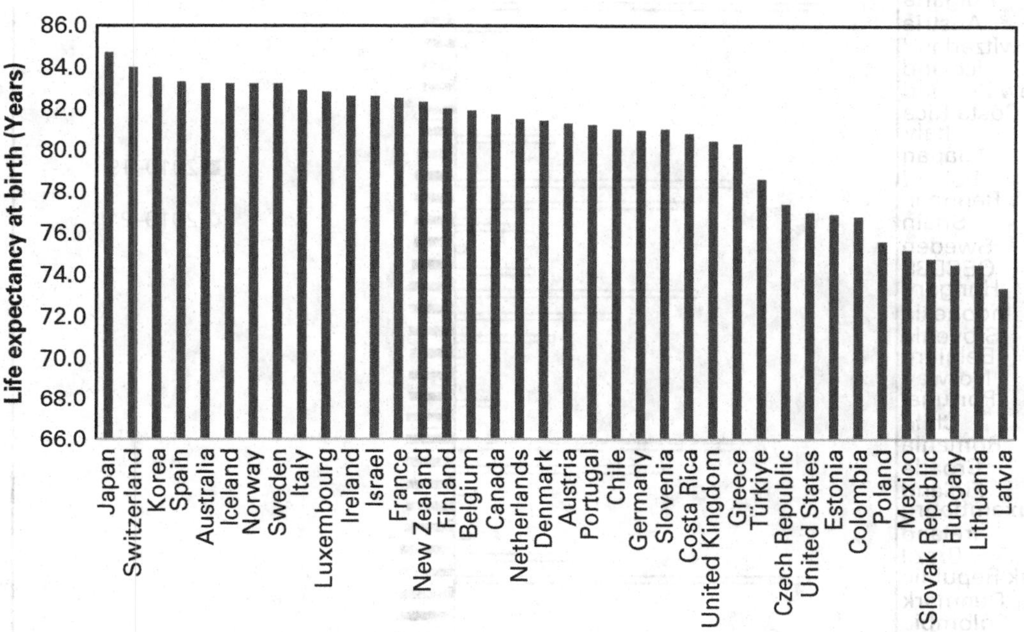

Figure 3.5 Life expectancy at birth (years), OECD member countries, 2021 (or nearest year available) (3)

Now imagine you would like to look at the impact the COVID-19 pandemic had on the mortality experience of populations globally. Again, you could do this with rates, but a more powerful way would be to look at life expectancy gains in the period prior to the emergence of this disease and compare these with what happened after it had spread globally. Figure 3.6 presents an OECD analysis of average life expectancy changes between 2010 and 2019 compared with those between 2019 and 2021. This shows that all 49 countries in the analysis experienced life expectancy gains in the nine years prior to COVID-19, ranging from 0.01 years per year in the United States to 0.9 years per year in South Africa (average of 0.2 years per year). In the two years after its emergence, however, 34 of the 49 countries experienced declines in life expectancy by an average of 0.14 years per year; the remainder experienced an average increase of only 0.02 years per year. Only two countries experienced higher annual life expectancy gains after the emergence of COVID-19 than before (Australia and Mexico).

Given the widespread use of life expectancy as a measure of health attainment globally, it is important to understand how it is calculated. The most common approach is with an **abridged life table**, the origins of which can be traced back to John Graunt, one of the founders of demography in seventeenth-century England. An abridged life table is distinct from a **complete life table** in that it only requires mortality data by age groups not single years of age. This lessens the computational load without compromising precision to any

Abridged life table: The essential inputs are age-specific mortality rates and the median age of death in each age group. From this information, an artificial cohort is exposed to the implied mortality risks and the average amount of time spent at each age is determined. This is distinct from a *complete life table* in that it only requires mortality data by age groups, not single years of age.

Complete life table: The same as an *abridged life table* but requires mortality data by single years of age.

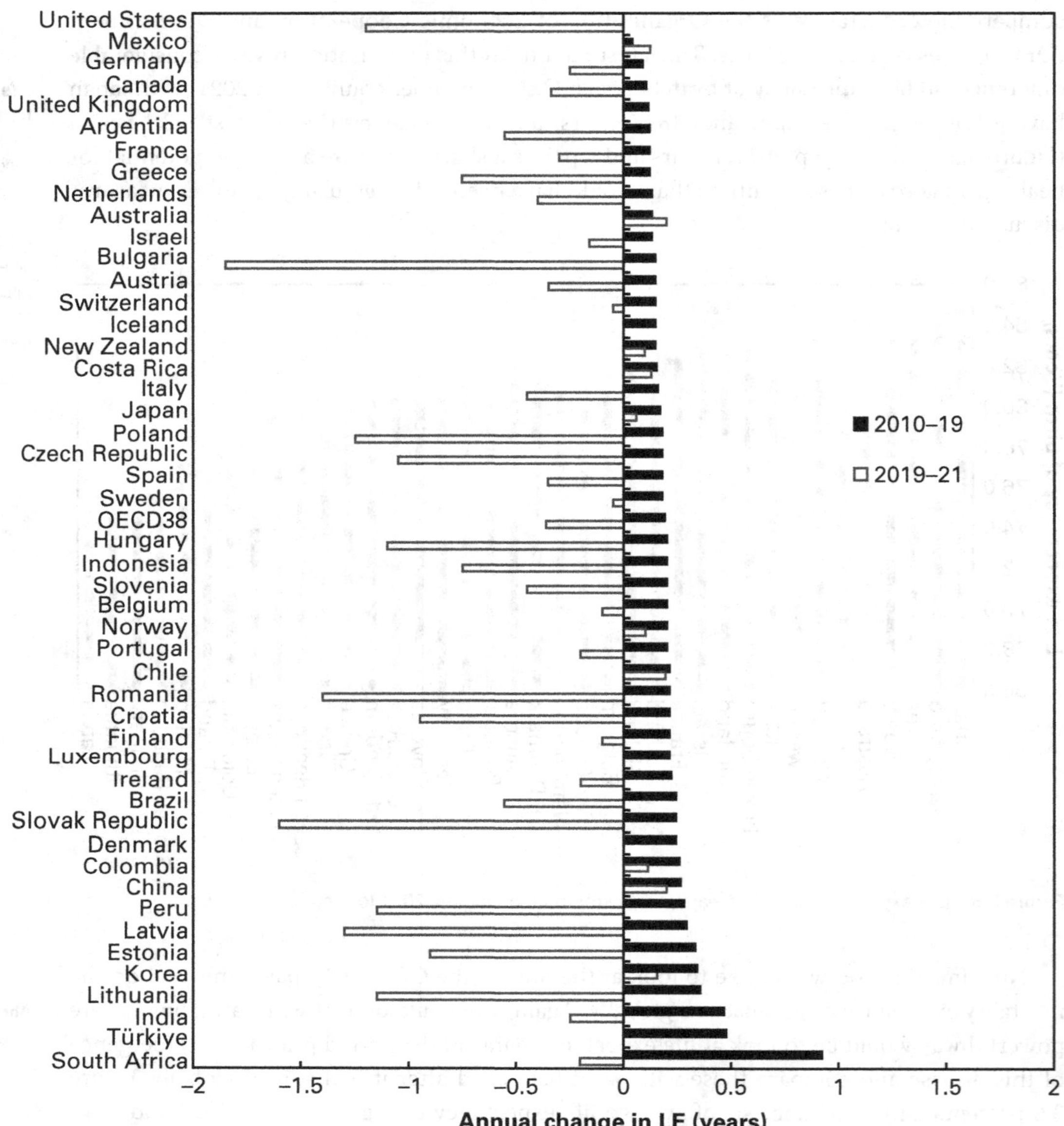

Figure 3.6 Changes in life expectancy, 2019–21 and 2010–19 (4)

Period life table: A life table that uses *mortality* rates for a given period (usually a year) and assumes that these apply without change into the future.

Cohort life table: A life table that uses projected *mortality* trends into the future.

significant extent. The essential inputs are age-specific mortality rates and the median age of death in each age group. From this information, an artificial cohort is exposed to the implied mortality risks and the average amount of time spent at each age is determined.

There are two basic approaches: the **period life table** and the **cohort life table**. The period life table approach is the most common because it uses mortality rates for a given period (usually a year) and assumes these apply without change into the future. This assumption is reasonable if trends in mortality are flat – that is, not increasing or decreasing – but for many populations, this isn't the case. The cohort life table approach, on the other hand, seeks to overcome this limitation by assuming past trends in mortality will continue into the future. This is a more realistic assumption in many cases but means the calculations are more complicated and uncertain because they include an element of forecasting.

For our purposes, we will focus on the period life table because it is the one used by statistical and health authorities when compiling life expectancy results such as those presented above. It is also easier to calculate and feeds more directly into our discussion of heath-adjusted life expectancy below. Example 3.5 shows how to calculate a period life table using age-specific mortality rates for an artificial population.

EXAMPLE 3.5

Table 3.5 Example of life expectancy calculations for an artificial population

Column A	Column B	Column C	Column D	Column E	Column F	Column G	Column H	Column I	Column J
x	n	a	${}_nM_x$	${}_nq_x$	l_x	${}_nd_x$	${}_nL_x$	T_x	e_x
0	1	0.1	0.0131	0.0130	100 000	1 297	98 833	6 710 000	67.1
1	4	0.4	0.0008	0.0032	98 703	317	394 052	6 611 167	67.0
5	5	0.5	0.0003	0.0014	98 386	140	491 581	6 217 115	63.2
10	5	0.5	0.0004	0.0018	98 246	177	490 788	5 725 534	58.3
15	5	0.5	0.0009	0.0047	98 069	461	489 193	5 234 746	53.4
20	5	0.5	0.0019	0.0093	97 608	908	485 770	4 745 553	48.6
25	5	0.5	0.0023	0.0115	96 700	1 114	480 715	4 259 784	44.1
30	5	0.5	0.0028	0.0141	95 586	1 345	474 569	3 779 069	39.5
35	5	0.5	0.0053	0.0261	94 242	2 463	465 050	3 304 499	35.1
40	5	0.5	0.0062	0.0303	91 778	2 784	451 934	2 839 449	30.9
45	5	0.5	0.0086	0.0423	88 995	3 763	435 567	2 387 516	26.8
50	5	0.5	0.0126	0.0612	85 232	5 219	413 112	1 951 949	22.9
55	5	0.5	0.0178	0.0852	80 013	6 821	383 012	1 538 837	19.2
60	5	0.5	0.0231	0.1090	73 192	7 980	346 010	1 155 825	15.8
65	5	0.5	0.0424	0.1917	65 212	12 504	294 800	809 815	12.4
70	5	0.5	0.0632	0.2730	52 708	14 388	227 571	515 015	9.8
75	5	0.5	0.0930	0.3774	38 320	14 464	155 442	287 443	7.5
80	5	0.5	0.1418	0.5235	23 856	12 490	88 058	132 002	5.5
85+	n.a.	n.a.	0.2587	1.0000	11 367	11 367	43 943	43 943	3.9

Columns A and B tell you the starting age of the age interval (x) and its width (n), respectively. So the first line of data relates to the <1-year-olds, the second to the 1- to <5-year-olds, the third to the 5- to <10-year-olds, and so on up to the 85+ year-olds. Column C tells you the proportion of the interval n alive by those who died in that interval. So, in the first age group, it is 1 × 0.1 = 0.1 years. In the second, it is 4 × 0.4 = 1.6 years, and so on. Column D is where you enter the age-specific mortality rates for the population. In this example, they

EXAMPLE 3.5 Continued

have been expressed per unit of population rather than some other multiplier such as 1000 or 100 000. Column E converts the age-specific mortality rates in Column D into age-specific probabilities of dying using the formula ${}_nq_x = (n \times {}_nM_x) / (1 + n \times {}_nM_x \times (1 - a))$ for all age intervals except the last, where the probability of dying is 1. There are other approaches for adjusting M_x values to q_x values, but the results are similar. Column F (l_x) is a hypothetical cohort of 100 000 babies (called the radix) who are progressively exposed to the relevant age-specific probability of dying (${}_nq_x$) as they age. Column G is the expected number of deaths at the end of n years in each age interval using the formula ${}_nd_x = {}_nq_x \times l_x$. Column H is the number of person years alive in each age interval using the formula ${}_nL_x = (l_{x+n} \times n) + ({}_nd_x \times a \times n)$. Column I ($T_x$) is the cumulative years lived by the hypothetical cohort in the age interval and all subsequent age intervals. And finally, Column J is an estimate of life expectancy at the beginning of each age interval using the formula $e_x = T_x / l_x$.

Several points are worth noting about the table in Example 3.5. First, it can be set up as a template in which the only figures you need to enter are the age-specific mortality rates in Column D. This makes life expectancy calculations much easier than they look for populations with reliable and complete mortality data. A range of demographic techniques are required where mortality data are unreliable or incomplete. Second, Column J provides life expectancy estimates for each age interval in the life table. While the figure typically reported in the literature is life expectancy at birth (i.e. e_0 or the first row in Column J), you will also see life expectancy at older ages being reported. The OECD, for example, publishes tables for both e_0 and e_{65}. Finally, a note on interpretation. The first row of Column J represents the average number of years a hypothetical newborn child could be expected to live if they were to experience the age-specific mortality rates in Column D for the rest of their life. However, if there are declining mortality trends in the population (as has been the case in many populations over the last century) and these are expected to continue, then Column D will over-estimate the mortality risk of an actual child born when Column D was collected and Column J will under-estimate their life expectancy. The reverse is true if mortality trends are expected to increase into the future (although this is less common). Thus, the period life table approach doesn't reflect the actual life expectancy of a population in most situations, but it is widely used nonetheless because the alternative (the cohort life table approach) requires you to first predict what mortality will be in the future (a task filled with inherent uncertainty).

Hugo: Right, so it's a compromise?

Author (Stephen): Exactly! And there's a saying that comes to mind here: never let the best get in the way of the good. As we will see, this is not the only compromise people make when developing ways to summarise data.

Potential years of life lost

Another measure that relies exclusively on mortality data is called **Potential Years of Life Lost (PYLL)**. PYLL is calculated by summing up deaths occurring at each age in a population and multiplying this by the number of remaining years that could have been lived up to an agreed limit. We discuss this measure here for several reasons. First, it represents one of the earliest attempts to combine epidemiological data with **normative values** when comparing the mortality experience of entire populations and therefore serves as a useful bridge to other more elaborate measures, which we discuss later in this chapter. Second, it remains in widespread usage today, despite several shortcomings.

Potential Years of Life Lost (PYLL): Calculated by summing up deaths occurring at each age in a population and multiplying this by the number of remaining years that could have been lived up to an agreed limit.

Normative value: A value judgement about how the world *should be*, rather than how it actually is.

Rachael: Hang on, what do you mean by 'normative values'? That doesn't sound very epidemiological.

Author (Stephen): You're right, it doesn't. Let me explain.

EXPLANATION 3.1: Normative values in epidemiology

Until now, we have been talking about epidemiological data such as incidence, prevalence and mortality, and how we can transform these data to help us compare populations in ways that do not stray too far from the underlying numbers. So, for instance, there is not a lot of debate about how to calculate numbers of deaths, crude and age-specific mortality rates and life expectancy. And while we pointed out that there is an element of arbitrariness to the value of an age-standardised rate because it is influenced by which standard population we choose, this doesn't affect the conclusions we might reach if we are careful about not mixing standards when making comparisons. Even with life expectancy, the decision about which approach to use is more about practical concerns rather than other considerations. PYLL is thus different in this respect because the conclusions we draw are directly affected by the decisions we make. This is because it contains a value judgement about how the world *should be*, rather than how it is. This is a normative statement.

Let's unpack this a bit further. The steps you would typically follow to calculate PYLL for a specific population or group are as follows:

1. Identify the threshold age below which you would consider a death to be premature.
2. Collect data on the number of deaths in the population, stratified by age groups.
3. For each death in the dataset, subtract the age at which the person died from the predetermined threshold. This gives you the number of years that person 'lost' by dying prematurely.
4. Sum up all the years lost for each death to calculate the total PYLL for the population.

EXAMPLE 3.6

Table 3.6 illustrates PYLL calculations for an artificial population using two different thresholds with respect to Step 1. Other decisions could equally have been made.

Table 3.6 Example of PYLL calculations using two thresholds in an artificial population

Column A	Column B	Column C	Column D	Column E	Column F	Column G
			Years lost per individual		PYLL	
Age group	Deaths	Average age of death	Threshold = 65	Threshold = 75	Threshold = 65 [B x C x D]	Threshold = 75 [B x C x E]
0	206	0.1	64.9	74.9	13 369	15 429
1–4	37	2.6	62.4	72.4	2 309	2 679
5–9	23	7.5	57.5	67.5	1 323	1 553
10–14	23	12.5	52.5	62.5	1 208	1 438
15–19	105	17.5	47.5	57.5	4 988	6 038
20–24	162	22.5	42.5	52.5	6 885	8 505
25–29	268	27.5	37.5	47.5	10 050	12 730
30–34	314	32.5	32.5	42.5	10 205	13 345
35–39	413	37.5	27.5	37.5	11 358	15 488
40–44	584	42.5	22.5	32.5	13 140	18 980
45–49	954	47.5	17.5	27.5	16 695	26 235
50–54	1 359	52.5	12.5	22.5	16 988	30 578
55–59	1 912	57.5	7.5	17.5	14 340	33 460
60–64	2 824	62.5	2.5	12.5	7 060	35 300
65–69	4 507	67.5	0	7.5	0	33 803
70–74	5 851	72.5	0	2.5	0	14 628
75–79	7 117	77.5	0	0	0	0
80–84	8 192	82.5	0	0	0	0
85+	14 187	85	0	0	0	0
Total	49 038				129 916	270 186

Hugo: Wait a minute – that can't be right. These answers are very different. Which one is correct?

Author (Stephen): Which one, indeed. This is a very good question.

As should be apparent by now, there is no 'correct' answer when it comes to PYLL. It all depends on your response to the question of what should be considered a premature death? (Note the word *should* here.) Were you to respond by saying any death below the age of 65, then the PYLL in this population would be 129 916 years of life lost due to premature mortality. However, this figure more than doubles to 270 186 years if you raise the threshold to 75 years of age instead. Such sensitivity to a key parameter in the calculations is a central criticism of the measure as a way of comparing the mortality experience of different populations (5). Another is that the PYLL calculation is essentially a weighting mechanism that gives greater weight to certain ages relative to other ages. In this sense, it is similar to the direct age-standardisation procedure; however, unlike with age-standardisation, the PYLL weights are applied to age-specific numbers of deaths, not rates. Thus the total PYLL value for a population does not consider its size or age structure and you will rarely see this figure in the literature; instead, you will see crude or age-standardised PYLL values, adding a further layer of complexity to both the calculations and the interpretation.

Despite these limitations, PYLL estimates continue to be provided regularly by statistical and health authorities around the world. For example, the Australian Institute of Health and Welfare (AIHW) consistently publishes annual PYLL estimates for Australia, using a threshold of 75 years, with mortality data dating as far back as 1907. These estimates are available both as raw numbers and as crude rates. Figure 3.7 reveals that, in 2021, there were 893 170 PYLLs in Australia, representing a 43 per cent reduction from 1 576 383 PYLLs in 1907. Over the same period, Australia's population grew by more than 475 per cent, resulting in a crude PYLL rate of 38 PYLLs per 1000 people in 2021 compared with 382 PYLLs per 1000 people in 1907. This represents a 90 per cent decrease over the years, although the impact of population ageing cannot be determined from these data as the PYLL rates are not age-standardised.

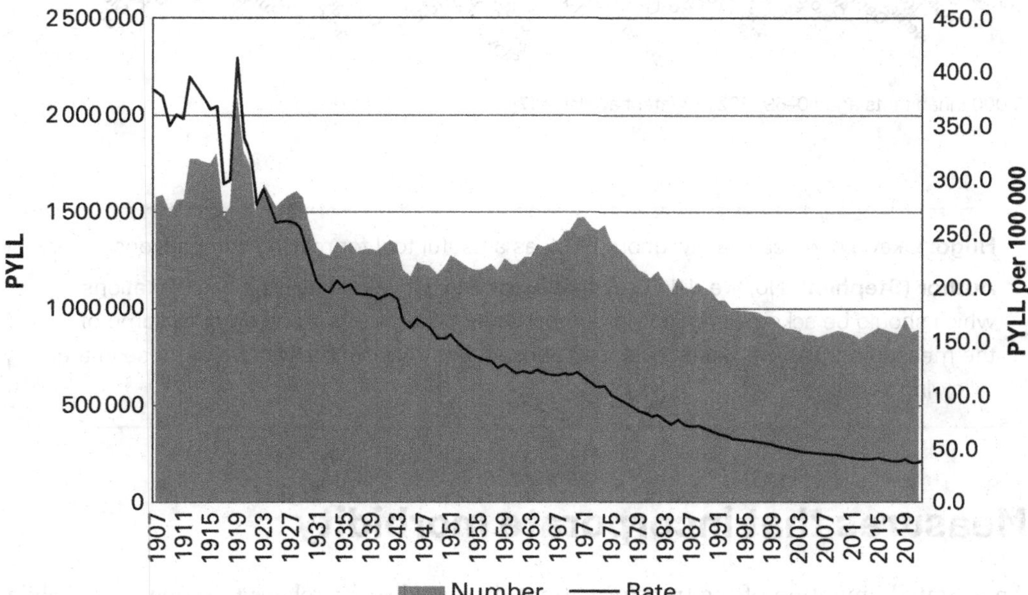

Figure 3.7 Potential years of life lost, number and crude rate (person-years per 1000 population) before age 75, Australia, 1907–2021 (6)

Another example comes from the OECD, which publishes annual PYLL tabulations for 46 countries using 75 as the threshold and age-standardised to the OECD population in 2010. Estimates for 2021 or the latest year available are presented in Figure 3.8. These data indicate low rates of premature mortality of between 2800 and 4100 PYLL per 100 000 across Western Europe, Australia, New Zealand and Canada, and higher rates of between 5000 and 12 500 PYLL per 100 000 across Eastern Europe and the Americas, with South Africa having the highest PYLL rate per 100 000 of 18 000. Other than saying that there appears to be scope for reducing premature mortality in all countries, but particularly in Eastern Europe, the Americas and South Africa, it is not clear what other conclusions can be drawn from such an analysis.

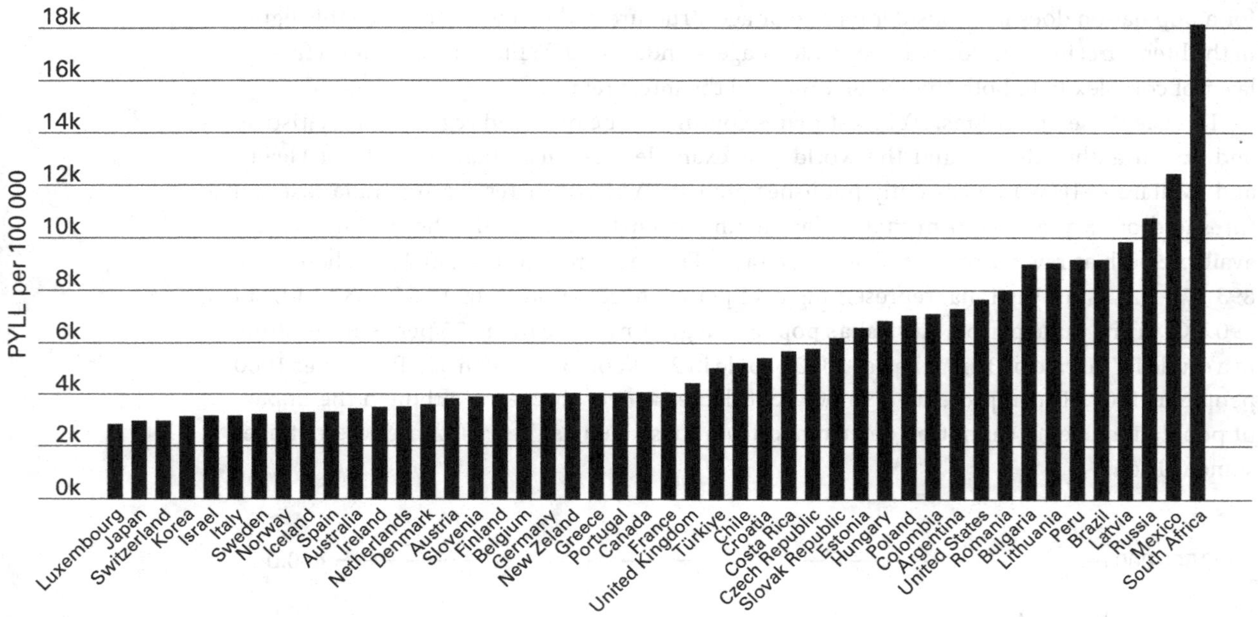

Figure 3.8 PYLL per 100 000 inhabitants aged 0–69, 2021 or latest available (7)

Hugo: Okay, so we can safely ignore PYLL as a useful tool for making comparisons.

Author (Stephen): No, we didn't say that exactly. What we did say is it has limitations which should be acknowledged. More importantly, though, it is a precursor to some of the measures that have been developed subsequently. We will cover two of these in the following section.

Measures that incorporate morbidity

An unstated limitation of the transformations discussed so far relates to scope. Thus, while each represents a way of transforming raw frequency counts into measures of varying degrees of usefulness for making comparisons within and between entire populations or groups, none attempts to bridge the conceptual divide between comparisons of mortality and those relating to morbidity. In other words, none provides us with the tools for combining information on deaths with incidence or prevalence data. Instead, we start with data from one of these sources and proceed from there, without reference to the others. So, for example, age-standardised rates allow us to assess whether the incidence of dementia is increasing or decreasing over time or whether its mortality is increasing or decreasing, but not whether the total burden of dementia in the population is increasing or decreasing. Likewise, a life table allows us to assess whether the total mortality experience in one population is greater or less than another, but not whether the combined impact of illness and disease prior to death is greater or less in one than the other. On the surface, this is understandable. It is not immediately clear, for instance, how one might combine information on deaths with information on incident or prevalent cases. What is the common link that connects these fundamentally different concepts? And even if there is a common link, what might such a composite measure look like? In this section, we explore two approaches to answering these questions: one that builds on what we have learnt about life expectancy, the other on what we have learnt about premature mortality.

Health-adjusted life expectancy

As we noted above, life expectancy is something most people understand easily because they can relate it to their own experience. This is one reason for its popularity as an indicator of overall population health globally. Having seen how a life table is constructed, however, we now know that the picture it paints is incomplete. Being based solely on mortality data, it tells us in a relatable way about a population's longevity but not about the quality of people's lives before they die. Historically, epidemiologists have tended to regard this limitation as not their concern; measuring health-related quality of life was something for practitioners from other disciplines, such as health economics and health psychology, to explore. Epidemiology was about describing patterns of disease using traditional measures such as crude and standardised rates, rate ratios or even life expectancy before moving on to the more important task of determining relationships between exposures and outcomes. Certainly, this is one of the discipline's major contributions to improving the health of populations around the world, and one that we will explore in extensive detail in coming chapters. But to ignore important advances that have been made over the last 30 years in the ways we understand and describe the health of populations is to miss the significance of descriptive epidemiology as a distinct sub-discipline and the contributions it has made to health policy and priority setting globally.

A case in point is **Health-Adjusted Life Expectancy (HALE)**, the origins of which can be traced to calls for more comprehensive assessments of population health than longevity alone, particularly in an ageing world (8). HALE extends the concept of life expectancy and reflects the average length of time a person at a specific age can expect to live in full health. Some of the earlier work in this area includes measures such as Disability-Free Life Expectancy (DFLE) and Healthy Life Expectancy (HLE) and can be linked to broader concerns with understanding not only how long people live but how long they can expect to live in good health, free from disabilities and limitations in daily activities. HALE can be thought of as the best of these efforts for several reasons. First, unlike with some of the other attempts there is no assumption with HALE that health is an all or nothing concept; rather, it is regarded as lying somewhere on a continuum from perfect health to death, with an infinite number of

Health-Adjusted Life Expectancy (HALE): Extends the concept of life expectancy and reflects the average length of time a person at a specific age can expect to live in full health.

possibilities in between. Second, if calculated in a particular way, HALE shares many of the attractive features of an alternative approach to resolving these issues known as **Disability-Adjusted Life Years (DALYs)**, which we discuss in the next section. Example 3.7 describes how to calculate HALE from a life table in four steps.

Disability-Adjusted Life Years (DALYs): A common health indicator used to assess the burden of disease, injury or disability in a population. It takes into account not only deaths but also the impact of non-fatal conditions on the quality of life. One DALY means the loss of one year of healthy life, and it is calculated by combining the years of life lost due to premature death and the years of life lived with illness or disability.

EXAMPLE 3.7

At its most basic, the calculation of HALE involves the following steps:

1. Construct an abridged period life table from age-specific mortality rates.
2. Obtain data on the proportion of a year people lose, on average, to illness at different ages.
3. Reduce the ${}_nL_x$ column in the life table to reflect the data collected in Step 2.
4. Proceed with calculating the T_x and ex columns as if you were calculating life expectancy.

Table 3.7 sets out these steps for the same example population we used previously. The first three columns are taken directly from Table 3.5. Column D (${}_np_x$) is the proportion of a year people lose, on average, to illness. Column E is the number of person years live in each age interval in full health using the formula ${}_nL'_x = {}_nL_x \times (1 - {}_np_x)$. Column F ($T'_x$) is the cumulative years of healthy life lived by the hypothetical cohort in the age interval and all subsequent age intervals. Column G is an estimate of health-adjusted life expectancy at the beginning of each age interval using the formula $e'_x = T'_x / l_x$. Columns H and I are life expectancy (e_x) from Table 3.5 and the difference between e_x and e'_x, respectively. The prime symbol (') has been used to identify columns in Table 3.7 that perform the same function as in Table 3.5, but with different values because of the health loss adjustment that has been applied to ${}_nL'_x$.

Table 3.7 Example of health-adjusted life expectancy calculations for an artificial population

Column A	Column B	Column C	Column D	Column E	Column F	Column G	Column H	Column I
x	l_x	${}_nL_x$	np_x	${}_nL'_x$	T'_x	e'_x	e_x	Diff.
0	100 000	98 835	0.1752	81 516	6 244 595	62.4	67.1	4.7
1	98 705	394 064	0.0336	380 833	6 163 079	62.4	67.0	4.5
5	98 390	491 581	0.0355	474 154	5 782 246	58.8	63.2	4.4
10	98 243	490 722	0.0386	471 757	5 308 093	54.0	58.3	4.3
15	98 046	489 131	0.0587	460 396	4 836 336	49.3	53.4	4.1
20	97 606	485 723	0.0614	455 884	4 375 940	44.8	48.6	3.8
25	96 683	480 652	0.0553	454 073	3 920 056	40.5	44.1	3.5
30	95 578	474 566	0.0517	450 052	3 465 983	36.3	39.5	3.3
35	94 249	465 082	0.0542	439 889	3 015 931	32.0	35.1	3.1
40	91 784	451 915	0.0551	427 021	2 576 041	28.1	30.9	2.9
45	88 982	435 546	0.0625	408 326	2 149 020	24.2	26.8	2.7
50	85 236	413 167	0.0705	384 032	1 740 694	20.4	22.9	2.5

Column A	Column B	Column C	Column D	Column E	Column F	Column G	Column H	Column I
x	l_x	$_nL_x$	np_x	$_nL'_x$	T'_x	e'_x	e_x	Diff.
55	80 030	383 104	0.0773	353 496	1 356 662	17.0	19.2	2.3
60	73 211	346 070	0.0982	312 086	1 003 167	13.7	15.8	2.1
65	65 217	294 833	0.1180	260 042	691 081	10.6	12.4	1.8
70	52 716	227 617	0.1433	194 994	431 039	8.2	9.8	1.6
75	38 331	155 500	0.1718	128 785	236 045	6.2	7.5	1.3
80	23 869	88 111	0.1856	71 754	107 260	4.5	5.5	1.0
85+	11 375	43 970	0.1925	35 506	35 506	3.1	3.9	0.7

Hugo: Hmm, this is complicated, but not as complicated as it was before. Does this mean a baby will live 67.1 years but lose 4.7 years due to illness?

Author (Stephen): Exactly! Another way of saying the same thing is that a baby can expect to live 62.4 years in full health. This is why it is called *health-adjusted* life expectancy. The same interpretation applies to any age in the life table. For example, a 60-year-old can expect to live another 15.8 years but will lose 2.1 of these years due to illness. In other words, they can expect to live another 13.7 years in full health.

Rachel: Okay, I get this. But I still feel like I'm missing something here. Where did $_np_x$ come from again?

Author (Stephen): Ah yes, we glossed over that bit. Let's rewind a bit.

As you can see now, the only difference between an ordinary life table and one that has been modified to calculate HALE instead of LE is the inclusion of an extra column containing the proportion of a year people lose to illness ($_np_x$), which is used to adjust the number of person years lived in each age interval ($_nL_x$) downwards. Everything else is the same. So what is this extra column and where does it come from? It turns out that there are two ways to derive this element of HALE. The short way first. In the explanation above, we noted that $_np_x$ is the proportion of a year people lose, on average, to illness. One way to assess this would be to ask a **representative sample** of the population how healthy they felt at the time of the survey on a scale from 0 'perfect health' to 1 'as good as dead'. We could then stratify the responses by age and calculate averages for each age group. Since this is point prevalence data, we can assume it is representative of all time points across a year and is therefore a reasonable estimate of the proportion of a year people lose, on average, to illness (the parameter we are seeking). There are variations to this basic approach, some of which involve asking people more than one question to determine their overall health state; whichever is adopted, however, their responses must ultimately be summarised into a single number on a scale of 0 to 1 in order to derive age-specific averages of health loss and complete the calculations.

Representative sample: A subset of a large population that accurately reflects the sociodemographic characteristics of the target population. The selection process of a representative sample often involves a probability sampling method (e.g. random sampling) to select members from the target population to form the study sample.

A key limitation of this approach, aside from any of the response biases inherent in self-reported data, is that it does not allow you to unpack the causes of illness that might lead people to respond in particular ways. This is an important omission since it prevents you from saying, for example, how much heart disease or diabetes contributes to the loss of health you have quantified. This is the type of information you might want if you were setting priorities, understanding trends or determining the drivers of health disparities. It is not that it is not possible at all, it is just that it is not possible having derived an overall health state for an individual without attributing this to whichever illness or combination of illnesses they might be experiencing. Of course, such an attribution would be easier where a person has only one illness, but the chance of this decreases with age, and it gets more complicated to untangle what proportion of overall health loss is caused by which illness when two or more are present.

The solution to this problem is to derive the extra column (i.e. ${}_{n}p_{x}$) the long way. This involves developing a comprehensive list of possible causes of illness and injury that might affect a population, determining a severity weight ranging from 0 to 1 for each cause and multiplying this by plausible estimates of the prevalence and average duration of each cause. This results in cause-specific values that can be summed to create all-cause values and used together with all-cause mortality rates as in the example in Table 3.7. Alternatively, they can be combined with the corresponding **cause-specific mortality** rates to create cause-specific life tables that, when added together, represent all causes. This is more computationally intensive and often requires extensive corrections for misclassification and under-reporting biases but allows you to both calculate HALE and decompose by cause any differences you might observe over time or between populations (9) – in other words, determining the contribution of heart disease or diabetes, for example, to such differences.

Cause-specific mortality: A measure of *mortality* that includes the number of deaths from the phenomenon of interest over a specified period.

Hugo: That sounds like a lot of work.

Author (Stephen): It is. But it's being done on a regular basis by organisations such as the Institute of Health Metrics and Evaluation (IHME) and the AIHW, so it is possible. Let's look at some examples.

Figure 3.9 presents an analysis of the latest IHME data on life expectancy and health-adjusted life expectancy for the World Bank's four income regions in 2019. This analysis shows a strong economic gradient in life expectancy across the world, with the wealthiest region experiencing lives that are almost 16 years longer on average than the poorest. The economic gradient for HALE is in the same direction but not as strong, with the wealthiest region experiencing healthy lives that are 12.2 years longer than the poorest. The combination of these trends means that 11.8 years of life (or 14.6 per cent of the expected lifespan) are lost to illness in the wealthiest region compared to only 8.5 years (13 per cent) in the poorest; in other words, as longevity increases with wealth, so too does the time that is lost to illness, both in absolute terms (years) and as a proportion of people's lives. This challenges popular notions of economic progress as it suggests that wealth creates conditions that are better at keeping people alive than keeping them healthy.

In another example, recent work suggests that in 2011, HALE was 62.0 years in Indigenous Australians compared with 73.7 years in other Australians. Figure 3.10 presents an analysis of which diseases and injuries contribute most to this gap of 11.7 years. This shows that more than half of the Indigenous health gap (5.8 years) is explained by just four diseases (type

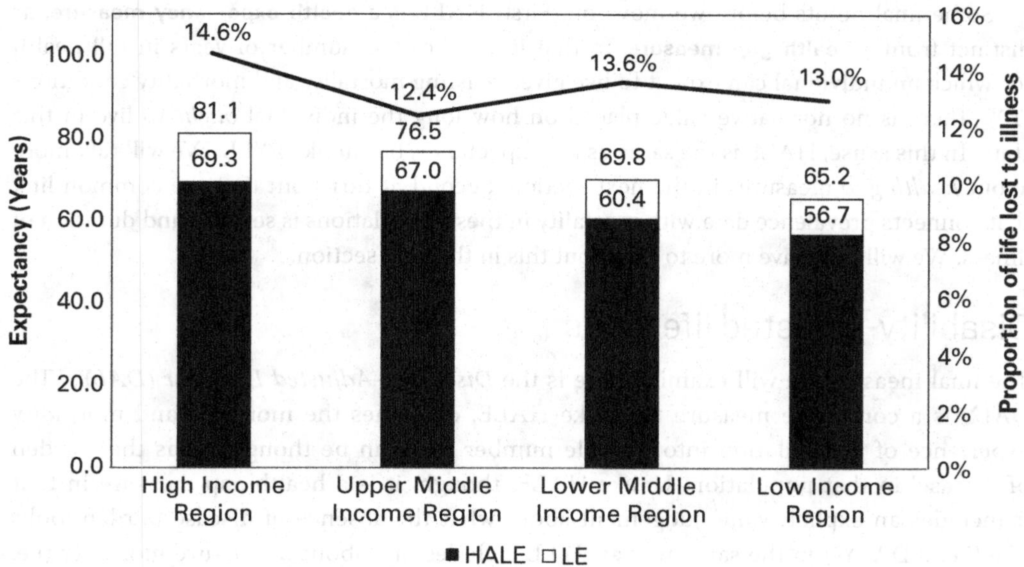

Figure 3.9 Life expectancy and health-adjusted life expectancy, World Bank regions, 2019 (2)

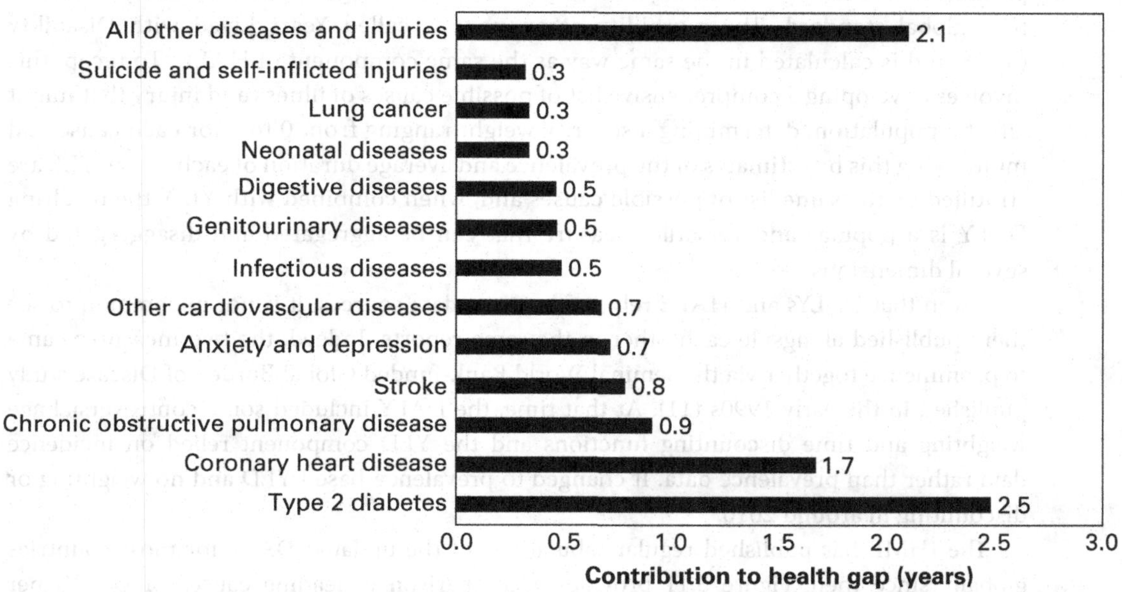

Figure 3.10 Decomposition of health-adjusted life expectancy gap between Indigenous and other Australians, 2011

2 diabetes, coronary heart disease, chronic obstructive pulmonary disease and stroke). In other words, if rates of mortality and morbidity from type 2 diabetes, coronary heart disease, chronic obstructive pulmonary disease and stroke in Indigenous Australians were reduced to be the same as in other Australians, the health gap between these two groups would be more than halved. This provides a clear picture of where prevention and treatments efforts could most effectively be targeted.

Health expectancy measures: Measures such as HALE that assess the number of years in full health for which an individual can expect to live given existing mortality and morbidity conditions. Distinct from a health gap measure.

Health gap measures: Measures such as the DALY that include an explicit value judgement about what the absence of disease burden looks like.

Some final points before we move on. First, HALE is a **health expectancy measure**, as distinct from a **health gap measure**, in that it assesses the number of years in full health for which an individual can expect to live given existing mortality and morbidity conditions (10). There is no normative value placed on how long the individual *ought* to live in this state. In this sense, HALE is the same as life expectancy, but unlike PYLL. We will talk more about *health gap* measures in the next section. Second, it turns out that the common link that connects prevalence data with mortality in these calculations is severity and duration of illness. We will also have more to say about this in the next section.

Disability-adjusted life years

The final measure we will examine here is the *Disability-Adjusted Life Year (DALY)*. The DALY is a composite measure that, like HALE, combines the mortality and morbidity experience of a population into a single number that can be thought of as the 'burden of disease' in that population. Unlike HALE, though, it is a health gap measure in that it includes an explicit value judgement about what the absence of disease burden looks like (i.e. 0 DALYs) in the same way as PYLL includes one about premature mortality (i.e. 0 PYLL). The mortality component of the DALY is even called Years of Life Lost (YLL) and is calculated in a similar way: deaths at each age are multiplied by a measure of premature mortality – in this case, life expectancy at that age as determined by reference to a global standard. The morbidity component is called Years Lived with Disability (YLD) and is calculated in the same way as the same component of HALE. To recap, this involves developing a comprehensive list of possible causes of illness and injury that might affect a population, determining a severity weight ranging from 0 to 1 for each cause and multiplying this by estimates of the prevalence and average duration of each cause. YLL are stratified by the same list of possible causes and, when combined with YLD, the resulting DALY is a popular and versatile measure that can be aggregated and disaggregated by several dimensions.

Given that DALYs and HALE rely on the same data sources, it is not uncommon to see them published alongside each other in the same reports. Indeed, the two measures came to prominence together via the seminal World Bank-funded Global Burden of Disease study published in the early 1990s (11). At that time, the DALY included some controversial age weighting and time discounting functions and the YLD component relied on incidence data rather than prevalence data. It changed to prevalence-based YLD and no weighting or discounting in around 2010.

The IHME has published regular tabulations of the updated DALY for most countries globally since then. Figure 3.11 provides a comparison of leading causes of DALYs per 100 000 globally in 1990 compared with 2019 using data from the IHME Global Burden of Disease data-visualisation tool. This shows that neonatal causes remained the leading cause of burden in both 1990 and 2019, whereas lower respiratory infections dropped from second to fourth and diarrhoeal disease from third to fifth. On the other hand, ischemic heart disease increased from fourth to second and stroke from fifth to third. These changes are consistent with a general decline in communicable diseases and an increase in non-communicable diseases globally over this period.

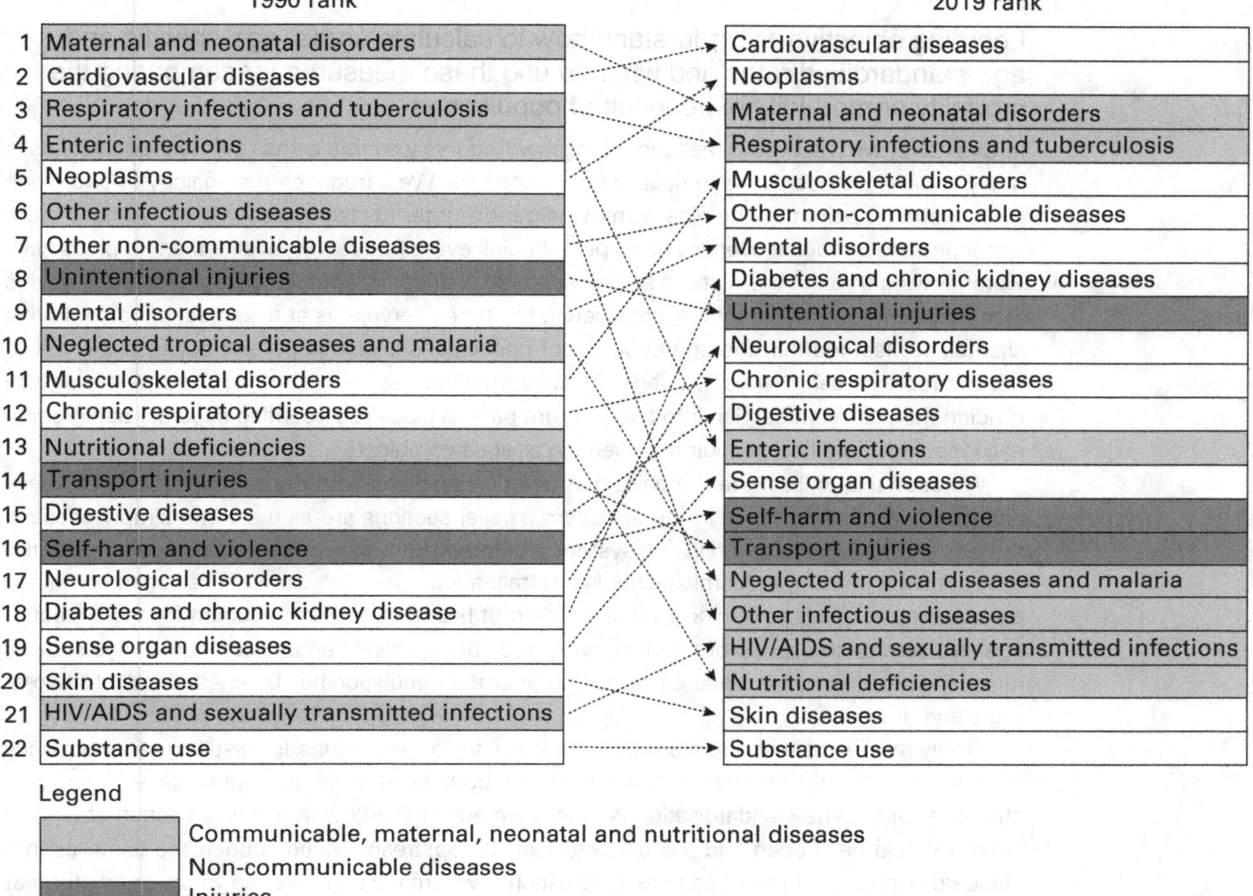

Figure 3.11 Leading causes of DALYs per 100 000 globally, 1990 and 2019 (2)

Several points on the DALY before we finish up. First, like PYLL, the raw DALY value for a population does not consider its size or age structure and you will rarely see this in the literature; instead, you will see crude or age-standardised DALY values, adding a further layer of complexity to both the calculations and the interpretation. Second, also like PYLL, DALY calculations are sensitive to key normative assumptions such as which standard life expectancy to use, whether to base YLD on incidence or prevalence data and whether to age-weight and discount; comparing old publications with new is problematic because of changes in each of these areas. Finally, like HALE, the common links that connect prevalence and mortality data in DALY calculations are severity and duration of illness. The incorporation of this information into the equations allows epidemiologists to say, for example, whether diabetes contributes more or less than suicide and self-inflicted injuries to any differences in overall health between populations or groups. In other words, this allows them to compare apples with oranges. This represents one of the major advances of descriptive epidemiology over the last 30 years.

Conclusion

Learning objective 1: Understand how to calculate crude, age-specific and age-standardised rates and when to use these measures for comparing the mortality or morbidity experience of populations

In Chapter 2, we discovered that comparing raw frequency counts across different populations is rarely informative due to the impact of population size. We introduced the analogy of two pipes to illustrate the point that the pipe with the larger diameter (think population size) will have more water passing through it over any given period (think event frequency), even if the two pipes have water flowing through them at the same speed (think underlying force). One way to address this is to rescale frequency counts by considering the time everyone is at risk, creating rates. In this chapter, we learned that the age structure of populations is also important because the risk of health problems can change with age. To accommodate this, we extended the pipe analogy by dividing the upstream section into two or more parallel pipes representing separate age groups, each feeding into a final section representing all ages combined.

We used this to illustrate the point that two final sections with the same diameter can have different flows even if flows in the upstream parallel sections are all the same simply because the diameter for an age group in one system is different from the corresponding age group in the other. For this reason, epidemiologists like to talk about rates calculated for all ages combined as *crude* rates. This is to remind us that no attempt has been made to account for the impact of age structure on the speed of the underlying force being calculated and compared. *Age-specific* rates, on the other hand, are rates calculated after the population has been stratified into two of more age groups.

Finally, we learnt that age-standardisation is a set of techniques for distilling raw frequency counts into a single number that accounts for both differences in population size *and* age structure. Direct age-standardisation is where we adjust the flow in the final section of pipe to what it would have been had the diameters of the upstream sections been the same as in a standard population. Indirect age-standardisation is where we compare the volume of water that has flowed through the final section with what it would have been had the flows in the upstream sections been the same as in a standard population, but with the diameters unchanged. Both methods allow as to compare the underlying force of mortality and morbidity data between different populations of groups, or within one population or group over time.

Learning objective 2: Describe life expectancy and potential years of life lost as two measures other than rates that are commonly used for comparing the mortality experience of populations

We then explored two measures other than rates that are commonly used for comparing populations that can only be used with mortality data and that do not have an incidence or prevalence equivalent. The first is life expectancy, which we learned is calculated with a life table in which an artificial cohort is exposed to the implied mortality risks from observed mortality data and the average amount of time spent at each age is determined. A period life table approach is the most common because it uses mortality rates for a given period (usually a year) and assumes these apply without change into the future. The last column of the first row of a life table represents the average number of years for which a hypothetical newborn child could be expected to live if they were to experience the observed age-specific mortality rates for the rest of their life. If there are declining mortality trends, and these are expected to continue, then this approach will over-estimate the mortality risk of an actual child born when the data were collected and under-estimate their life expectancy. The reverse is true if mortality trends are expected to increase into the future. The second exclusively mortality-based measure is Potential Years of Life Lost (PYLL), which is calculated by summing up deaths occurring at each age in a population and multiplying this by the number of remaining years that could have been lived up to an agreed limit. This measure involves making a value judgement about what constitutes a premature death and therefore serves as a useful bridge to other more elaborate measures, which we discuss next.

Learning objective 3: Identify the common links that allow mortality and morbidity data to be integrated and describe Health-Adjusted Life Expectancy (HALE) and Disability-Adjusted Life Years (DALY) as two popular measures that achieve this, thereby allowing us to compare the overall health of populations

Finally, we learnt that a common link that allows us to incorporate mortality and morbidity data into a single measure is severity and duration of illness. We explored two measures that adopt this approach. The first is HALE, which extends the concept of life expectancy by reflecting the average length of time a person at a specific age can expect to live in full health. HALE is calculated using a life table in which the average amount of time the artificial cohort spends at each age is adjusted downwards by the average amount of time people lose to illness at that age. Obtaining these data can be time consuming as it typically involves developing a comprehensive list of possible causes of illness and injury that might affect a population, determining a severity weight ranging from 0 to 1 for each cause and multiplying this by estimates of the prevalence and average duration of each cause. The second is the Disability-Adjusted Life Year (DALY), which is a composite measure that combines the mortality and morbidity experience of a population into a single number that can be thought of as the 'burden of disease' in that population. The mortality component of the DALY is called Years of Life Lost (YLL) and is calculated by multiplying deaths at each age by life expectancy at that age as determined by reference to a global standard. The morbidity component is called Years Lived with Disability (YLD) and is calculated in the same way as the same component of HALE. The incorporation of this information into the equations allows epidemiologists to compare apples with oranges and represents one of the major advances of descriptive epidemiology over the last 30 years.

Further reading

Murray CJL, Salomon JA, Mathers CD, Lopez AD. *Summary Measures of Population Health: Concepts, Ethics, Measurement and Applications*. World Health Organization; 2002.

Questions

Answers are available at the end of the book.

Multiple-choice questions

1. Why does the age structure of a population play a crucial role in influencing the frequency of health-related phenomena?

A – Because age structure directly determines the size of the population.

B – Because age structure is essential for creating population pyramids.

C – Because the risk of many health-related phenomena is dependent on age.

D – Because age structure has no significant impact on the occurrence of health-related phenomena.

2. What is the purpose of age-standardisation in epidemiology?
   A – To complicate the comparison process by introducing additional adjustments.
   B – To simplify comparisons by providing a single number for a population or group that accounts for both population size and age structure.
   C – To emphasise the differences in population size and age structure when comparing rates.
   D – To highlight the limitations of crude and age-specific rates in epidemiological studies.
3. Why might the period life table approach lead to under-estimating or over-estimating the actual life expectancy in certain situations?
   A – Because the period life table assumes that mortality rates will remain constant into the future, which may not reflect actual trends.
   B – Because the period life table relies on historical mortality data, which may not accurately represent current mortality patterns.
   C – Because the period life table approach is less common and, therefore, less reliable than the cohort life table approach.
   D – Because the period life table over-estimates mortality risk for a child born when the data was collected.
4. What distinguishes Health-Adjusted Life Expectancy (HALE) from a health gap measure?
   A – HALE assesses the number of years in full health an individual can expect to live, while a health gap measure places a normative value on how long an individual ought to live in a healthy state.
   B – HALE and health gap measures are essentially the same, both assessing the number of years in full health an individual can expect to live.
   C – HALE, like life expectancy, places a normative value on how long an individual ought to live in full health, while a health gap measure does not.
   D – HALE focuses on assessing the severity and duration of illness, while a health gap measure does not consider these factors.
5. Why is the raw DALY value for a population rarely seen in the literature?
   A – It is a less accurate measure of overall health.
   B – It does not account for differences in population size and age structure.
   C – It requires complex calculations that are rarely performed.
   D – It is only applicable to specific demographic groups.

Short-answer questions

1. What are some of the challenges in making comparisons between different populations in descriptive epidemiology?
2. How do both the size and age structure of a population influence the raw frequency count of a health-related phenomenon such as dementia?
3. What is the distinction between crude rates and age-specific rates, and why might age-specific rates pose a challenge when making comparisons?
4. What is age-standardisation and how does it address the limitations of crude and age-specific rates in epidemiology?
5. What is an age-standardised rate calculated using the direct method and what information is required for its application in epidemiology?
6. What is indirect standardisation and when is it typically employed in epidemiology?
7. How does an abridged life table differ from a complete life table and what are the essential inputs for constructing an abridged life table in epidemiology?
8. What does the first row of the last column in a period life table represent and why might it lead to under-estimation or over-estimation of life expectancy in a population?

9. What is Health-Adjusted Life Expectancy (HALE) and what is its purpose in population health assessment?
10. What is the Disability-Adjusted Life Year (DALY) and how does it differ from Health-Adjusted Life Expectancy (HALE)?

References

1. United Nations (Population Division). *World Population Prospects*; 2022. http://population.un.org/woo
2. Institute of Health Metrics and Evaluation. *Global Burden of Disease Data Visualisation Tool.* 2023. http://ihmeuw.org/68ri
3. Organisation of Economic Cooperation and Development. Health status. *OECD Health Statistics Database*; 2023. https://doi.org/10.1787/data-00540-en
4. Organisation of Economic Cooperation and Development. *Health at a Glance 2023: OECD Indicators.* OECD Publishing; 2023. https://doi.org/10.1787/7a7afb35-en
5. Gardner J, Sanborn J. Years of Potential Life Lost (YPLL)—What Does it Measure? *Epidemiology.* 1990;1(4):322–9.
6. Australian Institute of Health and Welfare. Supplementary tables [Excel spreadsheet]. In: *Deaths in Australia*; 2024. www.aihw.gov.au/getmedia/a3bd1a2f-a596-4f5b-8f00-091dc9bddaa4/AIHW-PHE-229-report-supplementary-tables.xlsx
7. Organisation of Economic Cooperation and Development. Potential years of life lost; 2024. https://doi.org/10.1787/193a2829-en.
8. Sullivan DF. A single index of mortality and morbidity. *HSMHA Health Reports.* 1971;86(4):347-54.
9. Nusselder WJ, Looman CW. Decomposition of differences in health expectancy by cause. *Demography.* 2004;41(2):315–34.
10. Murray CJ, Salomon JA, Mathers C. A critical examination of summary measures of population health. *Bulletin of the World Health Organization.* 2000;78(8):981–94.
11. Murray CJ. Quantifying the burden of disease: The technical basis for disability-adjusted life years. *Bulletin of the World Health Organization.* 1994;72(3):429–45.

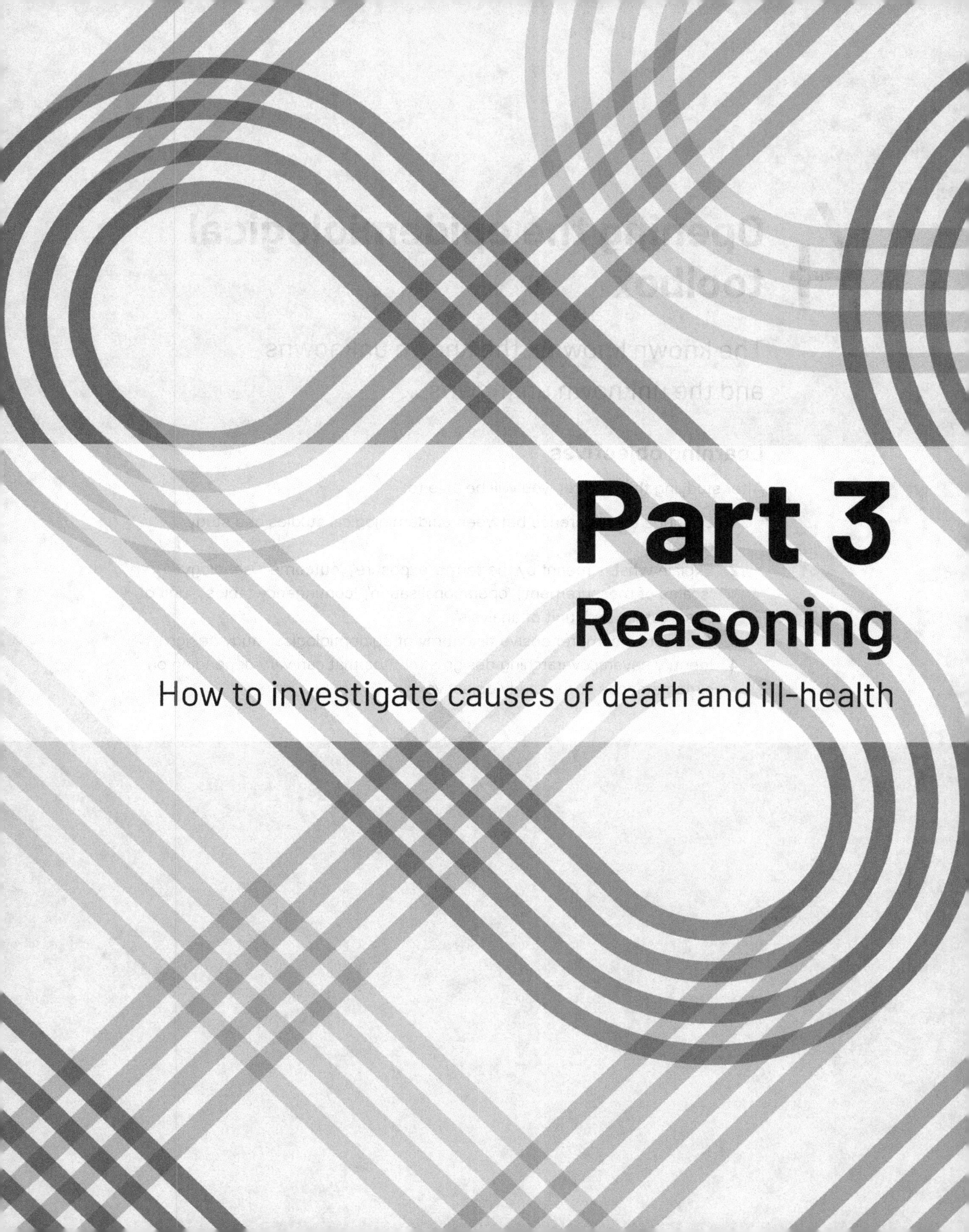

Part 3
Reasoning
How to investigate causes of death and ill-health

4 Opening the epidemiological toolbox

The known knowns, the known unknowns and the unknown unknowns ...

Learning objectives

After studying this chapter, you will be able to:

1. Describe the difference between epidemiological studies and study design
2. Explain what is meant by the terms 'exposure', 'outcome', 'aetiology', 'scales of measurement', 'operationalisation', 'contingency tables', 'unit of observation' and 'unit of analysis'
3. Articulate a comprehensive taxonomy of epidemiological study design
4. Identify several overarching design attributes that can vary depending on circumstances or the study objective

Introduction

Congratulations again: you've made it to Part 3 of this textbook on how to investigate causes of disease and ill-health. As we progress through this part and the next, you will be introduced to the different ways in which epidemiologists go about analysing the factors that are associated with people becoming ill or getting better. Each of these has a role to play in building up our knowledge about what influences human health. Our objective here is to provide an overview of the range of techniques that are available and to develop your understanding of which of these might be more appropriate in any given situation. One way to think about these techniques is as a set of tools for tackling a range of problems – much like a carpenter has a box full of tools for tackling different aspects of building a house. No one tool is useful in every situation, and some are more useful at certain stages of the construction process than others. Some even have features that make them useful in a variety of situations. Of course, context is everything, so even when a tool might not look like it's the 'right' one in a particular situation, if the results are robust and reliable then that might be all that matters (hands up if you've ever contemplated hitting a nail with a screwdriver). So, let's open the epidemiological toolbox and see what's inside.

Epidemiological studies and study design

We will start our inspection by reiterating the distinction between epidemiological *studies* and the concept of *study design*. Epidemiological studies are discrete attempts to pursue an epidemiological question, many of which get written up and published in the scientific literature or elsewhere. Study design, on the other hand, refers to the way such an attempt has been executed. As we noted in Chapter 1, there are vastly more published studies than there are types of study designs. In fact, the range of study design options that have evolved over the years can be summarised into just a handful of general approaches, most of which we have listed already under various headings in the tree diagram presented in Figure 1.2.

In this chapter, we will introduce you to various elements of study design using real examples to illustrate certain points as we go. These have been selected for both their significance to the field of epidemiology and because they have played an important role in shaping human health in some way. The first is Example 4.1, in which we introduce you to the British Doctors Study. This study was established in response to concerns at the time about increasing mortality from lung cancer in males (Figure 4.1) and the need to identify potential causes.

EXAMPLE 4.1

The British Doctors Study, initiated in 1951, is a pioneering epidemiological investigation that significantly contributed to our understanding of the relationship between smoking and lung cancer. Conducted by Sir Richard Doll and Sir Austin Bradford Hill, the study involved the analysis of smoking habits and health outcomes among British physicians, providing compelling evidence of the link between tobacco consumption and an increased risk of developing lung cancer.

EXAMPLE 4.1 Continued

The study's inception was driven by concerns about the rising mortality from lung cancer and the need to identify potential risk factors. The researchers targeted doctors as study participants due to their relatively homogeneous socioeconomic status and access to medical care, facilitating comprehensive data collection. Over 40 000 male doctors aged from 35 to 70 were recruited, and their smoking habits and health issues were meticulously documented over time using questionnaires and medical records.

The key findings of the British Doctors Study, published in a series of landmark papers starting in the early 1950s (e.g. 2), unequivocally established the association between cigarette smoking and lung cancer. The research revealed a striking dose–response relationship, with heavier smokers experiencing a significantly higher risk of developing lung cancer compared with non-smokers or light smokers. Moreover, the study demonstrated the cumulative effect of smoking over time, with the risk increasing with the duration of smoking.

The British Doctors Study also provided evidence of the association between smoking and other respiratory and cardiovascular diseases, further highlighting the broad-ranging health consequences of tobacco use. The comprehensive and long-term nature of the study allowed for the identification of specific diseases associated with smoking, contributing to the understanding of the overall health impact of tobacco consumption.

The impact of the British Doctors Study extended beyond the scientific community, playing a pivotal role in shaping public health policies and anti-smoking initiatives. The study's findings were instrumental in raising awareness about the dangers of smoking and served as a catalyst for tobacco-control measures globally. Smoking cessation campaigns and policies aimed at reducing tobacco use in various countries drew inspiration from the evidence presented in the British Doctors Study.

Subsequent analyses and follow-up studies reinforced and expanded upon the initial findings, solidifying the consensus within the scientific community about the causal relationship between smoking and lung cancer. The study's legacy is evident in the decline in smoking rates and the implementation of tobacco-control measures worldwide.

The British Doctors Study is considered a landmark in epidemiological research for several reasons. It was one of the first large-scale cohort studies, providing robust and reliable evidence through long-term follow-ups and careful data collection. The homogeneity of the study population, consisting of male doctors, helped control for potential confounding factors, strengthening the study's internal **validity**.

Validity: The extent to which a conclusion, concept or theory accurately reflects the true world. In studies, whether findings accurately reflect the characteristics of a study population (internal validity) or can be generalised to a broader population (external validity). In measurement, the extent to which the instrument measures what it intends to measure (involves content, construct and criterion validity).

In summary, the British Doctors Study significantly contributed to our understanding of the health risks associated with smoking, particularly its role in the development of lung cancer. The study's meticulous design, long-term follow-up and clear demonstration of the dose–response relationship between smoking and disease outcomes made it a ground-breaking and influential contribution to epidemiology. Beyond its scientific impact, the study played a crucial role in public health efforts to combat tobacco use and save lives by informing policies aimed at reducing smoking prevalence globally.

Source: www.ctsu.ox.ac.uk/research/british-doctors-study

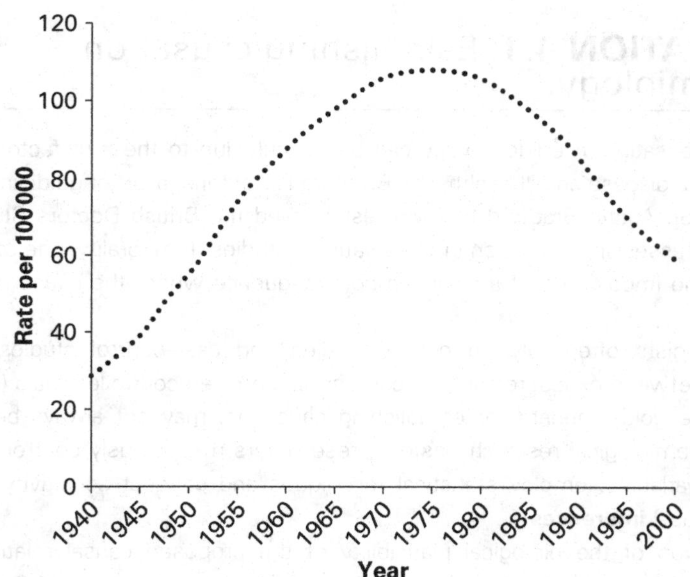

Figure 4.1 Age-standardised lung cancer mortality in males, England and Wales, 1940 to 2000. Adapted from (1)

The British Doctors Study is important in the history of epidemiology because of its contribution to what we know today about smoking as a major cause of lung cancer and because it is one of the earliest examples of a high-quality *cohort study*. You will learn all about the defining features of this type of study design in Chapter 8. For now, though, let's focus on how a study such as this sits alongside all the other tools in the toolbox.

If we return to Figure 1.2, we can see that, as a cohort study, the British Doctors Study is representative of a *non-experimental analytical* study design, along with cross-sectional and case control studies.

Hugo: How come?

Rachael: Yes – what makes all these designs so similar?

Author (Stephen): As we shall see, the answer to this lies in our motivation to undertake an epidemiological study in the first place.

One of the central preoccupations of epidemiologists since the early days has been to shed light on the underlying causes, or **aetiologies,** of human health-related phenomena. Explanation 4.1 introduces you to some of things we need to start considering when seeking to establish a causal relationship between two factors in epidemiology. We will expand on this topic in later chapters.

Aetiology: The science of causes.

EXPLANATION 4.1: Establishing causation in epidemiology

Establishing causation in epidemiology can be difficult due to the multifactorial nature of many causes of disease and ill-health. The Bradford Hill criteria, a set of guidelines proposed by the same Sir Austin Bradford Hill who established the British Doctors Study, offers a framework for assessing causation in observational studies. Temporality, one of the criteria, emphasises the importance of a clear temporal sequence where the cause precedes the effect.

Epidemiologists often rely on cohort studies and case-control studies to explore associations between exposures and outcomes. Randomised controlled trials (RCTs), while considered the gold standard for establishing causation, may not always be feasible or ethical in epidemiological research. Instead, researchers meticulously control for potential confounding variables, employ statistical techniques and conduct sensitivity analyses to strengthen causal **inferences**.

Inference: A conclusion reached about a subset (or sample) of the population that is applied to the whole population from which the sample was drawn.

Consideration of the biological plausibility of the proposed causal relationship adds another layer of evidence. Epidemiologists also assess the consistency of findings across different studies and populations, reinforcing the robustness of causation arguments.

Despite these efforts, establishing causation in epidemiology requires a cautious approach due to the inherent complexities of human health. Ongoing research, collaboration and methodological advancements continually refine our ability to draw meaningful causal inferences from an often-complex body of observational and (where possible) experimental evidence.

Of course, people can undertake epidemiological research for reasons other than establishing causation, such as describing the distribution of health in populations or informing health system priorities. Aetiological inquiry is the main one, however, and this is reflected in the way we group and classify different study designs (3). We will get to how this works in a moment. But first let's take a closer look, with the help of a simple thought experiment, at how you might go about researching causation as an epidemiologist.

Exposures, outcomes and aetiological research

Aetiological research begins by thinking about epidemiological phenomena in terms of just two dimensions: *exposures* and *outcomes*. Exposures are factors that are thought to contribute to a person experiencing one or more health states (either positive or negative). Outcomes are the different health states that a person might experience. In case you missed it, you thought about a health problem in this way in Example 1.1 in Chapter 1. Here the exposure was 'cold draught from open window' and the outcome was 'the common cold'. Other factors may also play a role in getting a cold, such as season or room density, and the common cold might even be a factor that contributes to someone getting a different outcome, such as more severe lower respiratory disease. But the simple classification of health phenomena into exposures and outcomes in the first instance still works.

Let's now say that after applying your newly acquired critical thinking skills to this problem, you have ruled out 'cold draught from an open window' as a cause. This is because you now suspect that sitting in a classroom with open windows might actually *protect* you from getting a cold. In other words, 'common cold' is still the outcome, but your exposure has become 'sitting in a classroom with inadequate ventilation'. Let's also say that you have been asked by your tutor to design a study to test this **hypothesis**. You now need to define these phenomena and work out how you might collect some data on them. Let's focus on the first of these tasks for a moment as it influences the second. It turns out that the most common cause of a cold is infection from a group of viruses called *rhinoviruses*. While this can be tested for in a laboratory setting, it is typically not worth the effort due to the costs involved compared with the duration and severity of the symptoms (less than a week; runny or stuffy nose, sore or scratchy throat, cough, sneezing, mild headaches, low-grade fever). Of course, these symptoms are very similar to those you get from other common ailments such COVID-19, for which there is a cheap and effective screening tool, the coronavirus Rapid Antigen Test (RAT).

One way to define your outcome, therefore, might be to say that it includes anyone who is observed to have one or more symptoms associated with rhinovirus infection while at the same time testing negative on a RAT. This would be something you could collect data on such that your observations would classify every person included in your study according to whether they had a cold (yes/no). This is an example of **operationalisation**. Operationalisation means turning an abstract conceptual idea into something that is measurable. And measurement is an activity that is fundamental to all scientific inquiry.

Hypothesis: A statement that proposes a relationship (or association) between two or more key variables, which the researcher intends to test in a study. In the context of an epidemiological study, a hypothesis often proposes a relationship between an exposure factor and a specific health outcome.

Operationalisation: Turning an abstract conceptual idea into something that is measurable. In so doing, researchers seek to define specific criteria, measurements or procedures that capture the essence of the concept in a tangible and measurable form. This process is essential for ensuring that the variables under study can be observed, measured and analysed reliably and consistently across different settings and studies.

Measurement

Usually, when we hear the word 'measurement', we picture checking how long something is (like the length of the line of students waiting for coffee) or counting some entity (maybe the number of students in the coffee queue), without putting much thought into the nature of the data we have just collected. But there's another way of looking at it. In epidemiology (and science more generally), we think of measurement in the context of a slightly broader term: **scales of measurement**. There are four distinct types – nominal, ordinal, interval and ratio – each with its own set of properties that determine the nature of the data collected and which statistical analyses are appropriate. The very act of measuring something necessarily involves adopting one of these scales, whether we like it or not. Thinking back to our toolbox analogy, it's a bit like having some very precise tools, one of which must be used when approaching a measurement task because none of the others can do the job. Explanation 4.2 introduces you to each of the scales and the properties that make them unique.

Scales of measurement: The different ways in which variables or data are categorised, ordered or measured in statistical analysis. These scales define the level of measurement and the properties of the data, influencing the types of statistical analyses that can be applied. There are four scales of measurement: nominal, ordinal, interval and ratio.

EXPLANATION 4.2: The four scales measurement

1. Nominal scales

Nominal scales are the simplest form of measurement and do not possess any arithmetic properties. Instead, they classify members of an entity such as a population into distinct categories without implying any order or hierarchy. The categories must be mutually exclusive and exhaustive, meaning that each member can be assigned to only one category. Since nominal scales lack arithmetic properties, there is no inherent ranking, and no mathematical operations beyond relative comparisons in terms of proportions can be applied. Let's say

Nominal scale: This is the simplest measurement scale and involves categorising data into distinct categories or groups without any inherent order. Examples include gender (male, female) and marital status (single, married, divorced). Nominal data cannot be ranked or ordered numerically.

EXPLANATION 4.2 Continued

you're doing a study and you're looking at gender. You might code Female as 1 and Male as 2 (or any other numbers if you like) when you are entering in the data on your computer. So, those numbers 1 and 2? They're just standing in for different categories of data, like a secret code for the computer to understand. Other examples include:

- hair colour (e.g. 1 for blonde, 2 for red, 3 for brown, etc.)
- marital status (e.g. 1 for single, 2 for married, 3 for de facto, 4 for divorced, etc.).

A good way to remember all of this is that *nominal* sounds a lot like *name* and nominal scales are like names or labels (4).

A special type of nominal scale has only two categories (e.g. exposed/not exposed) and is called a *dichotomous* scale. Variables for recording observations with only two categories are called **dichotomous variables**.

Dichotomous variables: Variables that have only two possible values.

Ordinal scale: In this scale, data are categorised into distinct groups with an inherent order or ranking, but the differences between categories are not consistent or quantifiable. Examples include survey responses indicating levels of agreement (strongly disagree, disagree, neutral, agree, strongly agree). While there is a clear order, the intervals between categories are not meaningful.

2. Ordinal scales

Ordinal scales arrange members of an entity in a specific order, either from most to least or vice versa. However, the values assigned to these ranks lack other mathematical properties such as equal intervals or a true zero point. This means that when dealing with ordinal data, we can only establish whether one member of an entity possesses more or less of a certain attribute compared with another member – the precise extent of this difference remains unknown (a known unknown!). For example, when Hugo comes first in a stats test and Rachael comes second, we can't determine how close their results were; we only know that Hugo outperformed Rachael. Likert-type scales, exemplified by questions such as 'On a scale of 1 to 10 with one being no pain and ten being high pain, how much pain are you in today?' are another example. A person may not necessarily be in half as much pain if they responded 4 than if they responded 8. All we can say is that an individual who responds 6 is in less pain than if they had responded 8 but in more pain than if they had responded 4.

Ordinal scales are typically measures of non-numeric concepts such as satisfaction, happiness and discomfort. Other examples include:

- level of education (e.g. 1 for high school certificate, 2 for bachelor's degree, 3 for master's degree, etc.)
- socioeconomic deprivation (e.g. 1 for most deprived, 2 for second most deprived, etc.).

Ordinal is easy to remember because it sounds like *order*, which is the only information you get from this type of scale.

Interval scale: These have ordered categories with consistent intervals between them, but there is no true zero point. Temperature measured in Celsius or Fahrenheit is an example of interval scale data. While differences between temperatures are consistent (e.g. the difference between 10°C and 20°C is the same as that between 20°C and 30°C), a temperature of 0°C does not represent the absence of heat.

3. Interval scales

Interval scales display the characteristic of not only order (like ordinal scales), but the presence of equal intervals between each successive point on the scale as well. This means that the difference between any two consecutive points on an interval scale is the same. Take temperature in degrees Celsius, for example. We know this is an interval scale because the difference between 50 and 51 degrees (i.e. 1 degree) is the same as the difference between 80 and 81 degrees. The useful feature about having these characteristics is that you can add and subtract (51°C minus 50°C makes sense), and you can calculate measures of central tendency such as mean, median or mode. More complex statistical analyses are also possible.

The only feature that differentiates this type of scale from the next (the ratio scale) is the absence of a true zero point. In other words, 0 on an interval scale does not mean the absence of value but is just another number such as 1 or 10. Negative numbers are also possible and have meaning on an interval scale. Why is this important? It means that you cannot say that the value of 40 on an interval scale is twice the value of 20. And in case you were wondering, some interval scales may appear to have zero points, but these are in fact arbitrary and do not signify the absence of the measured attribute. For example, a temperature of 0°C does not indicate the absence of heat; it simply indicates the freezing point of water at sea level. Water temperatures below 0°C are possible. It is therefore not accurate to say that 40°C is twice as warm as 20°C (even though it might feel that way!). Other examples include:

- altitude
- a clock.

One way to remember the key points of an *interval scale* is that *interval* means 'space in between'. Interval scales tell us not only about order, but also about the value between each item (4).

4. Ratio scales

Ratio scales are like interval scales in that they display both the characteristics of order and the presence of equal intervals between each successive point on the scale. What sets them apart from the other scales is the presence of an absolute zero – a point below which no numbers exist. In other words, zero on a ratio scale means the absence of value and that negative numbers have no meaning. For example, a person's weight is measured on a ratio scale because a zero weight means you don't exist and a negative weight makes no sense. This attribute allows us to treat ratio data as true numbers, meaning you can add, subtract, multiply and divide with ratio data. Why is this important? It means that if Hugo weighs 75 kilograms and Rachael weighs 50 kilograms, you can say with confidence that Hugo is 1.5 times heavier than Rachael. You can also calculate measures of central tendency such as mean, median or mode, and undertake more complex statistical analyses. Other examples include:

Ratio scale: Like the interval scale but with a true zero point, meaning that a value of zero represents the absence of the measured attribute. Examples include measurements of height, weight and time. On a ratio scale, it is meaningful to calculate ratios and perform mathematical operations like multiplication and division.

- income
- age
- height
- the number of individuals living in a respondent's household.

Table 4.1 summarises the fundamental differences between the four scales of measurement.

Table 4.1 The fundamental differences between the four scales of measurement

Scale	Indicates difference	Indicates direction of difference	Indicates amount of difference	Indicates ratio of difference
Nominal	✓			
Ordinal	✓	✓		
Interval	✓	✓	✓	
Ratio	✓	✓	✓	✓

Rachael: Okay, but I reckon I would have done better in stats, ordinally speaking …

Hugo: And I'm not sure that the weight ratio was strictly accurate!

Author (Stephen): All right, points taken. These were meant to be *hypothetical* examples to illustrate the four different measurement scales!

Returning now to our thought experiment, we can extrapolate from what we have learned in Explanation 4.2 that an observation made according to our operational definition of the outcome in this example is being measured on a special type of nominal scale called a dichotomous scale (i.e. there just two possible values – has the common cold, does not have the common cold) – and the outcome variable is therefore a dichotomous variable.

Let's now briefly turn to the exposure variable 'sitting in a classroom with inadequate ventilation.' This will take a bit more effort to operationalise because it is easy to think of different ways one might measure 'inadequate ventilation.' For example, if a classroom has windows that are not entirely closed, how closed do they have to be for ventilation to be regarded as inadequate? Is the degree of 'openness' important? What if there is a central ventilation system in place – how would you account for this? And so on. There is also another factor to consider, which relates to the amount of time students spend sitting in a classroom with inadequate ventilation. A time dimension is not uncommon with exposure variables, particularly those to do with the environment where length of exposure to an airborne pathogen such as rhinovirus is likely to influence your chances of getting infected.

Obviously, there are many ways to go here, and our intention is not to identify the best. Rather, it is to observe what effect different approaches might have on the type of data we end up collecting. If we ignore the time spent sitting in a classroom for the moment, a very crude measure of exposure might be to simply observe whether a classroom has open windows and/or a ventilation system. If this was coded as 0 = 'no ventilation,' 1 = 'open windows *or* a ventilation system,' 2 = 'open windows *and* a ventilation system,' the data would be ordinal because, while it has a natural order to it, there is no sense in which the intervals between 0 and 1 or between 1 and 2 are meaningful. At the other end of the spectrum, a very precise measure of ventilation might be the volume of air that passes through a classroom each minute, regardless of how it is circulated (e.g. via an open window and/or a central ventilation system). This would be ratio data because it has order (a volume of 2 m^3/min is more than 1 m^3/min), equal intervals between each successive point on the scale (the interval between 1 m^3/min and 2 m^3/min is the same as the interval between 2 m^3/min and 3 m^3/min) and a true zero point (negative volume does not make any sense). The accuracy of data collected in this way would be only limited by the precision of the instrument used to take the measurements (in this case, presumably an airflow meter).

Contingency tables

Clearly, both approaches would need further work to make them consistent with how we framed exposure in this thought experiment at the outset (i.e. 0 = 'adequate ventilation,' 1 = 'inadequate ventilation'). For example, with the crude approach we would need to decide which categories aligned with our notion of inadequate ventilation; with the precise approach we would need to decide on a threshold air flow volume below which we regarded ventilation to be inadequate. The advantage of arriving at exposure and outcome variables that are both recorded on a dichotomous scale, however, is that it allows us to summarise any data we might collect in the form of a **contingency table**, which is a cross-tabulation of data such that categories of one characteristic are represented horizontally (in rows) and categories of another are represented vertically (in columns). In epidemiology, exposures are typically presented in the rows and outcomes in the columns. Tables involving more than two dimensions and/or categories are possible, but the simple 2 × 2 contingency as depicted in Figure 4.2 for classroom ventilation and the cold is the most common. You will be introduced to how contingency tables are used to calculate measures of association like an odds ratio or relative risk in Chapters 7 and 8, respectively.

Contingency table: A cross-tabulation of data such that categories of one characteristic are represented horizontally (in rows) and categories of another are represented vertically (in columns). In epidemiology, exposures are typically presented in the rows and outcomes in the columns.

		Outcome	
		Has a cold	Does not have a cold
Exposure	Classroom with inadequate ventilation		
	Classroom with adequate ventilation		

Figure 4.2 A 2 x 2 contingency table using common cold and classroom ventilation as an example

A comprehensive taxonomy of study design

Now you have a better appreciation of how epidemiologists approach problems from an aetiological perspective, let's return to the relevance of this way of thinking to how we might want to classify different study designs.

Non-experimental and experimental study designs

The first distinction you will see in conventional taxonomies such as Figure 1.2 is between **experimental study designs** and non-experimental study designs. An experimental study design is one in which the objective is to investigate what happens to an outcome when an exposure is manipulated in some way. In other words, the epidemiologist is actively involved in conducting an experiment in the traditional sense. This is distinct from a non-experimental study design, in which data on exposures and outcomes is utilised without any intervention on behalf of those conducting the study, other than to analyse the data appropriately. Here, the role of the epidemiologist is to simply observe events unfold. The term 'observational study design' is also used here.

Experimental study design: A type of epidemiological study where the objective is to investigate what happens when exposure is manipulated.

While this distinction is a critical one to make, you might interpret it as implying that experimentation is at the apex of some sort of evidence hierarchy. This is not necessarily the case for one very important reason: experimentation in epidemiology is only possible when there is reason to believe that no harm will be caused to humans by your experiment. It would be unethical to commence or continue such research if you believed otherwise. So, for example, it would be difficult for you to justify conducting a study in which you asked people to sit for a period in a room with no ventilation if you suspected they might get the common cold or COVID-19 as a result. You could, however, justify observing people sitting in classrooms with different levels of ventilation and measuring what happens.

Indeed, the limited opportunity for using experiments to investigate many important health-related questions has led to claims that epidemiology is largely an observational science (5); you have already seen how this might work in the case of the British Doctors Study (Example 4.1). None of the insights we have gained from this study about the harmful effects of tobacco would have been possible had the investigators restricted themselves to an experimental study design. In Chapter 8, we introduce you to another influential study in the history of epidemiology, the Framingham Heart Study. Much of what we know about the risk factors for cardiovascular disease is due to this work. Again, experimentation would not have been an option in this instance.

Yet, despite observational research being central to many important success stories in epidemiology, it remains true that a carefully constructed experiment can provide high-quality evidence on causation since this is an inherent feature of its design. In this sense at least, the experimental branch of Figure 1.2 identifies the options we should consider if we want to undertake aetiological research, but only when our actions are likely to *improve* outcomes, not make them worse. In practice, this means research into the potential benefits of new therapeutic options (i.e. clinical trials) or population-wide interventions (i.e. community trials). The burgeoning field of evidence-based practice is replete with examples of the former. In Example 4.2, we introduce you to an example of the latter: the Community Intervention Trial for Smoking Cessation (COMMIT) study.

EXAMPLE 4.2

The Community Intervention Trial for Smoking Cessation (COMMIT) study, initiated in the late 1980s, is a landmark research endeavour that aimed to assess the effectiveness of community-wide interventions in reducing smoking rates. Led by the National Cancer Institute (NCI) and involving multiple communities across the United States, COMMIT sought to implement and evaluate comprehensive tobacco control programs, marking a significant shift from individual-focused cessation efforts to community-wide strategies.

The primary objective of COMMIT was to investigate whether community-level interventions, involving a combination of media campaigns, school programs, workplace initiatives and health system changes, could lead to a substantial reduction in smoking prevalence. The study adopted a community-randomised trial design, enlisting multiple intervention and control communities, and involving extensive collaboration between researchers, health professionals and community leaders.

The study's interventions were multifaceted, reflecting a recognition that addressing tobacco use required a comprehensive and community-based approach. This included mass media campaigns to raise awareness, smoking cessation programs in schools and workplaces, changes in healthcare delivery to incorporate anti-smoking messages, and policies to create smoke-free environments.

One of the distinctive features of COMMIT was its emphasis on community involvement and tailoring interventions to the specific needs and characteristics of each community. Local leaders, health organisations, and community members played active roles in shaping and implementing the anti-smoking initiatives. This collaborative approach recognised the importance of considering local contexts and fostering community ownership for the success of tobacco control efforts.

The study's evaluation framework involved collecting extensive data on smoking prevalence, cessation rates and changes in community norms regarding tobacco use. Researchers employed a variety of methods to assess the impact of interventions, including surveys, interviews and observational data.

The COMMIT study produced a wealth of findings that significantly contributed to the understanding of effective tobacco control strategies. One of the key outcomes was the demonstration that comprehensive, community-wide interventions could indeed lead to notable reductions in smoking rates. The communities that received the multi-component interventions experienced greater success in reducing smoking prevalence compared with the control communities.

The study also provided insights into the specific components of the interventions that were most effective. For instance, media campaigns that employed strong anti-smoking messages, coupled with community programs and policy changes, proved to be particularly impactful. Additionally, the COMMIT study highlighted the importance of sustained efforts over time, as communities that maintained their anti-smoking initiatives continued to see positive results.

The COMMIT study had a lasting impact on public health approaches to tobacco control. It emphasised the significance of addressing smoking at the community level and demonstrated that a combination of strategies, tailored to local contexts, could lead to meaningful reductions in tobacco use. The findings influenced subsequent tobacco control policies and interventions, and shaped the framework for comprehensive, community-based tobacco-control programs globally.

In summary, the COMMIT study was a ground-breaking research initiative that assessed the effectiveness of community-wide interventions in reducing smoking rates. Through its collaborative and comprehensive approach, COMMIT provided crucial insights into the success of multifaceted, community-based tobacco-control strategies. The study's findings influenced public health policies and interventions, emphasising the importance of tailored, community-driven efforts in the ongoing global fight against tobacco use.

Source: (6).

As you will have seen from this example, the COMMIT study is important in the history of epidemiology because it was one of the first to investigate the effectiveness of efforts to reduce smoking rates in a community-wide setting. We will explore experimental study designs such as this and their place in the evidence hierarchy in more detail in Chapter 9; of course, the tools covered in this chapter cannot be used to examine the effects of *increasing* potentially harmful exposures.

Rachael: I guess observational studies are best for looking at health effects of harmful exposures and experimental studies are best for working out how to prevent effects from harmful exposures.

Hugo: So, you can only wait and see what happens to people who smoke, but you can actively test anti-smoking strategies?

Author (Stephen): You've got it! Luckily, some ethical principles have evolved over time to help us here. A key one is non-maleficence, which requires us to avoid causing harm to study participants and to society more generally. Another is beneficence, which requires us to minimise potential risks and maximise potential benefits. You can read more about ethical obligations of epidemiologists in (7).

Unit of observation: The 'who' or 'what' for which data are measured, collected or acquired.

Unit of analysis: The 'who' or 'what' for which information is analysed and conclusions are reached.

The final point to make about the *experimental/non-experimental* dichotomy is that it is becoming increasingly dated because it does not account for the emergence of a group of tools for synthesising data from other studies and sources that do not sit comfortably under either of these headings. The key problem for these tools is that their **unit of observation** is neither individuals nor groups of individuals when the dominance of the aetiological perspective has conditioned us to regard one or the other as essential to 'doing epidemiology'. By unit of observation, we mean the 'who' or 'what' for which data are measured, collected or acquired. This is distinct from the **unit of analysis** of a study, by which we mean the 'who' or 'what' for which information is analysed and conclusions are made (8). We will return to these concepts at the end of the chapter, where we introduce two examples of non-traditional epidemiological research.

Descriptive and analytical study designs

Descriptive study design: A type of epidemiological study in which the analytical intent is not to explore causal relationships.

The second distinction you will see in conventional taxonomies such as Figure 1.2 is between *descriptive* and *analytical* study designs. A **descriptive study design** has a focus on the 'who, where, when and what' of exposures and outcomes, and is useful when little is known about a problem as it helps to draw attention to new and emerging issues or generate hypotheses about causation without necessarily generating the evidence needed to support such theories. Figure 1.2 lists case reports and cross-sectional surveys as relevant tools in this regard.

Take a closer look at this list, however, and you will notice cross-sectional surveys also being listed under the analytical heading, with an 'analytical' qualifier in parentheses. While this is not a mistake, nor does it indicate a fundamental difference in underlying design because, as you will learn in later chapters, a cross-sectional survey is a cross-sectional survey regardless of how you might decide to classify it. The distinguishing factor here is how data from this type of study are analysed *after they have been collected.* Let's see how this works using our thought experiment from Chapter 1. Since our purpose was to explore the relationship between inadequate ventilation and the common cold, we would be justified, according to convention, in classifying an analysis of this relationship based on data from a cross-sectional survey as 'analytical'. If, on the other hand, we had a non-aetiological purpose such as comparing the prevalence of the common cold in different populations, convention would have us classify this analysis 'descriptive'. The data can even be from the same survey in both examples and these conventions would still apply.

Several points need to be clarified here because it not as straightforward as we might like. First, while the 'analytical' label is entrenched in conventional taxonomies of study design, it does a poor job of describing the boundaries of this category since working with data invariably involves analysis of one sort or another, regardless of purpose. A better label might be 'aetiological', as this would at least indicate which type of analysis is being referred to. Second, even if such a label change was adopted, there is still the problem – at least in the case of cross-sectional surveys – of having to classify these studies according to analytical purpose rather than underlying design considerations. This appears insoluble, at least not without some degree of taxonomical redesign. In other words, we are stuck with these anomalies for the time being.

What we can say unequivocally is that all the tools listed under the analytical heading in Figure 1.2 have design features that enable aetiological research, albeit in an observational setting. Yet each does this in a slightly different way. Cross-sectional surveys and ecological studies share the common feature that measures of exposure and outcome are assessed at the same time. However, these data come from the same source in a cross-sectional survey but can come from multiple sources in an ecological study. (The unit of analysis is also different, but we will come back to this point in due course.) With case control studies, participants are recruited according to the outcome and then assessed for past exposures, while the opposite is the case for cohort studies, where at-risk participants are classified according to past or current exposures and then assessed for outcomes. Of course, clinical and community trials also enable aetiological research; however, as we have already discussed, these are experiments in which exposure is manipulated in some way and they are therefore classified as experimental. The timing of these different approaches to assessing exposure and outcomes in relation to a reference point in time is summarised in Table 4.2, in which we call the reference point 'time zero' and represent it as t_0, and any time after that as t_{0+n}.

Table 4.2 Timing of exposure and outcome assessments with reference to time zero for different types of aetiological study design options

Study design option	Exposure	Outcome
Ecological studies	t_0	t_0
Cross-sectional surveys	t_0	t_0
Case control studies	t_{0+n}	t_0
Cohort studies	t_0	t_{0+n}
Clinical and community trials	t_0	t_{0+n}

The ordering of the study designs options in Table 4.2 reflects a hierarchy, in increasing order of evidentiary strength, that we will expand upon in our discussion about causation in later chapters; it is also the reason why we have ordered the contents of Chapters 5 to 9 in the way we have. So, for example, information about a possible exposure/outcome association from a case series or case report (Chapter 5) is not regarded as highly as evidence from a cross-sectional or ecological study (Chapter 6), which in turn is not regarded as highly as evidence from a case control study (Chapter 7), which in turn is not regarded as highly as evidence from a cohort study (Chapter 8), and so on. If your purpose is aetiological, then this order will have intuitive appeal – at least theoretically. This is because it can be more difficult (although by no means impossible) to establish with certainty the correct sequence of events (i.e. exposure then outcome) when outcomes are assessed first or when exposures and outcomes are assessed simultaneously compared with when exposures are assessed first in a group of at-risk participants.

As always, a willingness to think critically and be pragmatic about your options is arguably much more important, particularly in a crisis. Example 4.3 provides a stark reminder of how the right tools for the job can be as simple as a single case series report and a half-finished case control study. As illustrated in this example, thousands of lives were ultimately saved, and many more birth abnormalities prevented, because of the speed with which these study designs could be deployed compared with the alternatives.

EXAMPLE 4.3

The thalidomide tragedy of the 1960s remains a haunting chapter in the history of medicine, underscoring the catastrophic consequences of inadequate drug safety testing. The story begins in the late 1950s with the emergence of an unusual epidemic in Germany, marked by a surge in severe limb defects among newborns known as *phocomelia*. This is a congenital condition that involves malformations of human arms and legs, resulting in a flipper-like appendage (Figure 4.3). The anomalies, which were once rare, began occurring more frequently, triggering various theories among the medical community reminiscent of the uncertainty during past epidemics such as cholera. Amid suspicions of impure water, nuclear testing or an unknown toxin, questions arose about a potential chemical warfare program originating in the Soviet bloc, given the concentration of cases in West Germany compared with the scarcity in East Germany (9).

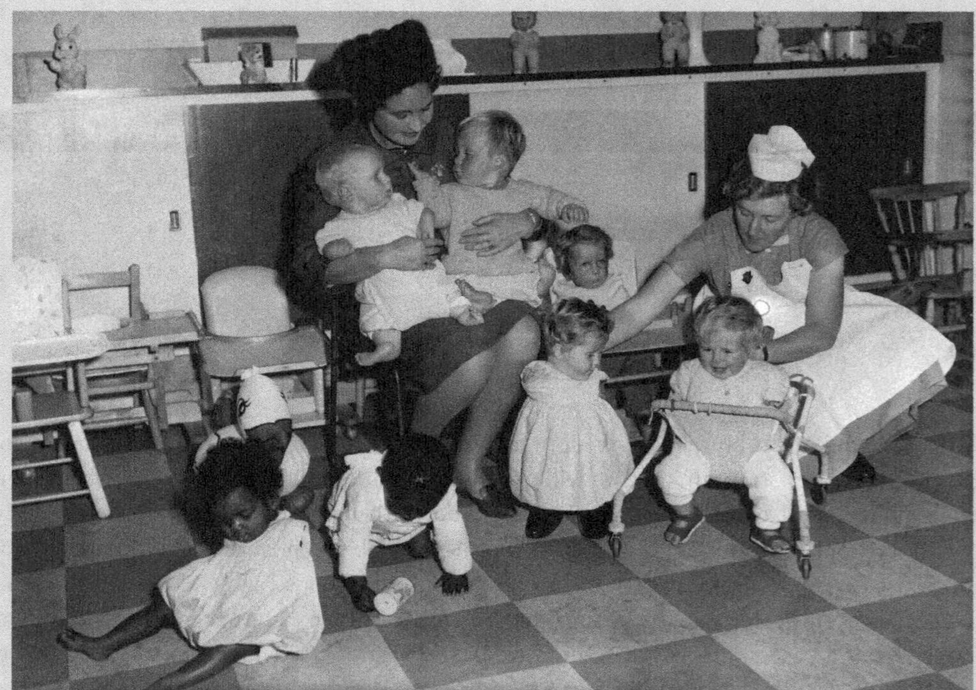

Figure 4.3 Children born with phocomelia, 1962

The cause of this tragedy was eventually discovered by a group of clinicians working as epidemiologists independently in different parts of the world. The initial sign that something unusual was occurring surfaced in Munich when a gynaecologist by the name of Dr Weidenbach reported in 1959 on a child displaying phocomelia in the arms and legs (10). Weidenbach recognised this as an exceptionally rare deformity, given the absence of comparable cases in the German literature and the records of the Bavarian Institution for Crippled Children since its establishment in 1913. Other isolated instances were subsequently reported, but evidence of a common cause didn't surface until a gathering of the German Society for Paediatrics in September 1960 where Drs Kosenow and Pfeiffer presented detailed information on two cases involving children born with phocomelia and additional deformities of the intestine and upper lip (11). Significantly, both children were born on consecutive days in the same small German town.

By the start of 1961, it was evident that a surge in limb deformities was occurring across the country. A Hamburg paediatrician by the name of Dr Lenz was convinced that a common cause underlay the epidemic and started interviewing the mothers of affected children about the use of any new or unusual drugs during pregnancy but found nothing unusual. By August, Lenz had estimated a tenfold increase in the incidence of phocomelia in Hamburg and potentially a 100-fold or more increase in certain towns in Rhineland and Westphalia. A month later, a paper by Dr Wiedemann documented a similar trend in his Krefeld clinic – only four cases of limb deformities were noted between 1950 and 1959, but an abrupt rise to 13 cases had occurred in the previous 10 months (12). Wiedemann too suspected that a recently introduced toxic element or some other common cause was responsible for the surge he was witnessing but rigorous investigation had ruled out infection, irradiation, contraceptive chemicals and attempted abortion as potential causes.

It was a paediatrician by the name of Dr Weicker who first identified the potential culprit of the crisis as it was emerging in Germany. Called thalidomide and sold as Contergan, this drug had been marketed aggressively as a harmless sedative since its synthesis by the German pharmaceutical company, Chemie Grünenthal, in 1956. Weicker spend every spare hour, including the weekends, locating the cause (13) and by August 1961 had gathered comprehensive histories on 20 pregnancies, with Contergan implicated in at least five (14, 15). However, he dismissed the link because of his mistaken belief that thalidomide was extensively used in the United States, where no occurrences of phocomelia had been reported. In fact, the drug had been blocked for use in that market due to concerns about inadequate testing. By 11 November, Lenz had confirmed the use of Contergan in 26 pregnancies and now strongly suspected that this was the cause of the epidemic of limb malformations (13). On 16 November, he wrote to Chemie Grünenthal requesting that the drug be taken off the market and then, on 18 November, spoke to Weicker about his suspicions, causing the latter to recheck his collection of case histories. Within a few days, Weicker had identified an additional 34 cases with clear evidence of thalidomide use by the mothers (13).

Over the next week, Chemie Grünenthal personnel spoke extensively with Lenz. The strength of the latter's case lay in his use of a simple case control study design and extensive case histories from numerous women, which ultimately showed that of 112 women with malformed babies, 90 had taken Contergan in the critical weeks of gestation, compared with none in a group of 188 women who had borne normal children (16). These data can be summarised in a 2 x 2 contingency table (see Table 4.3).

EXAMPLE 4.3 Continued

Table 4.3 2 x 2 contingency table of exposure to thalidomide vs number of malformed babies

		Malformed babies		Total
		Yes	No	
Exposure to thalidomide	**Yes**	90	0	90
	No	22	188	210
	Total	112	188	300

As you will learn in Chapter 6, the association between thalidomide and birth malformations implied by these data is very strong. Lenz later reflected:

> When I was in the process of collecting and checking this information, I reached a certain point of personal conviction. Theoretically I had to choose now between completing a respectable study, which would have meant that the malformation epidemic would go on for some time, or to rush into publicity in an attempt to speedily remove thalidomide not only from the market but from every household where it might still be the cupboard. In fact I felt there was no choice left (13).

In Australia, the link between thalidomide and foetal abnormalities was identified more quickly due to the astute observations and persistence of an obstetrician by the name of Dr William McBride. Dr McBride had encountered an unusual case on 4 May 1961 at the Sydney Women's Hospital, a large metropolitan hospital with an annual birth rate of 4000; a baby with bowel atresia (absence or narrowing of an opening) and phocomelia of both arms was delivered, marking the first instance of phocomelia he had witnessed in his seven years of experience in obstetrics. The emergence of another similar case 20 days later raised his suspicions, and by 8 June, with the arrival of a third case, Dr McBride became alarmed.

To solve the mystery, Dr McBride searched the literature on drug-induced malformations and scrutinised the case notes of the three pregnancies. The sole commonality was the administration of Distaval to the mothers – Distaval being the brand name of thalidomide in Australia. The drug had been manufactured and distributed in Australia, the United Kingdom and other Commonwealth countries under licence from Chemie Grünenthal since April 1958 by Distillers Company (Biochemicals) Ltd (Distillers), a UK pharmaceutical company with its head office in London. On 13 June, Dr McBride successfully urged the Medical Superintendent at the Women's Hospital to cease the use of the drug. He then set about attempting animal experiments using available mice and guinea pigs, despite having limited expertise in this area. He even sought the assistance of a professor of pharmacology at the University of Sydney who, despite being approached twice, remained unconvinced by McBride's circumstantial evidence, deeming the cost of an animal study unjustified.

By November, McBride had seen a further three cases associated with thalidomide, prompting him to convey his suspicions to Distillers' representatives in Australia. His letter arrived in the company's London office on 21 November, six days after Lenz's letter had been sent to Chemie Grünenthal in Germany. Distillers wrote to Chemie Grünenthal on 24 November outlining McBride's suspicions and, on Sunday 26 November, Chemie Grünenthal informed German health authorities of its decision to withdraw the drug from the market. On Monday 27 November 1961, thalidomide-containing medicines were taken off the West German market and Chemie Grünenthal informed its international distribution and licence partners of these actions. Drugs containing thalidomide were removed from Commonwealth markets including the United Kingdom and Australia on 2 December, and from other markets soon after.

McBride took the further step of sending a letter to the *Lancet*, one of the most prestigious journals in medicine both then and now. Published on 16 December 1961, this marked the first published record of the potential *teratogenic* effects of thalidomide. Teratogens are substances that cause congenital disorders in a developing embryo or foetus. Lenz's final results were published the following year in the *Archives of Environmental Health: An International Journal* (16).

Thalidomide and congenital abnormalities

Sir,—Congenital abnormalities are present in approximately 1.5% of babies. In recent months I have observed that the incidence of multiple severe abnormalities in babies delivered of women who were given the drug thalidomide ('Distaval') during pregnancy, as an antiemetic or as a sedative, to be almost 20%.

These abnormalities are present in structures developed from mesenchyme—i.e., the bones and musculature of the gut. Bony development seems to be affected in a very striking manner, resulting in polydactyly, syndactyly, and failure of development of long bones (abnormally short femora and radii).

Have any of your readers seen similar abnormalities in babies delivered of women who have taken this drug during pregnancy?

Hurstville, New South Wales.
W. G. McBride.

*** In our issue of Dec. 2 we included a statement from the Distillers Company (Biochemicals) Ltd. referring to "reports from two overseas sources possibly associating thalidomide ('Distaval') with harmful effects on the foetus in early pregnancy". Pending further investigation, the company decided to withdraw from the market all its preparations containing thalidomide.—ED.L.

Source: (17).

By the end of 1961, thalidomide-containing products had been withdrawn from most countries around the world, but not before having caused limb-reduction defects in over 10 000 children globally and a diverse range of systemic disorders. An unknown number of foetuses perished in utero because of the drug.

Hugo: It's great that epidemiology saved the day but really terrible that this was only after so many babies were affected!

Rachael: I guess they are more careful about medications used during pregnancy these days?

Author (Stephen): Yes, they are. In fact, these events prompted the introduction of much more rigorous and regulated approaches to drug safety testing globally. Drugs must now pass through three main phases of testing (preclinical trials using computer and laboratory models, animal trials and human trials) before being considered for release in most markets. It remains a tragic example of system failure that thalidomide was not required to be tested on pregnant animals prior to being marketed to pregnant women. Animal trials conducted in the months after its withdrawal demonstrated phocomelia and other systemic disorders of the embryo as likely risks.

The tools we have covered thus far represent those you would expect to see in conventional taxonomies of study design. As promised, we will complete the picture by mentioning some newer options that tend to be left off the list.

Synthesis study designs

As noted already, overlooked in Figure 1.2 is a class of tools that has emerged in recent decades for synthesising data from other studies and sources, of which the *systematic review* is arguably the most influential. You should be familiar with this type of study already from Chapter 1. Very briefly, in a systematic review, data on what others have reported on a topic are collected systematically and then inferences are made about the state of knowledge from these data. The topic can be aetiological in nature but does not have to be, and numerical findings can even be pooled across studies into what is called a **meta-analysis** when this is appropriate. In each case, however, the unit of observation is other studies, not individuals nor groups, making it difficult to classify this type of design according to conventional taxonomies, even though it is often held up as at the top of the evidence hierarchy in discussions about causation. We will return to the different ways in which systematic reviews can be used in epidemiology in later chapters.

Meta-analysis: Statistical methods used to pool the data from two or more quantitative studies to produce a single estimate of effect.

Another important example of a synthesis study design is the *burden of disease study*. Here, multiple sources of data including mortality and disease registers, health surveys, epidemiological studies and systematic reviews are rigorously accessed and synthesised into a detailed picture of the burden of disease and its causes in a population. The incorporation of aetiological research into this picture has been a central feature since the beginning and is used to quantify the proportion of disease burden that is attributable to a range of hazardous exposures. While the results are typically presented for discrete population groupings, the unit of observation is information sources, not individuals nor groups, again making it difficult to classify this type of study as epidemiological in the traditional sense, even though it is increasingly referred as the gold standard for descriptive epidemiological inquiry (18). Explanation 4.3 describes the impact of the burden of disease study on advancing the discipline and decision-making and public policy more generally, and in Chapter 5 we illustrate this with examples.

EXPLANATION 4.3: What is a burden of disease study?

The emergence of the burden of disease study marks a paradigm shift in descriptive epidemiology, providing a nuanced and quantitative lens through which the distribution and impact of diseases on populations are comprehensively understood. Descriptive epidemiology traditionally focused on characterising the occurrence and distribution of diseases within populations, but the advent of burden of disease metrics has elevated this sub-discipline to a new level.

The burden of disease study introduced a systematic framework, quantifying the impact of both fatal and non-fatal health outcomes on individuals and communities. By employing metrics such as Disability-Adjusted Life Years (DALYs), researchers can now holistically assess the burden imposed by specific diseases, considering both mortality and morbidity. This shift from a purely incidence-based approach to a more holistic, population-centred perspective has transformed how epidemiologists conceptualise and communicate the public health landscape.

The comprehensive nature of burden of disease metrics enables researchers to prioritise health issues based on their actual impact, guiding resource allocation and intervention strategies. This evolution in descriptive epidemiology not only enhances our understanding of disease patterns but also facilitates evidence-based decision-making, ultimately contributing to more effective public health policies and interventions worldwide.

In this section, we have highlighted the range of tools in our epidemiological toolbox that are likely to be useful when 'doing' epidemiology. By 'doing', we mean in the broadest sense of collecting or working with epidemiological data in one way or another. Of course, the options we have described come in many shapes and sizes, depending on the application, but these variations are unlikely to be so great as to render the basic taxonomy invalid. What remains, therefore, is to draw your attention to several design considerations that transcend these options in the sense that they can vary depending on the situation or study objective rather than necessarily being determined by the choice of tool.

Overarching design considerations

Primary and secondary data

A simple question that reveals much about the underlying design of a study is 'Where did the data come from?' If the answer is they were collected by those conducting the study for the purposes of the study, then it can be said that these data are **primary data**. In this case, the collection of new data is an inherent design feature of the study. Another term that is sometimes used here is primary research. This is distinct from **secondary data**, which are data that already exist because they have been collected for other purposes – usually by other people – but happen to be useful for the purposes of the study. In this sense, secondary data are acquired, not collected, and the acquisition process becomes an inherent design feature of the study.

Primary data: Data that are collected by those conducting a study for the purposes of that study.

Secondary data: Data used in a study that already exist because they have been collected for other purposes, usually by other people.

If collecting new data seems like the foundation of scientific inquiry, it may be surprising to learn that this is a requirement for only a small number of the study design options covered in the previous section: case reports, case series, RCTs and systematic reviews. These tools cannot be deployed successfully without collecting primary data of one sort or another. For the remaining options, however, this is not the case; some – such as ecological studies and burden of disease studies – rely heavily on secondary data while others – such as cross-sectional surveys, case control studies, cohort studies and community intervention trials – can be deployed successfully by relying on either primary or secondary data, or a mix of both. A simple example of the latter is a cohort study in which primary data about participants are supplemented with information from a census about the neighbourhoods in which they reside, such as population density or deprivation.

Research protocol: A detailed plan of your study, including how you will recruit participants, what data you will collect from them and how you will analyse these data.

When relying on primary data, this will most likely involve the submission of a **research protocol** to an ethics committee for approval before you can start. This is a detailed plan of your study, including the study design, how you will recruit participants, what data you will collect from them and how you will analyse these data. The advantage of going down this route is that you control how and what is collected. When resources are limited, however, it might be tempting to turn to secondary data sources instead, even if the way these have been collected is not ideal for your purposes. Thinking back to our thought experiment in Chapter 1, imagine we wanted to compare the prevalence of the common cold in different populations and, after a bit of searching, we discover a national health survey in which respondents are asked whether they have a cold. This is not exactly according to the operational definition we devised for assessing someone's cold status (i.e. one or more cold symptoms but a negative result on a RAT), so we would need to decide whether it is good compared with the alternative (i.e. conducting another survey using our definition). Suppose we decide in favour of using the survey. If this dataset is in the public domain, then acquiring it will be relatively straightforward; if not, and it is held by custodians, we will most likely have to agree to specific conditions around how it is to be used and who it can be shared with. These can be legally binding and sometimes even lengthy to negotiate.

Aggregated data: Secondary data that have been received for the purposes of a study in some form of a contingency table.

Micro data: (synonym 'unit record data') Secondary data that have been received as individual records that can be aggregated into custom contingency tables using statistical software.

Another potential pitfall when relying on secondary data relates to the granularity of the dataset in its received format. If, for example, the dataset is received as some form of contingency table such as the one presented in Figure 4.1, then these data can be said to be **aggregated data**. Data provided in this way cannot be disaggregated and reaggregated in other ways. If, on the other hand, the dataset is provided as individual records that can be aggregated into customised contingency tables using statistical software, then these data can be said to be **micro data**. 'Unit record data' is another term used. Clearly, micro data are more versatile than aggregated data, but often privacy or confidentiality considerations mean the underlying dataset cannot be released at this level of detail. A compromise is to allow researchers access to micro data in a controlled environment from which only certain aggregations of data or statistical results can be exported. Example 4.4 describes one such environment that allows access to health-related surveys in Australia. While restrictions such as these may not always be apparent at the outset of a study, they can influence the types of questions that can ultimately be asked of secondary data.

EXAMPLE 4.4

The ABS DataLab (www.abs.gov.au/statistics/microdata-tablebuilder/datalab), developed by the Australian Bureau of Statistics (ABS), offers a secure virtual workspace where approved researchers can analyse health-related datasets with precision while safeguarding the confidentiality of sensitive information.

Designed to ensure the privacy of individuals contributing to health datasets, the ABS DataLab incorporates strict security measures and access controls. Researchers benefit from a controlled environment that follows the principles of 'safe people, safe settings and safe data'. This commitment ensures that health data are handled responsibly and ethically.

The ABS DataLab allows researchers to explore and interpret a range of micro data, aiding in the analysis of health trends, demographics, and various factors impacting health and well-being. By offering a secure avenue for data analysis, the ABS DataLab contributes to informed decision-making in healthcare policies and research initiatives. This user-friendly platform thus serves as a valuable resource for researchers aiming to advance their understanding of health-related phenomena while upholding high standards of data security and privacy.

Single- and multi-level studies

Another design consideration that can vary depending on the situation rather than being necessarily determined by your choice of tool relates to the unit of analysis of a study. Ever since John Snow's famous Broad Street Pump study (see Examples 1.3 and 5.2), epidemiologists have been interested in the interplay between individual and contextual factors that influence health outcomes. In Snow's case, he was trying to determine the cause of a recent outbreak of cholera in the Broad Street area and suspected that the prevailing theories of infection were not explaining the patterns of disease he was observing. As it turned out, he was on the money: exposure to contaminated water from a particular water company was the ultimate source of the infection, not susceptibility to 'bad air'.

We mention the Broad Street Pump study here not just because of its enduring legacy in the annals of epidemiology but also because it is one of the earliest examples of a **single-level study** in which the unit of analysis is individuals. Remember that the unit of analysis of a study is the 'who' or 'what' for which information is analysed and conclusions are made. In a single-level study, the analysis is restricted to exposure and outcome variables analysed at the same level – in Snow's case, the level of the individual (e.g. where people lived, where they got their water). However, variables can just as easily be analysed at the level of the group, as is the case with an ecological study (see, we said we would return to this point!). An ecological study is a special type of single-level study in which the unit of analysis for both the exposure and outcome variables is groups, not individuals. Group level variables include attributes such as classroom immunisation rates, neighbourhood-level socioeconomic status and country-level mortality rates. In fact, anything that is expressed as an average across a group of individuals can be thought of as a group level variable.

Single-level study: A study in which the analysis is restricted to exposure and outcome variables measured at the same level.

Multi-level study: A study in which different units of analysis for the exposure variables are incorporated into one analysis.

Historically, most epidemiological studies have been like the Broad Street Pump study in that they are single-level studies. Increasingly, however, epidemiologists are turning to new statistical techniques for combining different units of analysis for the exposure variables into a single study (19). Called a **multi-level study**, this type of design is useful for teasing out the complex interplay between individual and group factors and their influence on individual-level outcomes. Nested groups are also possible, such as neighbourhoods within cities within countries.

Interaction: The independent operation of two or more factors on a causal pathway that enhance or prevent an outcome. The combined operation of these causal factors might increase or decrease the degree of the outcome to an extent that exceeds the sum of their individual effects.

To illustrate, consider a study examining the incidence of cardiovascular disease in a diverse urban population. The traditional approach would be to focus solely on individual-level risk factors, such as age, gender and lifestyle choices. However, a multi-level analysis expands the scope to include wider contextual factors. For example, we might want to investigate how neighbourhood-level characteristics such as socioeconomic status, access to healthcare and environmental factors contribute to variations in cardiovascular disease rates. By analysing exposures at both the individual and neighbourhood levels simultaneously, multi-level analysis can reveal whether the risk of cardiovascular disease is influenced not only by personal behaviours but also by the broader social and environmental context. This approach allows for a more thorough understanding of the **interactions** between individual- and group-level factors, guiding the development of more targeted and effective public health interventions to reduce cardiovascular disease in specific populations.

Ecological fallacy: Drawing misleading conclusions about individual behaviour from group-level data.

Individualistic fallacy: Drawing misleading conclusions about group behaviour from individual-level data. Also known as the 'atomistic fallacy'.

An interesting application of multi-level analysis techniques has been to revisit a seminal 1950 paper by Robinson, in which he demonstrated how the same datasets, when analysed at both the individual and group levels, can yield divergent results (sometimes wildly so) (20). These discrepancies prompted him to caution against drawing misleading conclusions about individual behaviour from group-level data and paved the way for the coining of the term **ecological fallacy** in 1958, which meant 'the invalid transfer of aggregate results to individuals' (21). Warnings about this methodological pitfall have appeared in epidemiological textbooks ever since, with much less attention being given to the reverse mistake: drawing misleading conclusions about group behaviour from individual level data, referred to at different times as the **individualistic fallacy** (22), also known as the 'atomistic fallacy' (23). Recent multi-level analyses of the same datasets used by Robinson have been able to demonstrate that both errors are to be avoided and that 'multilevel thinking, grounded in historical and spatiotemporal context, is ... a necessity, not an option' (24).

Hugo: Okay, so what would John Snow have done had he been alive today?

Rachael: Well, he wouldn't be studying water pumps, that's for sure!

Author (Stephen): No, he probably wouldn't. But it is interesting to speculate what he might have done after his initial success had he had access to multi-level techniques when he was alive. Would he, for example, have broadened the scope of his investigations to include housing conditions, water sources and levels of poverty across different neighbourhoods in London?

Conclusion

In this chapter, you have learnt about the different ways in which epidemiologists go about investigating the factors that cause people to become ill or get better. You will have seen how each of these has a role to play in building up our knowledge about what influences human health, much like a carpenter has a box full of tools for tackling different aspects of building a house. The key points you have learnt about the contents of this epidemiological toolbox are summarised below.

Learning objective 1: Describe the difference between epidemiological studies and study design

At the start of this chapter, you were introduced to the British Doctors Study as an example of both a famous and influential epidemiological study and a particular type of epidemiological study design (i.e. a cohort study). You were then introduced to other important epidemiological studies to illustrate the range of study design options that have evolved over the years.

Learning objective 2: Explain what is meant by the terms 'exposure', 'outcome', 'aetiology', 'scales of measurement', 'operationalisation', 'contingency tables', 'unit of observation' and 'unit of analysis'

Throughout this chapter, you were introduced to several new terms to add to your vocabulary, each with its own specific meaning. You discovered that terms such as 'exposure', 'outcome' and 'aetiology' are important to understanding the underlying objective of an epidemiological study, while terms such as 'scales of measurement', 'operationalisation', 'contingency tables', 'unit of observation' and 'unit of analysis' help us to break a study down into its individual components so we can better understand how it was designed.

Learning objective 3: Articulate a comprehensive taxonomy of epidemiological study design

Central to this chapter was the development of a comprehensive taxonomy of study design that builds on conventional distinctions, such as experimental versus non-experimental designs and descriptive versus analytical designs, but that accommodates newer synthesis study designs such as systematic reviews and burden of disease studies. These newer design options may not fit neatly into conventional taxonomies, but they are becoming increasingly influential in advancing epidemiological knowledge and informing public health debate.

Learning objective 4: Identify several overarching design attributes that can vary depending on circumstances or the study objective

This chapter concluded by highlighting several design considerations that can vary depending on the situation or study objective rather than necessarily being determined by the choice of tool. One such consideration is whether to use primary or secondary data. You learnt that while the collection of primary data is inherent to some study designs and others rely almost exclusively on secondary data, some can be deployed successfully with a reliance on either primary or secondary data, or a mix of both. Another consideration is deciding on an appropriate unit of analysis. You learned that while most epidemiological studies have historically been single-level studies in which the unit of analysis for both the exposure and outcome variables is individuals, epidemiologists are increasingly turning to new statistical techniques to explore the interplay between personal behaviours and broader social or environmental contexts and their effect on health.

Further reading

Gouda H, Powles J. The science of epidemiology and the methods needed for public health assessments: A review of epidemiology textbooks. *BMC Public Health*; 2014;14:139.

Questions

Answers are available at the end of the book.

Multiple-choice questions

1. Which of the following best defines operationalisation in the context of epidemiological research?
A – Turning abstract conceptual ideas into concrete hypotheses
B – Converting complex epidemiological phenomena into simple dichotomous variables
C – Transforming exposure and outcome variables into measurable quantities
D – Generating hypotheses based on observations of epidemiological phenomena

2. Which of the following statements best characterises the key property of ordinal scales of measurement?
A – They allow for precise arithmetic operations and have a true zero point.
B – They classify members of an entity into distinct categories without implying any order or hierarchy.
C – They display the characteristic of both order and the presence of equal intervals between each successive point on the scale.
D – They arrange members of an entity in a specific order but lack other mathematical properties such as equal intervals or a true zero point.

3. Which of the following best describes the relationship between exposures and outcomes in aetiological research?
A – Exposures refer to positive health states, while outcomes refer to negative health states.
B – Exposures are factors contributing to specific health outcomes, while outcomes represent the different health states experienced by individuals.
C – Exposures and outcomes are interchangeable terms used to describe various health phenomena.
D – Exposures and outcomes are unrelated concepts in aetiological research, each representing distinct aspects of epidemiological phenomena.

4. Which type of study has the unit of analysis for both exposure and outcome variables at the group level?
A – Cohort study
B – Cross-sectional study
C – Ecological study
D – Case control study

5. What cautionary lesson can we learn from the seminal paper by Robinson (1950) and subsequent research on multi-level analysis?
A – Drawing conclusions about individual behaviour from group-level data is always reliable.
B – Multi-level analysis techniques have no significant impact on data interpretation.
C – Both individual and group-level data analysis are prone to errors if considered in isolation.
D – The ecological fallacy only occurs when analysing individual-level data.

Short-answer questions

1. What was the thalidomide tragedy and which epidemiological study designs contributed to its cause being identified?
2. What was the primary objective of the Community Intervention Trial for Smoking Cessation (COMMIT) study and how was it conducted?
3. What was the primary objective of the British Doctors Study and how was it conducted?
4. What distinguishes the Broad Street Pump study in epidemiology and why is it significant?
5. Explain the distinction between analytical and descriptive study designs in the context of cross-sectional surveys and provide an example to illustrate this difference.
6. Describe the systematic review study design, including its key components and its significance in epidemiological research.
7. Describe the burden of disease study design, highlighting its key components and its role in epidemiological research.
8. Explain the role of data collection in different epidemiological study designs, highlighting examples where primary data collection is necessary and where secondary data can be utilised.
9. What is a multi-level study in epidemiology and why is it increasingly being utilised?
10. What cautionary lesson does the 1950 seminal paper by Robinson (20) and subsequent research on multi-level analysis teach us?

References

1. Griffiths C, Brock A. Twentieth century mortality trends in England and Wales. *Health Statistics Quarterly*. 2003;18:5–17.
2. Doll R, Hill AB. The mortality of doctors in relation to their smoking habits: A preliminary report. *British Medical Journal*. 1954;1(4877):1451–5.
3. Gouda HN, Powles JW. The science of epidemiology and the methods needed for public health assessments: A review of epidemiology textbooks. *BMC Public Health*. 2014;14:139.
4. Anonymous. Types of data & measurement scales: Nominal, ordinal, interval and ratio. www.mymarketresearchmethods.com/types-of-data-nominal-ordinal-interval-ratio
5. Webb P, Bain C, Page A. *Essential Epidemiology: An Introduction for Students and Health Professionals*. 3rd ed. Cambridge University Press; 2017.
6. Lichtenstein E, Wallack L, Pechacek TF. Introduction to the Community Intervention Trial for Smoking Cessation (COMMIT). *Community Health Equity Research & Policy*. 1990;11(3):173–85.
7. American College of Epidemiology Ethics Guidelines. *Annals of Epidemiology*. 2000;10(8):487–97.
8. Sedgwick P. Unit of observation versus unit of analysis. *British Medical Journal*. 2014;348:g3840.
9. Avorn J. Learning about the safety of drugs: A half-century of evolution. *New England Journal of Medicine*. 2011;365(23):2151–3.
10. Weidenbach A. Total phocomelia. *Zentralbl Gynakol*. 1959;81:2048–52.
11. Kosenow W, Pfeiffer R, eds. Mikromelie, Haemangiom und Duodenalstenose. *Mschr Kinderheilk*. 1960;109:227.
12. Wiedemann HR. Indications of a current increase of hypoplastic and aplastic deformities of the extremities. *Med Welt*. 1961;37:1863–6.
13. Lenz W. The thalidomide hypothesis: How it was found and tested. In: Kewitz H, ed. *Epidemiological Concepts in Clinical Pharmacology*. Heidelberg Springer-Verlag; 1987: p. 3–10.
14. Weicker H, Bachmann KD, Pfeiffer RA, Gleiss J. Thalidomide embryopathy. II. Results of individual anamnestic findings in the areas of inquiry of the universities of Bonn, Cologne, Muenster and Duesseldorf pediatric clinics. *Dtsch Med Wochenschr*. 1962;87:1597–607.

15. Botting J. The history of thalidomide. *Drug News Perspectives*. 2002;15(9):604–11.

16. Lenz W, Knapp K. Thalidomide embryopathy. *Archives of Environmental Health*. 1962;5:100–5.

17. James Lind Library. McBride WG (1961). www.jameslindlibrary.org/mcbride-wg-1961/?

18. The Lancet. GBD 2015: from big data to meaningful change. *Lancet*. 2016;388(10053):1447.

19. Diez Roux AV. The study of group-level factors in epidemiology: Rethinking variables, study designs, and analytical approaches. *Epidemiological Review*. 2004;26:104–11.

20. Robinson W. Ecological correlations and the behaviour of individuals. *American Sociological Review*. 1950;15:351–57.

21. Selvin H. Durkheim's suicide and problems of empirical research. *American Journal of Sociology*. 1958:607–19.

22. Alker H. A typology of ecological fallacies. In: Dogan M, Rokkan S, eds. *Quantitative Ecological Analysis*. MIT Press; 1969: p.69–86.

23. Susser M. *Causal Thinking in the Health Sciences*. Oxford University Press; 1973.

24. Subramanian SV, Jones K, Kaddour A, Krieger N. Revisiting Robinson: The perils of individualistic and ecologic fallacy. *International Journal of Epidemiology*. 2009;38(2):342–60; author reply 70–3.

5

Describing the problem

Will I be late for my class because of the unusual traffic congestion on my way to the university?

Learning objectives

After studying this chapter, you will be able to:

1. Examine the patterns of health-related issues by answering who, what, when and where questions
2. Be aware of the major sources of data and their uses for assessing the frequency and patterns of health events
3. Understand the importance and application of descriptive epidemiology to public health practice

Introduction

As mentioned in the previous chapters, epidemiology is a useful tool to address health issues, identify determinants of a specific health condition and provide information to promote health in populations. It can be applied to almost all fields in the health sciences. Importantly, the journey of learning epidemiology equips you with knowledge and skills essential to critical thinking and problem-solving in your study or future career. These will help you make scientifically informed decisions to improve population health. They include designing a study and applying quantitative research methods to collect data and identify 'problems'. The data collected in the process will allow you to assess the measures of disease morbidity and mortality and make comparisons across populations, geographic locations or different time points. Such comparisons allow us to determine potential 'health problems' in a relative way, which leads to further epidemiological investigations to search for possible 'clues' for 'problem-solving'. In this chapter, we will explore this basic function of epidemiology: describing patterns of health problems, known as descriptive epidemiology.

Rachael: It sounds logical, but I still don't know how I can start finding a problem.

Hugo: I couldn't agree more! Not sure where to begin … how can we find morbidity and mortality data to make comparisons?

Author (Patricia): Very good points, Rachael and Hugo. Identifying problems can start from your routine work or any day-to-day observations. For example, if you notice that the traffic on the way to the university is much slower than usual, you might be wondering what has caused it. Is there an accident somewhere down the road? Or is there some roadwork going on? Similarly, we can find health problems through the observation of some changes or differences in disease frequency (in the form of morbidity and mortality) shown in surveillance data, published literature or informed by community members. For instance, you discovered in Chapter 1 that the influenza case numbers reported in South Australia in 2022 (we can calculate influenza incidence using the given number of cases and the population of South Australia) were much larger than the numbers in the previous years, especially during the COVID-19 pandemic. In this example, we observed an 'unusual pattern' of cases based on the data of continuous monitoring of influenza. This comparison is based on the observation of influenza incidence in the same population over time.

Identifying what, who, when and where

Chapter 4 presented the key items in the epidemiological toolbox, including the two major categories of epidemiological study – descriptive and analytical studies – and various study designs under these categories. When it comes to descriptive epidemiology, we often begin our inquiry by asking a few 'W' questions to describe what, who, when and where of a health issue of concern to provide a general understanding of the distribution of the issue (1). These 'W' questions help us to determine the distributions and patterns of health issues in terms of person, place and time characteristics. We can break down the investigation activities of descriptive epidemiology into specific 'data-collection' concepts to ascertain a disease or health event in response to the four 'W' questions.

Descriptive studies focus on describing the health status of populations. Health status being studied in epidemiology includes a broad range of health-related events or conditions, including deaths, disabilities, communicable and non-communicable diseases, mental health issues, zoonotic diseases, injuries, environmental and occupational health concerns and any factors that may impact the health and well-being of populations. When we are asking a 'what' question in an epidemiological investigation, it can be targeting any of these health issues. Apart from answering what is occurring or has happened in our investigation, we also need to know 'how many' cases have been found. To quantify the magnitude of the issue, we may calculate a measure of disease frequency to determine the morbidity or mortality in a specified population. But how do we know the issue has reached a level that is considered a 'problem'? We then ask 'who', 'when' and 'where' questions to assess the 'patterns' of the issue in relation to person, place and time in descriptive epidemiology. We want to know how the disease rates vary between different groups of people or by geographic location or over time. The pattern of a health event is presented in a comparative matter. For example, a study examined the data on coronary heart disease (CHD) and stroke mortality in the populations of 26 countries from 1980 to 2010 (2). It found that CHD and stroke mortality rates decreased substantially over the study period and mortality was higher among men than women. However, the magnitude of variation between men and women varied by age across the selected countries.

Rachael: Wow! I can imagine there would be a lot of 'W' questions to answer when investigating an epidemiological event. Do we have to look for all different patterns of disease at the same time?

Hugo: I guess that, to be an epidemiologist, you need to have a brilliant mind to see any changes happening in whatever populations – does that rule me out?

Author (Patricia): Well, learning epidemiology will definitely train your brain to pay attention to detail. To your question, Rachael, it is not necessary to identify different patterns of disease in an epidemiological study or investigation. As a student, you can focus on one particular characteristic in your small study – for example, how the distribution of seasonal influenza varies across different age groups. However, it also depends on the type of event. For example, in a public health emergency, such as in the early stages of the COVID-19 pandemic, epidemiologists had to gather all possible information to describe the spread of the disease because so little was known about it.

Descriptive epidemiology is often performed in the early phase of an investigation when data are collected to depict the patterns of health-related events. It forms an important basis for analytical studies, which are developed to look for underlying 'determinants' to explain the observed patterns of a health event. In epidemiological practice, we often use tables, graphs/charts and maps to summarise descriptive data and visualise the patterns of health-related events in relation to person, place and time characteristics. These visual tools help epidemiologists to communicate epidemiological data with policy-makers and the lay public more effectively. In the following sections, we will discuss these characteristics in more detail.

Personal characteristics

In epidemiology, when asking 'who' questions, we are more interested in populations, not individual patients. The population can be defined in multiple ways, not limited to people living within a geographic location (such as a country or a city) with clearly defined boundaries. It can be a group of people with specific demographic characteristics such as sex, age, education or race/ethnicity, or people in a particular occupation (i.e. construction workers). In addition, social and economic classifications or groupings are recognised as important personal attributes that can influence the occurrence and distribution of many diseases and health-related conditions, or even risk factors of diseases such as smoking and overweight/obesity (3). Social epidemiology is a branch of epidemiology that places interest in understanding the effect of social structures, institutions and relationships on health, as well as the influence of social inequality on health (4).

Age and sex are common demographic characteristics that influence disease morbidity and mortality. For example, Figure 5.1 presents the age and sex distribution of public hospital admissions due to influenza, and the age-specific hospital admission rate per 1000 influenza notifications. Hospitalisation rates are a common health indicator used to assess the severity of a disease. The bar chart shows that the numbers of hospital admissions varied by age and sex. As population sizes vary in different sub-groups (sex and age), using simple counts (numbers of hospital admissions in this example) to make comparisons may not truly reflect the magnitudes of health issues in different population groups. Using relative measures of disease frequency such as percentages or rates (i.e. age-specific hospital admissions, depicted by the continuous

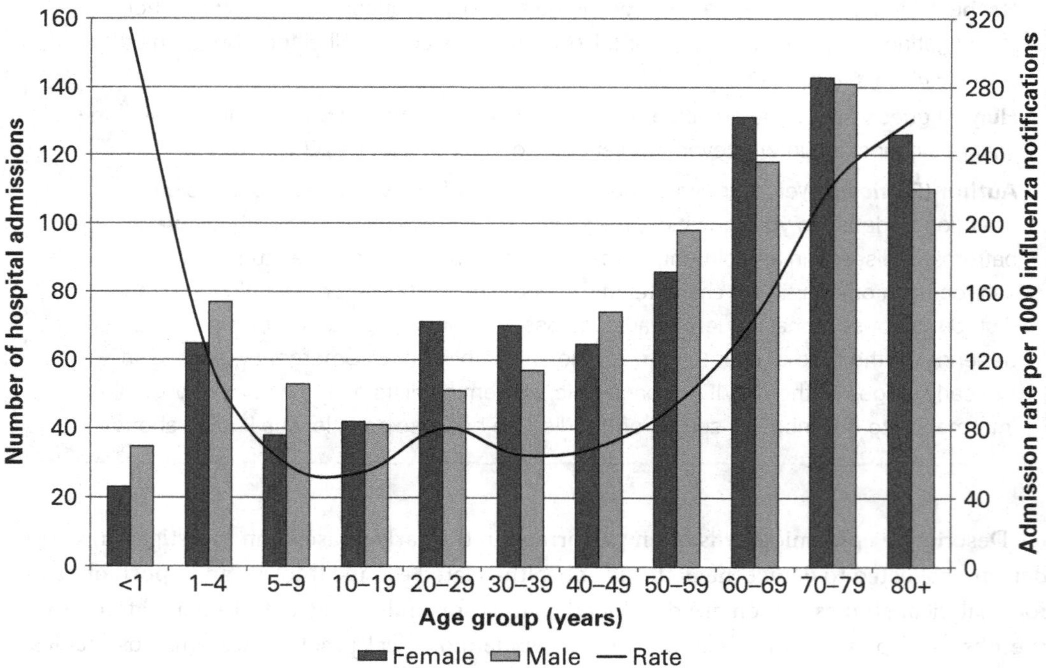

Figure 5.1 Laboratory-confirmed influenza admissions to Queensland public hospitals by age group, sex and age group, 2018 (5)

line in Figure 5.1) is more valid for such comparisons. The age-specific admission rate was highest in children < 1 year, followed by people aged 80+ years. However, the bar graph shows that children <1 years were one of the age groups with the lowest levels of hospital admissions (5). The descriptive data displaying the age difference in influenza hospital admission rates is valuable for influenza prevention such as prioritising annual vaccinations for young children and the elderly, and public health campaigns to protect these high-risk groups.

EXPLANATION 5.1: How can descriptive data be used to assess the patterns and determinants of health inequality?

As discussed in Chapter 3, life expectancy is a basic public health indicator commonly used to assess population health status. It is one of the key indicators for the health-related Sustainability Development Goals (SDGs), aiming to address issues of health inequality in disadvantaged populations such as women, children and people in low- and middle-income countries (6). According to the World Health Organization (WHO), the global estimate of life expectancy at birth increased from 66.8 years in 2000 to 73.4 years in 2023 (7). This increase can be attributed to improvements in social and economic conditions, advances in healthcare and medical technology and global disease prevention and health-promotion efforts. Australians are among the longest living populations, reaching an overall life expectancy of 83 years. However, the data of recent AIWH report revealed disproportionate distributions of life expectancy in some sub-populations within Australia (8). Figure 5.2 compares the data of life expectancy at birth by sex, Indigenous status and remoteness. We can see that, overall, women have longer life expectancy than men (three to five years' difference) and people living in major cities generally have longer life expectancy than those who live in regional and remote areas. Importantly, there seems to have a pattern of social gradient among Indigenous people living in metropolitan, regional and remote areas (a difference of up to seven years). It is striking that the discrepancy in life expectancy is even greater among Indigenous Australians living in remote areas compared with non-Indigenous Australians and people living in metropolitan areas. The life expectancy among Indigenous Australians in major cities is seven to nine years less than among non-Indigenous people. However, the gap between these two sub-population groups in remote areas is much greater, with 14 years of difference in life expectancy between Indigenous and non-Indigenous Australians for both men and women. These figures clearly illustrate the health gap between Indigenous and non-Indigenous Australians, especially those who live in remote areas.

The use of descriptive data helps to identify underlying determinants leading to the variations in disease occurrence between population groups. For example, the Australian Government conducts regular population surveys to examine the distributions of common social determinants and health risk factors, and address health inequalities in sub-populations. According to the AIWH (9), the disparity in health outcomes between Indigenous and non-Indigenous Australians is associated with unevenly distributed social determinants, including factors such as education attainment, household income, housing conditions and unemployment rate. There are also differences in the distributions of behavioural risk factors such as risky alcohol consumption, cigarette smoking, overweight/obesity and high blood pressure. Access to health services also differs, along with cultural and historical influences. All these factors contribute to the gap in overall health between Indigenous and non-Indigenous populations. These issues are complex and require fundamental social and policy changes to improve the health of socially disadvantaged people.

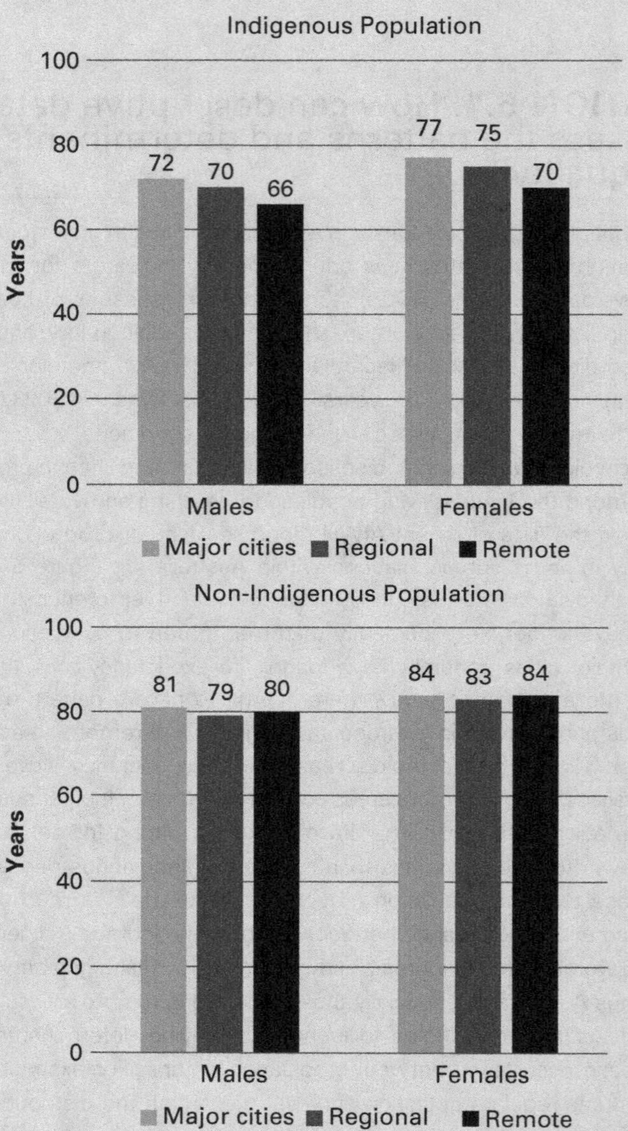

Figure 5.2 Life expectancy at birth by sex, Indigenous status and remoteness in Australia (2015–17). Data from (8)

The next example of comparing population health data to describe personal patterns involves applying the WHO's recent analysis on leading causes of death to describe the variations between countries in different levels of income groups. The overall statistics show that seven out of 10 global leading causes of death were due to non-communicable diseases. In fact, all non-communicable diseases together accounted for 74 per cent of deaths globally in 2019 (10). Figure 5.3 demonstrates differences in the leading causes of death in low-income and high-income countries in 2019 and 2000. The four levels of income-groups follow the World Bank's classification based on the gross national income: low, lower-middle, upper-middle and high. The graphs below only compare the leading causes of death between the highest and the lowest income groups. Based on the 2019 figures, in low-income countries communicable diseases or related conditions such as neonatal conditions, low respiratory infections and diarrhoeal diseases remained the major killers. In contrast, the leading causes of death in high-income countries were largely (nine out of 10 major causes of death) due to non-communicable diseases or conditions. Compared with the leading causes of death in 2000, we can see that the deaths due to communicable diseases in low-income countries had reduced significantly. In contrast, the rankings of leading causes of death in 2000 and 2019 were similar in high-income countries. It is noted that the number of people suffering from Alzheimer's disease and other dementias had risen dramatically in these countries. Overall, there was a growing trend in mortality due to non-communicable conditions in both low- and high-income country groups.

Hugo: The causes of death are so different in richer and poorer countries!

Rachael: It looks like communicable disease deaths improved a lot between 2000 and 2019 in low-income countries, but deaths from non-communicable disease got worse!

Author (Patricia): You are absolutely right, Rachael! Because of advancements in medical science and technology, as well as improving living standards, there has been a significant reduction in communicable disease deaths in the past 10 years in low-income countries. On the other hand, due to lifestyle changes and population ageing in high-income countries, the burden of non-communicable has worsened.

Comparing the differences in the key health indicators, including leading causes of death, helps us understand the levels of health inequality between high- and low-income countries and evaluate the effectiveness of existing health systems and how resources can be directed to help the most disadvantaged populations, such as people in low- and middle-income countries. More specifically, data can help focus activities and resource allocation among sectors such as transportation, food and agriculture, and the environment, as well as health (10).

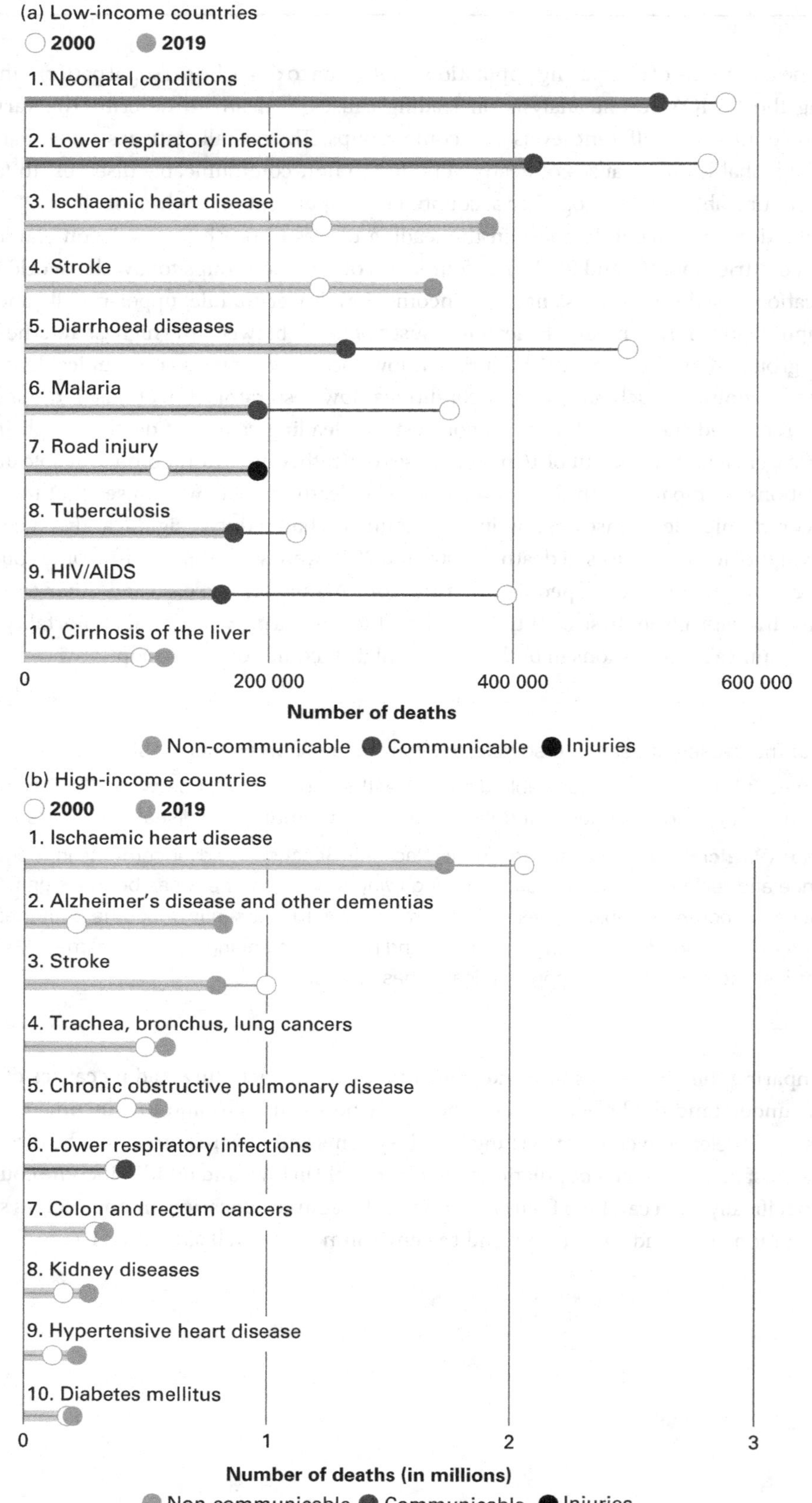

Figure 5.3 Leading causes of death by income group (10)

EXAMPLE 5.1

Over the last decade, there has been growing concern about the risk of developing silicosis among workers in the artificial stone industry, which involves the production of stone benchtops, tiles and other products made from artificial stone (11). Silicosis is a progressive fibrotic lung disease caused by prolonged exposure to respirable crystalline silica dust (12). Due to the irreversible and incurable nature of silicosis, several case reports and case series were carried out to describe the clinical features of the disease among patients. Epidemiological investigations revealed that workers in this specific industry had been exposed to high levels of silica dust from cutting and polishing the artificial stone to produce stone benchtops, tiles and other products. Studies also showed that the dust generated during the cutting and polishing of artificial stone contained high levels of silica particles, which can penetrate deep into the lungs and cause irreversible lung damage.

These studies highlighted the urgent need for increasing awareness of this health issue. Importantly, silicosis is preventable. The preventative measures require individual and collective actions involving all stakeholders, such as government agencies (especially occupational health and safety and health departments), owners of businesses in the artificial stone industry, workers' unions and workers themselves. Effective workplace exposure controls are crucial. The control measures can include limiting the duration of exposure, improving ventilation, implementing exposure control and monitoring, providing adequate personal protective equipment (PPE) and training of workers to ensure proper use of PPE, regular health screening for at-risk workers and introducing national silica exposure standards.

Source: (11–13)

Place characteristics

When examining 'place characteristics', we need to consider geographic variation in the mortality or morbidity of a disease or health-related event. The geographic variation includes different countries/regions, rural and urban differences, differences between communities, and specific locations such as workplaces, schools and childcare centres. The presentation of certain health issues in terms of occurrence and severity can vary greatly from country to country or location to location. As discussed above, for example, differences between urban and rural locations can have a significant impact on the health of populations. In rural areas, people are more likely to live in poorer housing, have less infrastructure and have limited access to social and health services. On the other hand, people living in urban areas or large cities may experience health challenges or risk factors such as air pollution, overcrowding and limited access to green spaces. For example, Figure 5.2 not only presents the variation in life expectancy between different population groups (by sex, Indigenous status and personal characteristics) but also addresses geographical differences (level of remoteness, place characteristics). In addition, the location of the workplace can also influence workers' health – for example, through exposure to occupational hazards increasing the risks of illness or injury. By examining various characteristics of 'place', we can investigate further to identify possible underlying factors contributing to the differences. When assessing variation in 'place' characteristics, we often use 'maps' to visualise the geographic differences. The earliest example of using a map as a tool to assist in epidemiological investigations in the history of epidemiology dates back to the mid-nineteenth century (Example 5.2). More recently, advanced technologies such as geographic information systems (GIS) and satellite maps like Google Maps have been used for high-quality data presentation in descriptive epidemiology.

EXAMPLE 5.2

As presented in Example 1.3 in Chapter 1, Dr John Snow investigated the source of the cholera outbreak in London during August and September 1854. He collected data from the death register and created a spot map of the affected area, then marked the locations of cholera cases on the map with small dots. Figure 5.4 illustrates the street map of the Golden Square Area and the distribution of cholera cases created by Dr Snow.

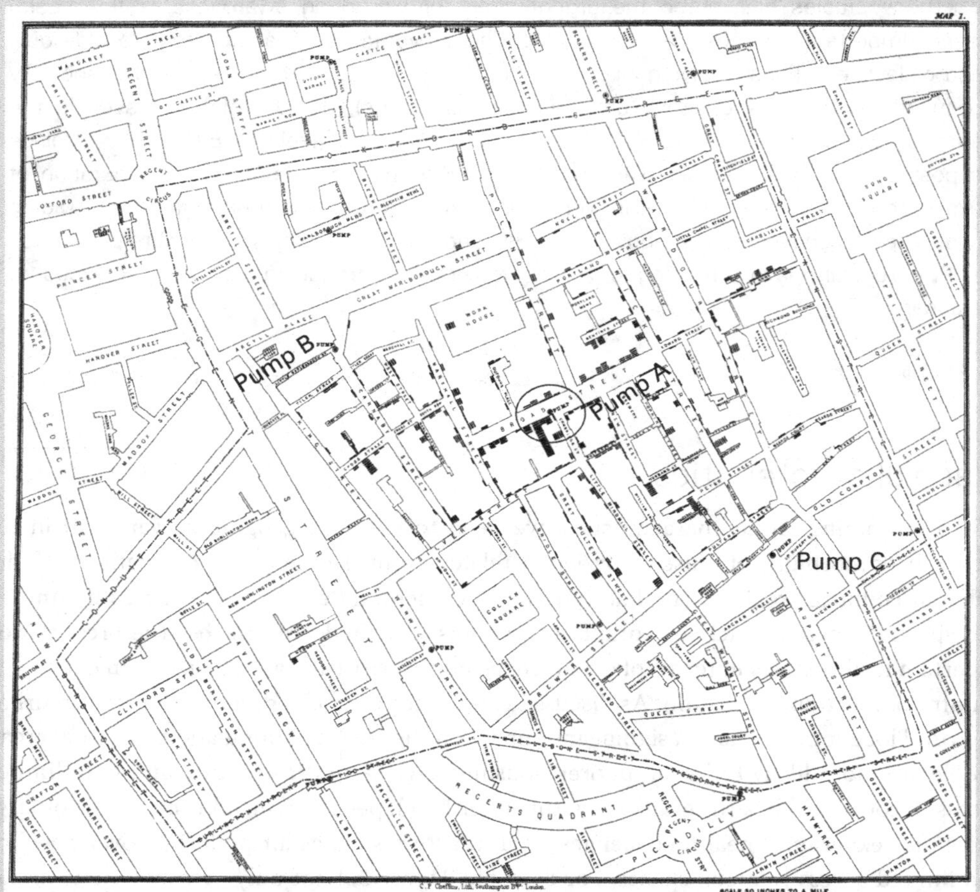

Figure 5.4 Distribution of cholera cases in the Golden Square Area of London, 1854 (by John Snow) (14)

Snow highlighted the locations of the key water pumps (A, B and C) and detailed the density of case distribution (with larger dots indicating five or more cases). By analysing the map, he found out that many cases were concentrated around the Broad Street Pump (Pump A), while areas served by other pumps (including Pumps B and C) had fewer cases.

Dr Snow immediately suspected the Broad Street Pump was responsible for spreading the disease, as it was a widely used source of water in the region where the outbreak affected the most people. He then carried out a series of investigations to support his hypothesis. He interviewed the residents and relatives of those deceased and discovered that many of them had been obtaining drinking water from the Broad Street Pump. He was also able to associate some victims with the pump even though they lived far away from Broad Street (they preferred getting water from the Broad Street Pump for drinking). In addition, he learned that a nearby brewery (only a block away from Pump A) had its own water source and therefore the workers in the brewery had not been affected by the outbreak.

Dr Snow used the information from his investigation to convince the local authorities to remove the handle from the pump to prevent the further spread of the disease. His use of spot maps and collecting descriptive data to identify the source of the cholera outbreak was a ground-breaking example of epidemiological investigation and was considered the founding event of epidemiology.

Figure 5.5 presents a weekly update of the COVID-19 situation summary using the world map published on the WHO's COVID-19 Dashboard. The graph represents the total COVID-19 cases recorded in all countries around the world (nearly 800 million cases). The greater the number of cases reported, the bigger the dot in each location. You can visit the WHO COVID-19 Dashboard and use the interactive feature to find out exactly what numbers were reported for each country, but for now we can see that the biggest dots are in the United States followed by China – where around 103 million and 99 million cases, respectively, had been reported to date (September 2024). Note that these were simply accumulative counts of COVID-19 cases reported by different countries. When making country comparisons, we need to adjust

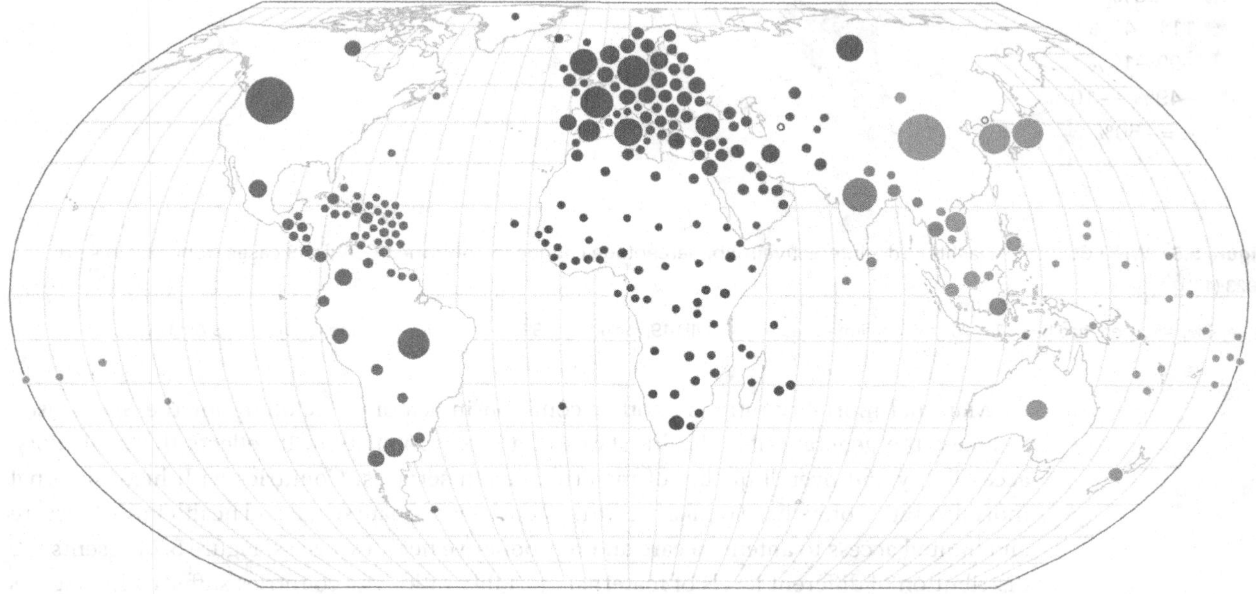

Figure 5.5 Cumulative global total of COVID-19 cases reported to WHO (15)

for the variation in population size. Such global data are pivotal to understanding how well control measures are working to contain the spread of disease; they were reported regularly by the WHO and other world bodies during the height of the pandemic.

Figure 5.6 summarises the percentages of case number change in confirmed COVID-19 cases globally using data published on the WHO COVID-19 Dashboard. For instance, although most European countries had relatively large cumulative case numbers (see Figure 5.5), the situation appeared to be improving, with most of those countries (except Spain) showing a reduction in case numbers from ≤−50 per cent to −10 per cent in April 2023. In contrast, there was an alarming 11 per cent to ≥50 per cent increase in case numbers in some low- to middle-income countries such as Mongolia, Nepal, India and several African countries (darker blue), even though their overall accumulated cases were relatively low (as shown in Figure 5.5). As middle and low-income countries have the least capacity and limited resources to manage disease outbreaks, global efforts and resources are required to assist those countries to tackle large-scale population health challenges.

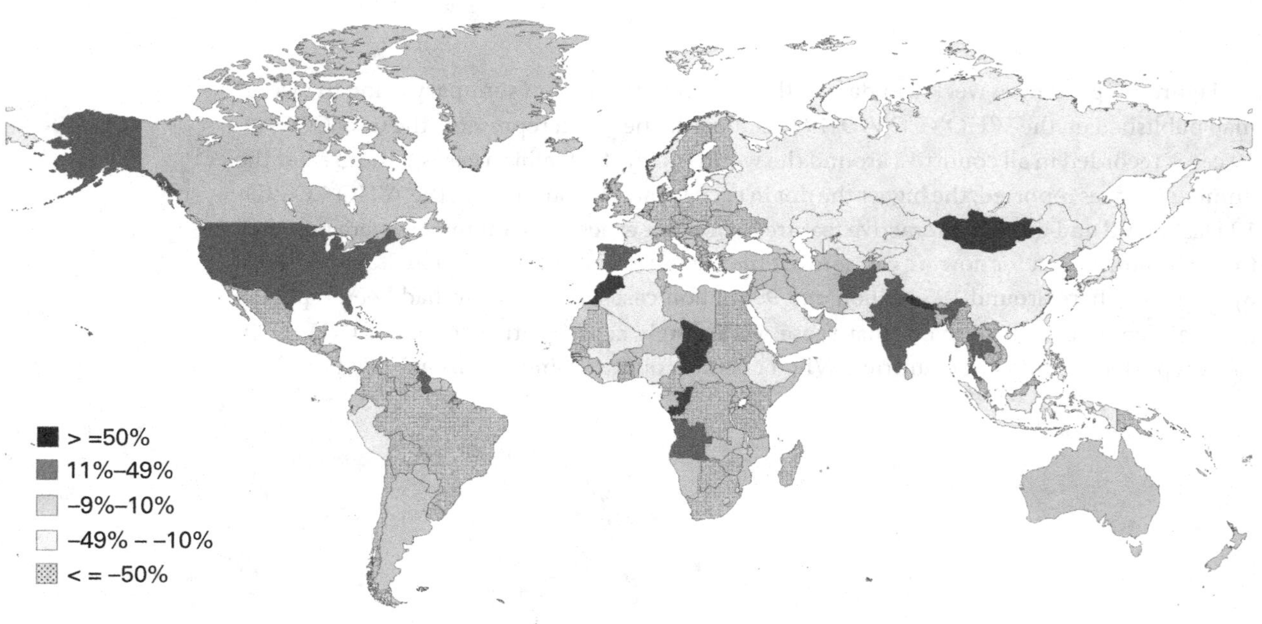

Figure 5.6 WHO COVID-19 Dashboard – interactive map, percentage change in confirmed COVID-19 cases (reported in April 2023 (15))

Note: Globally, there had been 762 201 169 confirmed cases of COVID-19, including 6 893 190 deaths, reported to WHO on 3 April 2023.

Maternal mortality ratio is another common indicator – including for the SDGs used to assess the general public health status of a given population. It reflects the availability, accessibility and overall quality of maternal health services. Countries with high maternal mortality ratios often have weaker health systems, inadequate social and health infrastructure and limited access to antenatal care and reproductive health services. Figure 5.7 presents the distribution of different levels of maternal mortality ratio. The countries suffering high levels of maternal mortality ratio (220–1500 deaths per 100 000 live births) are mainly situated in the Sub-Saharan African region. Global efforts are needed to improve access to and quality of reproductive and maternal healthcare services in these countries.

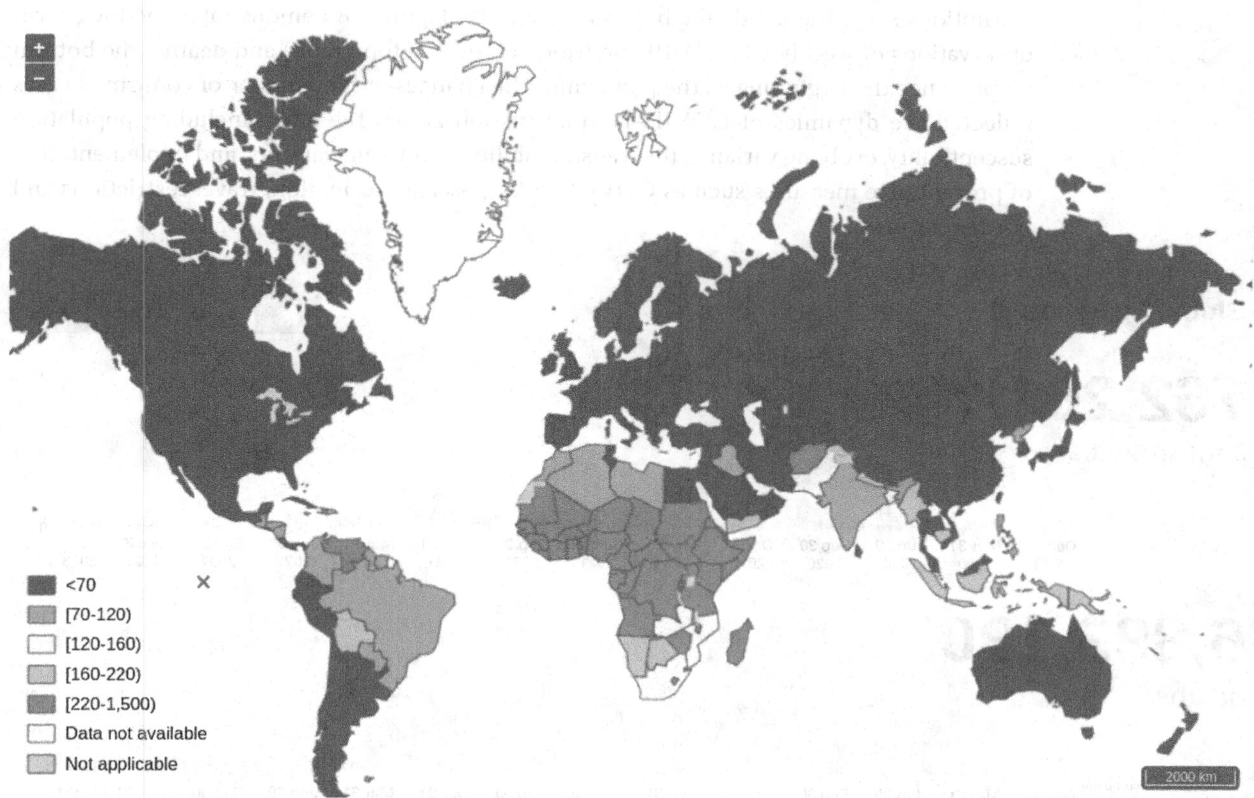

Figure 5.7 Global distribution of maternal mortality ratio (per 100 000 live births, based on 2020 data) (16)

Time characteristics

Time characteristics are useful for identifying changes in the patterns of health-related events over time. Monitoring such changes is essential for early detection of potential disease outbreaks and disease prevention. The time characteristics to be considered depend on the type of disease or health-related issue. Some diseases may display annual or seasonality patterns, while others may present short-term changes in occurrence on a daily or hourly basis, particularly during epidemics. For instance, seasonal influenza often peaks in the colder months, whereas food poisoning is common in the hot summer months. Some acute food poisoning epidemics can occur within days or even hours. In the early phase of the COVID-19 pandemic, the virus spread rapidly, resulting in an exponentially growing number of cases. On the other hand, the changes in the patterns of non-communicable diseases may appear for a much longer duration (in years). Constant monitoring of diseases over time (such as surveillance programs) enables us to see unusual temporal patterns or detect a rising trend, which is important information for disease control and early detection of potential outbreaks. Descriptive epidemiology involving time characteristics can also be observed by life events such as birth, childhood, puberty, pregnancy or menopause. Understanding the temporal patterns of diseases and health-related events can contribute to a prompt response to emerging health threats and effective disease prevention and control strategies.

COVID-19 has posed significant public health challenges and social and economic disruptions since the pandemic began in late 2019. Figure 5.8 demonstrates the long-term observations of weekly COVID-19 confirmed cases (the top graph) and deaths (the bottom graph) since the beginning of the pandemic. The changes in the number of confirmed cases reflected the dynamics of COVID-19 transmission across the globe including population susceptibility, evolving variants, the transmissibility of different variants, and implementation of preventative measures such as COVID-19 large-scale vaccination, travel restrictions and border closures.

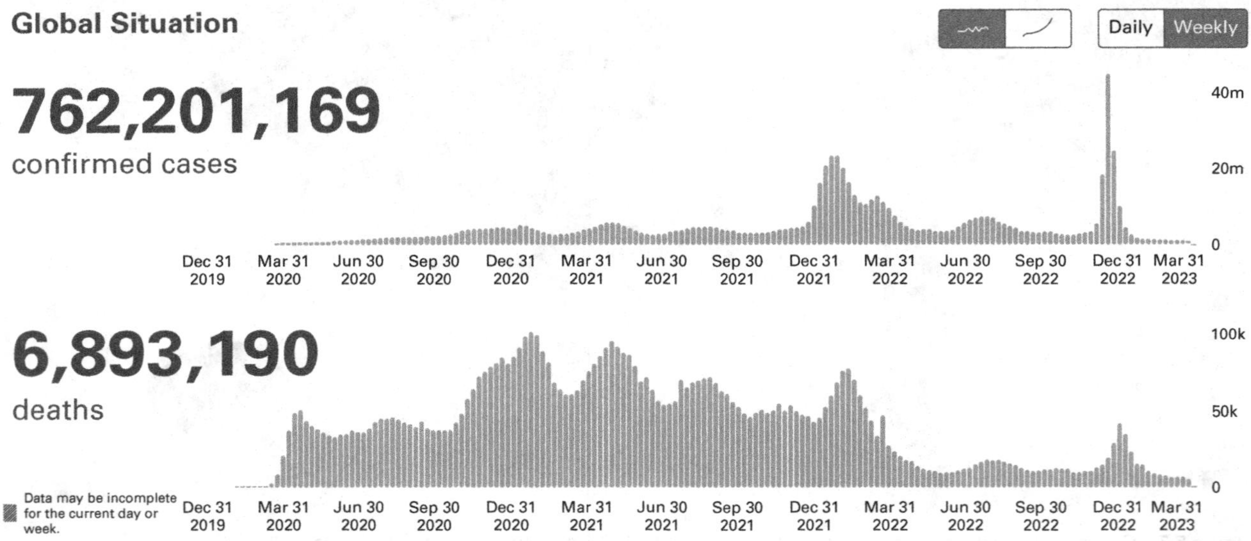

Figure 5.8 WHO COVID-19 Dashboard – COVID-19 confirmed cases and deaths from December 2019 to March 2023 (15)

For example, in the early stage of the pandemic, we can say that the entire human population was susceptible as COVID-19 was a new disease and no one was immune. As the virus continued to spread across countries and continents, we can see a steady rise in case numbers until early 2021. Although the vaccine rollout and non-pharmaceutical interventions started to take effect in some high-income countries in the first quarter of 2021, a new wave of cases due to the Delta variant soon followed. The emergence of the highly contagious Omicron variant and the relaxation of public health control measures around the world could have contributed to the latest large waves. As shown in the bottom graph, the patterns of COVID-19 deaths basically followed the waves of confirmed cases, except in the early stage of the pandemic (due to the high population susceptibility). Because of the increasing distribution of the vaccine rollout, there had been a decline in COVID-19 deaths since early 2022. When interpreting these findings, it is important to note that different scales are used for confirmed cases (20 million per unit) and deaths (50 000 per unit). This is because the daily numbers of confirmed cases across the globe were much larger in quantity compared with the daily numbers of deaths. The choice of measurement unit is made to enhance the visual presentation for examining long-term trends of health events.

The 'epidemic curves' (or histograms of frequency of case distributions) of incident cases of infectious diseases by time intervals (as shown in the top graph of Figure 5.8) are useful tools for **outbreak investigations**. The patterns of epidemic curves can provide clues for identifying transmission modes, and potentially determining the possible infectious agents. The content of outbreak investigation is beyond the scope of this book. Further details regarding various types of epidemic curves and examples can be found in the US CDC's *Field Epidemiology Manual* (1). Please see this reference under 'Further reading' at the end of this chapter.

Outbreak investigation: The process of gathering information to identify the cause and aetiology of a disease epidemic within a community and a specific timeframe, as well as to implement control measures to limit the spread of the disease.

Long-term monitoring of health data can also be used to evaluate the effect of disease-prevention interventions or health-promotion programs targeting populations. The effect may appear in the changing trajectory of disease occurrence following a specific intervention. Figure 5.9 shows that the case-fatality rate of COVID-19-related deaths in Australia has declined since October 2020. Despite several relatively large waves of Omicron variant transmission in 2022, the case-fatality rate remained low (around 0.1 per cent in April 2022). Figure 5.9 also highlights a few key milestone events of COVID-19 vaccination. The AIHW report *Australia's Health: Data Insight* suggested that the continuous fall of the case-fatality rate seemed to correspond with the rollout of the vaccination program (17, 18). Of course, we cannot rule out antiviral drugs and other medical treatments, as well as non-pharmaceutical interventions such as mask wearing, social distancing and travel restrictions playing a role in the reduction of case fatality.

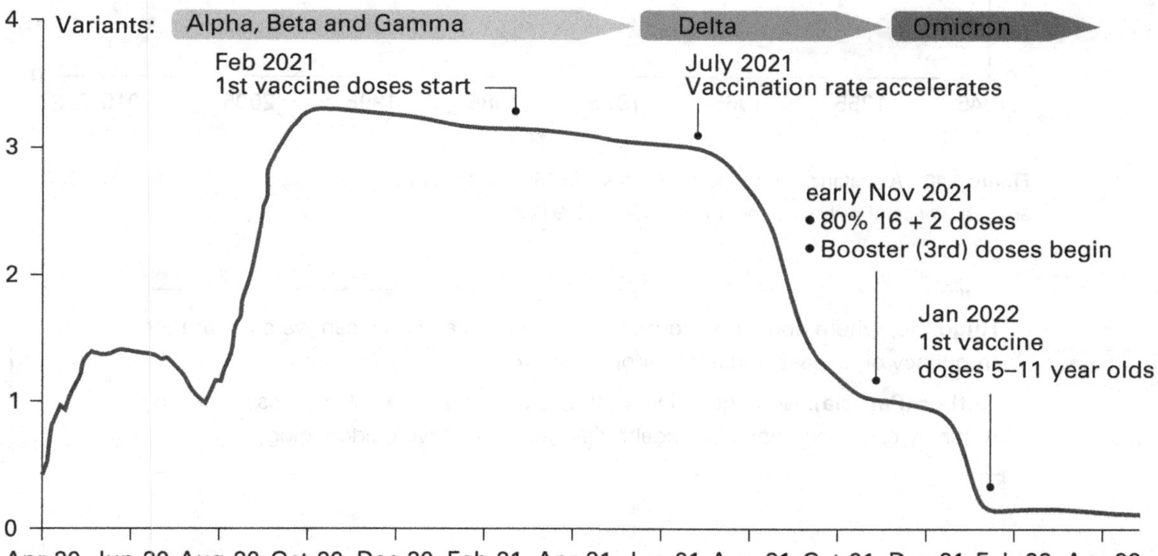

Figure 5.9 Case-fatality rate of COVID-19-related deaths in Australia from April 2020 to April 2022 (17)

We have examined disease patterns in terms of person, place and time characteristics using several examples of infectious diseases, especially COVID-19. The next example will turn our focus to a non-communicable disease: lung cancer. Figure 5.10 displays the changes in the age-standardised mortality rates from lung cancer by sex, together with the prevalence of smoking in Australia from 1964 to 2019. As you can see, the trends in lung cancer mortality rates seem to reflect the long-term prevalence of smoking in Australian males and females, with a time lag of around 20 to 30 years (19). The prevalence of smoking among males reached the highest level of around 70 per cent in 1945 and has been declining steadily (20). As a result, the mortality of lung cancer in males peaked in the 1980s and has since fallen sharply, almost paralleling the trend of smoking (with a lag of 20–30 years). Similarly, we can see that the smoking rate in females was rising from the early 1960s until it reached a peak in the mid-1970s, then started to drop in the mid-1980s, while female lung cancer morality was in gradual increase until 2010 and has since started to decline. The narrowing differences in smoking rates and lung cancer mortality between males and females over time also follow similar trends (19).

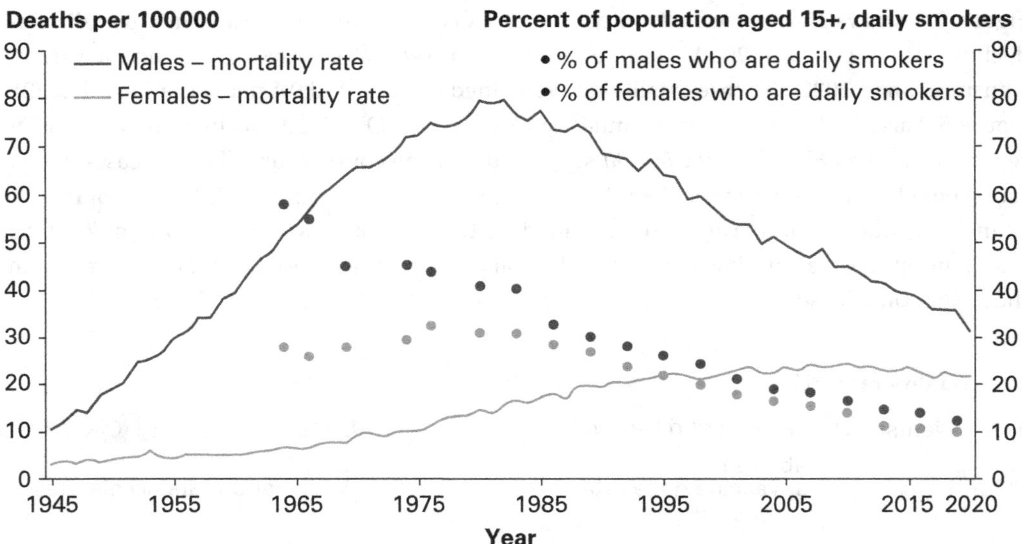

Figure 5.10 Age-standardised mortality rates (per 100 000 population) from lung cancer, by sex, 1945–2020, and prevalence of daily smoking, by sex, 1964–2019 (19)

Hugo: So, where does the information come from and how can we compare the frequency of disease in different populations?

Author (Patricia): Good question. In the next section, we will discuss where to find routinely collected population health data for descriptive epidemiology.

Collecting data for descriptive epidemiology and interpreting findings

There are two ways of obtaining data for epidemiological studies: collecting the data ourselves or making use of data that have already been collected by someone else, such as government agencies or other institutions/researchers. The former are called primary data, and the latter are secondary data. Collecting primary data on a small scale can be done in clinical settings such as through case reports and case series. For population-based descriptive studies, primary data collection is usually coordinated by government agencies due to the costs and resources involved to collect data from a large number of people (such as national health surveys and disease outbreak investigations) to describe population patterns of health conditions. The major sources of secondary data used in descriptive epidemiology are also collected by government agencies such as health or statistical agencies, especially routinely collected population demographic and health data. Secondary data can also be sought through other sources – for example, health records collected by insurance companies.

Interpreting the findings of descriptive epidemiology involves analysing and making sense of the data that have been collected. When analysing descriptive data, we often look for patterns in the occurrence of a specific disease or health condition in terms of person, place and time characteristics to answer *who, where and when* questions. We can use tables, graphs and maps to display the patterns in relation to these characteristics and interpret the patterns (such as the graphs demonstrated in previous sections). The identification of patterns will include making comparisons to find differences in disease rates between different population groups (such as sex or age groups) and different locations (such as countries and different time points). We can then come up with explanations based on the differences we have found. These explanations will help us to generate hypotheses that can be tested further in analytical studies to find possible causes of the disease.

The following section presents the sources of both primary and secondary data for the use of descriptive epidemiology and examines how they are collected; it also uses real-world examples to demonstrate how these data are used and interpreted to assess the patterns and trends of health-related events.

Studies used to collect primary descriptive data

Case reports and case series

Case reports and case series are collected through a process of reviewing and compiling information from patient medical records and relevant documents on a specific disease or health event in clinical settings. Case reports are unusual medical events or adverse effects following medical procedures or treatments, while case series consist of collections of case reports documented by physicians describing unusual conditions or atypical clinical features presented in a group of patients. These collections of cases of unique or rare events inform evidence-based medicine, and they are useful in the formation of new research questions/hypotheses. Case reports and case series can lead to further empirical inquiries (such as analytic epidemiological investigations) and novel discoveries of emerging diseases such as COVID-19.

Once patients have been identified, data are collected from their medical records and other relevant documents such as demographic information, medical history, physical examination findings, laboratory test results and treatment plans. The collected data are entered into a computerised database for analysis. The analysis results, including patient characteristics, clinical features and treatment outcomes, are interpreted and presented in a written report; any adverse effects are also reported. Sometimes case reports or case series are published in scientific journals to share information about such unusual cases across the globe. Example 5.1 demonstrates the use of case series to prompt further investigations of the risk of silicosis among artificial stone workers and interventions to protect these workers from excessive silica dust exposure. Example 5.3 presents another example of analysing case series to describe the clinical features of patients with monkeypox infection in an infectious disease centre in London.

Endemic: The persistent presence of a given disease in a specified population or arvea.

EXAMPLE 5.3

In 2021–22, monkeypox cases and localised outbreaks were reported in several countries. The origin of the outbreaks was unclear. Monkeypox is a zoonosis that is usually **endemic** to Central and West Africa. In the United Kingdom, monkeypox is classified as a 'high consequence infectious disease' (HCID). The 2022 outbreak began in May with an individual returning from West Africa, with six further infected people (without travel history to West Africa) identified in the following week. In the period from May to July 2022, a rapid community spread was observed. A total of 1735 monkeypox cases were identified in the United Kingdom, predominantly (96 per cent) occurring in gay and bisexual men, or other men who have sex with men. Around the same period, many monkeypox cases were also reported in several non-endemic countries in Europe and the Americas. As the observed clinical features of monkeypox infection in this outbreak differed from those in historical reports, a case series study was carried out to describe the patient characteristics and clinical features among people infected with monkeypox who were managed through a single HCID centre in South London.

Of the 295 cases referred to the south London HCID centre between 13 May and 1 July 2022, 197 (66.8 per cent) tested positive to the monkeypox virus by polymerase chain reaction (PCR). Those PCR-confirmed cases received a telephone consultation about their result and were included in a risk assessment. Clinical data collected through electronic healthcare systems included personal characteristics, signs and symptoms reported at presentation, mucocutaneous manifestations, risk factors, HIV status, and sexual health screen results. The findings indicated that all 197 infected individuals were men and the median age of the cases was 38 years (interquartile range 32–42 years). Of the 197 infected participants, 196 (99.5 per cent) identified as gay or bisexual, or as men who have sex with men; 170/177 (96.0 per cent) reported sexual contact with a male partner within 21 days of symptoms developing. Only 41 participants (26.5 per cent) reported having close contact with someone who showed symptoms of or was confirmed with monkeypox. Some 27.4 per cent of participants reported travelling abroad (especially to destinations within Western Europe) prior to the onset of monkeypox symptoms. The study described novel presentations of monkeypox infection in the participants that had not previously been reported. Some symptoms, such as rectal pain and penile oedema, were severe and required hospital admission. Importantly, the study suggested that these additional clinical presentations should be included in public health messaging to enhance early detection of cases and reduce potential community transmission.

Source: (21).

Prevalence surveys

Population prevalence surveys are conducted to estimate the overall health and well-being, and the prevalence of particular health conditions such as chronic diseases and common health risk factors, within a defined population. These surveys are usually coordinated by public health or statistical agencies to collect data from a representative sample of the population. The information collected in these surveys is important for decision-making for local communities, such as decisions about health programs and policies, and for better resource allocation for people in need. The timing and data collection methods can vary between different countries. In Australia, National Health Surveys (NHS) are conducted cross-sectionally every three years by the Australian Bureau of Statistics (22). The 2017–18 NHS involved around 21 000 respondents randomly selected from the population. The information collected from the survey included:

- sociodemographic characteristics
- prevalence of long-term health conditions
- health risk factors such as smoking, overweight and obesity, alcohol consumption and physical activity
- geospatial data
- information on the health literacy of respondents (22).

The NHS data are analysed and released by AIWH. The results are organised by topic and can be found on AIWH website, such as *Australia's Health Reports*, which are published biennially to present an overview of the health of Australians (23). Cross-sectional studies can also be developed to collect data for analytical studies; however, they are conducted in the same way as population prevalence surveys. The details of cross-sectional studies will be discussed in Chapter 6.

Common sources of secondary data for descriptive epidemiology

The following section introduces some common sources of routine data that provide information for descriptive epidemiology. The choice of data source will depend on the research question being asked and the availability and quality of data. It should also be noted that many routinely collected population or health data are aggregated in nature (i.e. total number of patients without personal details of each individual) and may have varying measurement units (e.g. monthly or annual data) and levels of representativeness. These issues need to be taken into consideration when employing different sources of data for epidemiological studies to yield meaningful comparisons.

Census data and vital statistics

Census data are information collected through periodic population surveys by government agencies of a country, territory or area. It is recommended that census surveys should be conducted at least once every 10 years (24), although some countries collect census data more frequently. For example, Australia and New Zealand conduct their national surveys every five years. Census surveys collect data on basic demographic, social and economic aspects of a population. Unlike prevalence surveys, which usually select a representative 'sample' of the target population to investigate health issues, census surveys involve the entire population in a country. As all members of the population are required to respond to these surveys, we can rule out the possibility of selection bias in census surveys. In contrast, we often use **probability sampling** methods to choose representative samples for prevalence surveys. Selection bias can occur when we try to select a 'representative' sample for our survey but certain groups of people in the intended list of individuals decline to

Probability sampling: A sampling method used in quantitative studies that involves randomly selecting a sample from a large population in a way that ensures that every member of the population has an equal chance or a predetermined probability of being selected for the sample. Common random sampling techniques include simple random sampling, systematic random sampling, stratified sampling and cluster sampling.

participate. The details of sampling and major sources of bias, including selection bias, will be covered in Chapter 6 and Chapter 11.

Census data can be used to inform policy, planning, governance and research concerning a wide range of issues such as public health, education, migration, welfare, housing, transport and other social services. The most common use of census data is to illustrate the numbers of people in terms of spatial distribution, age and sex structure, and other socioeconomic characteristics of a population. For instance, the ABS publishes the overall findings of the latest census survey (conducted in 2021), which outline the profile of the Australian population: a median age of 38 years, 50.7 per cent females, 80 per cent of residents living in eastern Australia, a long-term increase in specific population groups such as Aboriginal and Torres Strait Islander people, and people with culturally and linguistically diverse backgrounds. The census also initiated a simple health survey, including 10 common long-term health conditions in Australia. The result indicated that over eight million (32 per cent) Australians had been diagnosed with a long-term health condition. The information is useful for the projection of the burden of disease and planning for healthcare and disease prevention (25). For example, due to the continual fall in fertility and rising life expectancy in Europe and East and Southeast Asia, population decline and ageing are common challenges for countries in those regions. The government authorities in these countries need to prepare for the shifts in demographic structures and seek strategies to mitigate the increasing burden of disease and ageing populations (24). Many countries publish their census findings, with downloadable population data, on their statistical agencies' websites to enable easy access to these data. Some developed countries such as the United States or the United Kingdom produce interactive tables, graphs and maps to allow viewers to explore data in further detail by topic, theme or geography/community (26, 27).

Vital statistics are collected by government agencies responsible for maintaining records of births, deaths and marriages. The registration of these events is typically mandated by law. The collection of these data is through a country's civil registration system, although the exact process may vary by country and jurisdiction. When a vital event occurs (such as a birth or death), it is required to be registered with the appropriate government agency. After the event is registered, a certificate is issued by a medical or legal professional to certify the details of the event (i.e. the date and the cause(s) of death). The government agency responsible for maintaining vital statistics collects the registered information and compiles the data into statistical reports on a regular basis (e.g. monthly). The collected data are then analysed to identify trends and patterns in vital statistics, such as changes in birth rates or the major causes of death. The collection of vital statistics is important for understanding the general health and well-being of a population. Census data and vital statistics are crucial to determining a country's population sizes and demographic structures. These data constitute the 'population denominators' for the calculations of mortality and morbidity data, as well as many key health indicators.

Globally, the United Nations Statistics Division (UNSD) collects and collates census and vital statistical data from its member states and undertakes the subsequent analysis and interpretation to provide up-to-date statistics on the levels of and trends in fertility and mortality at the national, regional and international levels. Despite the importance of these data, there is an urgent need to improve the availability and quality of vital statistics in many countries. For instance, only 68 per cent and 73 per cent of countries/territories register ≥ 90% of the occurred deaths and births respectively due to deficiencies in capacity and resources (28).

The data of census and vital statistics are utilised by the health sector to identify emerging health risks and vulnerable population groups and provide an essential evidence base for determining health priorities and resource allocation (28). For example, these data are the key source for the numeric indicators of the UN SDGs. The WHO is responsible for monitoring health-related SDGs, as well as compiling and releasing data for the indicators used to assess the specific targets of the health-related SDGs (6). The indicators of life expectancy, maternal mortality, newborn and child mortality (SDG 3.1 and 3.2) are typical examples of such indicators. In addition, the WHO utilises data from multiple sources, including national vital statistics, to produce 'Global Health Estimates' using the latest available data on the causes of death and disability. These estimates provide crucial insights into mortality and disability patterns and trends, and can support informed decision-making on health policy and resource allocation. The Global Health Estimates platform features data visualisations for leading causes of death; key health indicators (such as infant mortality and maternal mortality); burden of disease and other cases of deaths by country, year, sex and country income group; and downloadable datasets (29). These data files can be used for descriptive data comparisons between countries, males and females, and over time.

Burden of disease and morbidity data

On the WHO's web page 'Life expectancy at birth', you can see the visual summary of country distribution, from the longest to the shortest life expectancy. You can also switch to **scatter plots** or a map to see the global distribution of life expectancy by WHO region/country. You can explore the details of obtaining WHO life expectancy data in 'Further reading'. Table 5.1 shows an extracted example of life expectancy data (at birth and at age 60) by country in the Global Health Estimates data hub.

Scatter plot: A graph in which each individual is presented by a single dot that demonstrates their position in relation to two variables shown on the x- and y-axes. A scatter plot graphically represents the relationship between the two variables across multiple individuals.

Table 5.1 WHO Global Health Estimates: Extracted data of life expectancy at birth and at age 60 by country (29)

Indicator Location	Life expectancy at birth (years)			Life expectancy at age 60 (years)		
	Both sexes	Male	Female	Both sexes	Male	Female
Argentina						
2019	76.58	73.51	79.5	21.11	18.84	23.08
2015	76.17	72.92	79.3	20.98	18.63	23.04
2010	75.44	72.14	78.63	20.62	18.27	22.70
2000	74.09	70.34	77.83	20.18	17.58	22.52
Armenia						
2019	76.03	72.49	79.16	20.41	18.24	22.15
2015	74.51	70.88	77.83	19.42	17.32	21.17
2010	73.12	69.39	76.61	18.79	16.76	20.52
2000	71.88	68.59	74.91	18.81	17.08	20.23
Australia						
2019	83.04	81.25	84.84	25.62	24.37	26.83
2015	82.28	80.41	84.17	25.01	23.72	26.27

Table 5.1 Cont.

Indicator Location	Life expectancy at birth (years)			Life expectancy at age 60 (years)		
	Both sexes	Male	Female	Both sexes	Male	Female
2010	81.90	79.84	83.99	24.74	23.29	26.13
2000	79.69	77.13	82.24	23.11	21.22	24.85
Austria						
2019	81.65	79.44	83.78	24.09	22.43	25.60
2015	80.98	78.60	83.29	23.59	21.8	25.21
2010	80.39	77.65	82.99	23.43	21.44	25.16
2000	78.17	75.09	80.98	21.95	19.73	23.69

Rachael: Can you explain the difference between life expectancy at birth and at age 60 years, Patricia?

Author (Patricia): Sure. This is a great question, Rachael! Life expectancy at birth is a measure of how long a newborn today is expected to live, while life expectancy at age 60 is a measure of how long a person who has already survived to age 60 is expected to live from that point forward. These measures are purely hypothetical and are calculated assuming that current mortality rates remain constant over their lifetime. If you take a look at the life expectancy data in 2019 in Australia in Table 5.1, the total length of life expectancy estimated at age 60 (both sexes: 60 + 25.62 = 85.62 years) is longer than the life expectancy expected at birth (both sexes: 83.04 years). The calculations of these measures take into account the higher mortality during infancy and early childhood compared with later adulthood. In other words, once an individual has survived through the early years, their chance of living to older years will increase. Therefore, life expectancy at birth tends to be shorter than life expectancy estimated at age 60.

EXPLANATION 5.2: How can we assess the changing patterns of the burden of disease over time using health data?

You can use the Global Health Estimates data to make comparisons between countries at different time points. You can also examine the shifts of the top 10 causes of death or burden of disease using disability-adjusted life years (DALYs) by age and sex from 2000 to 2019 in any selected countries. As mentioned in Chapter 3, DALYs are a common indicator used to assess the burden of disease, injury or disability in a population. They take into account not only deaths but also the impact of non-fatal conditions on the quality of life. Figures 5.11 and 5.12 compare the top 10 cases of DALYs in Brazil between 2000 and 2019.

In 2000, neonatal conditions and lower respiratory infections (classified as communicable diseases/conditions) were the first and fifth burdens of disease. However, these two conditions

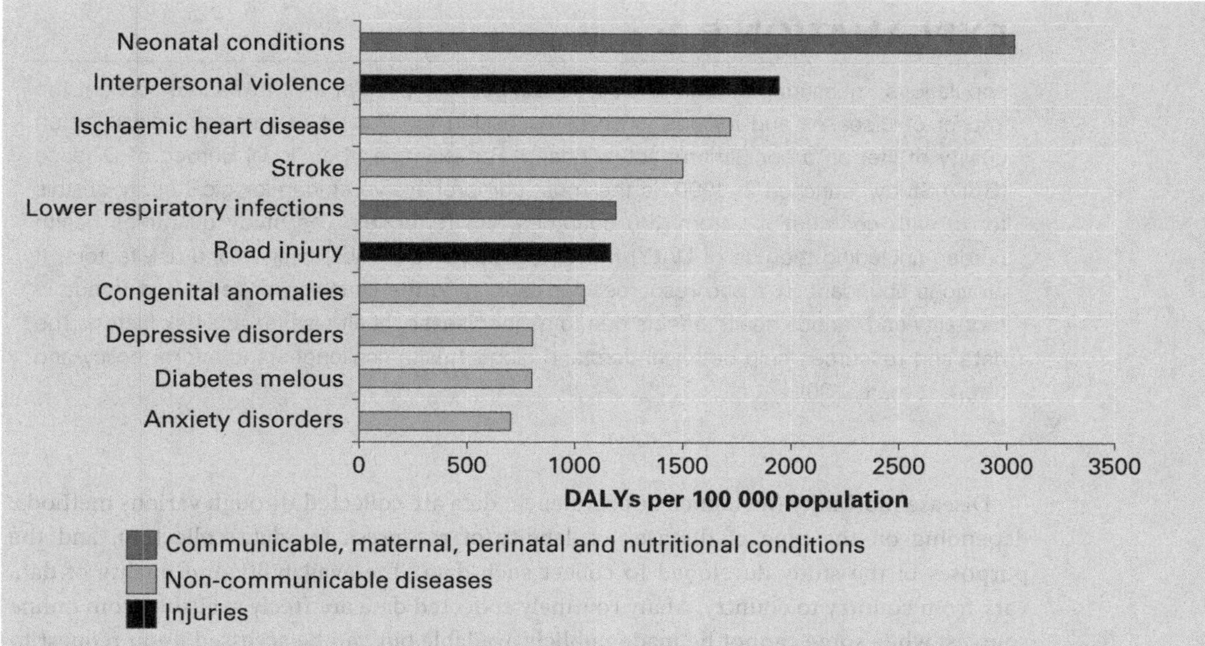

Figure 5.11 WHO Global Health Estimates visual summary: Top 10 causes of DALYs in Brazil in 2000 (29)

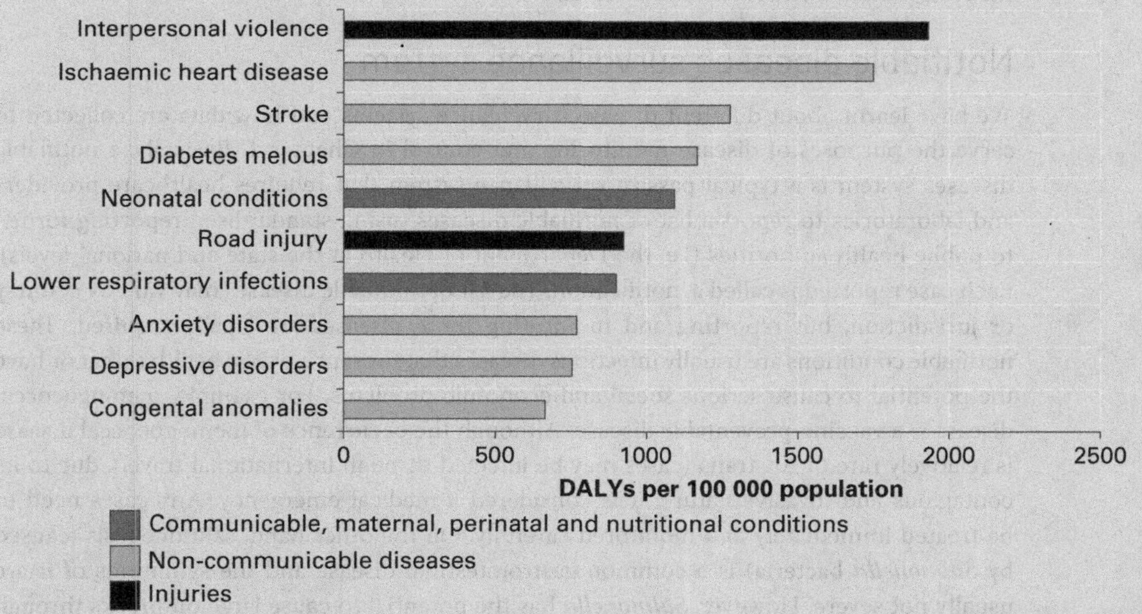

Figure 5.12 WHO Global Health Estimates visual summary: Top 10 causes of DALYs in Brazil in 2019 (29)

were ranked the fifth and seventh in 2019. It is noted that DALYs attributed to communicable diseases have halved since 2000. On the other hand, injuries and non-communicable diseases accounted for a large proportion of the country's burden of disease (29). Although mortality data are commonly used as a key indicator to compare general public health status in different

EXPLANATION 5.2: Continued

populations, measuring burden of disease has become popular as it takes into account the impact of diseases and injuries (such as assessing the impact of long-term disability on quality of life) on a population's actual health. For example, the Global Burden of Disease (GBD) Study, launched in 1990, is the most comprehensive epidemiological study on this topic, with contributions from 160 countries and territories. The study quantifies health burden (including the use of DALY) from hundreds of diseases, injuries and risk factors. It provides abundant data and resources for estimating the changing patterns and trends in mortality and various health effects due to major disease, health issues and risk factors. The data and resources help better understand global health challenges and inform policy and future research (30).

Disease morbidity (incidence or prevalence) data are collected through various methods, depending on the type of disease, availability of resources for data collection, and the purposes of the study developed to collect such data. The availability and quality of data vary from country to country. Many routinely collected data are freely available from online sources, while some cannot be made publicly available but can be accessed upon request to the responsible agencies. This section presents several common sources of morbidity data at the local, national and international levels.

Notifiable diseases surveillance system

We have learnt about different disease surveillance systems and how data are collected to serve the purposes of disease monitoring and control in Chapter 1. Basically, a notifiable diseases system is a typical passive surveillance system that requires healthcare providers and laboratories to report a list of notifiable diseases (using standardised reporting forms) to public health authorities (i.e. the Department of Health at the state and national levels). Each case reported is called a 'notification'. The list of notifiable diseases may vary by country or jurisdiction, but reporting and monitoring these diseases are legally required. These notifiable conditions are usually infectious diseases that present a public health threat or have the potential to cause serious social and economic problems. For example, meningococcal disease is a vaccine-preventable disease. Although the occurrence of meningococcal disease is relatively rare in Australia (cases may be infected through international travel), due to its contagious and invasive nature, it is considered a medical emergency. Any cases need to be treated immediately and monitored carefully. On the other hand, salmonellosis (caused by *Salmonella* bacteria) is a common gastrointestinal disease and the symptoms of it are usually not severe. However, *Salmonella* has the potential to cause large outbreaks through contaminated food, especially in warmer seasons. In Australia, the National Notifiable Diseases Surveillance System (NNDSS) coordinates national surveillance data for more than 70 diseases. The state and territory health authorities report new cases of these diseases to NNDSS (31).

Rachael: So COVID-19 is also part of a country's notifiable disease surveillance system?

Author (Patricia): Yes, COVID-19 is included in most countries' notifiable diseases surveillance as it is very contagious and poses a strong public health risk. The WHO declared COVID-19 a public health emergency of international concern on 30 January 2020; since then, most countries have included it in their notifiable diseases surveillance systems. According to the International Health Regulations, countries must notify the WHO of any events that may constitute a public health emergency of international concern (PHEIC) within 24 hours of the identification of the event, and thus the WHO had been updating COVID-19 cases and deaths since the PHEIC was declared, until it ended on 5 May 2023. The list of notifiable diseases in each country needs to be reviewed regularly. A new disease may be added to the list depending on its importance and potential health risk to the population.

As described in Chapter 1, a notifiable diseases system can help public health officials respond rapidly to outbreaks and take necessary action to prevent the further spread of disease. Public health officials use the data collected through a notifiable diseases system to monitor disease trends, investigate outbreaks and develop public health policies and disease-prevention and control interventions. This information can also be used to identify populations at risk for certain diseases and to target public health education and prevention efforts. As notifiable diseases surveillance requires continuous data collection, analysis, interpretation and feedback of collected data, the responsible health authorities provide regular reports on the monitoring of the notifiable diseases. For instance, NNDSS Australia generates fortnightly reports and tables to summarise the frequencies of notifiable diseases reported by disease group, disease name/code and jurisdiction. Datasets of reported cases are also available for selected diseases (influenza, meningococcal disease, pneumococcal disease and salmonellosis) from 2009 onwards (31). In the United States, the Centers for Disease Control and Prevention (32) compile weekly and annual notifiable disease tables and historical data detailing the frequencies of cases reported by disease (and subtype) and jurisdiction. These reports and tables are organised by calendar week/fortnight. Notifiable disease case reporting and monitoring at the state/territory level follow similar requirements and procedures.

EXPLANATION 5.3: How can the data of cases with notifiable conditions be used to monitor potential epidemics?

As mentioned above, healthcare providers are required to report cases with notifiable diseases to state or national health authorities. The data are collated and analysed for continuous monitoring of these conditions. For example, Queensland Health provides weekly updates of the total numbers of various notifiable conditions and summarises the trends of frequencies of these diseases in the past four weeks. Table 5.2 presents four weekly counts of selected notifiable diseases from 13 March to 3 April 2023 and year to date (YTD) comparisons. YTD refers to the period of time between the beginning of the

EXPLANATION 5.3: Continued

current calendar year and the present date. For example, the YTD of reported influenza cases in Table 5.2 was from 1 January to 9 April 2023. Let's focus on the reported numbers of influenza as an example to understand how the surveillance data can be interpreted. There was a surge of influenza cases in late March and early April (cases increased from 661 in mid-March to over 1000 in late March). Alarmingly, the total counts of reported cases (6374 cases) YTD 2023 (from the start of the year to 3 April) had exceeded the average counts (3463 cases) YTD in 2018–22. The ratio of YTD compared to YTD for the previous five years is 1.8, meaning a 1.8-fold increase in case numbers compared with the average number of the same period in the previous five years. In Australia, laboratory-confirmed influenza is included in the country's NNDSS. As we learnt in Chapter 1, there is a tendency for under-reporting in passive surveillance systems. Similarly, there is an under-estimate of influenza cases as only patients with moderate to severe symptoms would seek medical attention, and thus be tested and reported. Nevertheless, surveillance data remain useful for monitoring long-term trends when data are presented for the same population/location.

Table 5.2 Example of weekly statistics of notifiable conditions (33)

Disease	Weekly totals (week commencing)				Year to date (YTD) comparisons 1 Jan – 09 Apr 2023		
	Mon Apr 03 2023	Mon Mar 27 2023	Mon Mar 20 2023	Mon Mar 13 2023	YTD 2023	YTD mean: 2018–2022	Ratio YTD 2023: (YTD mean)
Mycobacterial diseases							
Leprosy	0	0	0	0	0	0	*
Nontuberculous Mycobacteria (M. ulcerans)	0	2	0	0	2	1	1.4
Nontuberculous Mycobacteria (other and unspecified)	20	29	32	18	375	388	1.0
Tuberculosis	3	4	2	2	50	42	1.2
Other vaccine preventable diseases							
Diphtheria	0	0	0	0	1	4	0.3
Influenza (lab confirmed)	1021	1041	814	661	6374	3462	1.8
Measles	0	1	0	1	2	5	0.4
Mumps	0	0	1	0	6	50	0.1

Disease	Weekly totals (week commencing)				Year to date (YTD) comparisons 1 Jan – 09 Apr 2023		
	Mon Apr 03 2023	Mon Mar 27 2023	Mon Mar 20 2023	Mon Mar 13 2023	YTD 2023	YTD mean: 2018–2022	Ratio YTD 2023: (YTD mean)
Pertussis	1	3	2	2	18	261	0.1
Poliomyelitis	0	0	0	0	0	0	*
Rotavirus	10	20	19	22	342	186	1.8
Rubella	0	0	0	0	0	0	*
Tetanus	0	0	0	0	0	0	*
Varicella	141	213	200	210	2876	2608	1.1

* The ratio of YTD compared to YTD for the previous five years is not calculated when the average YTD number of cases in the previous five years is less than 1.

EXAMPLE 5.4

Considering the importance of influenza and its potential to become a widespread pandemic, the WHO established the Global Influenza Programme and the Global Influenza Surveillance and Response System (GISRS) for influenza surveillance data reporting and analysis, and to provide guidance on outbreak response activities to mitigate pandemic threats to populations. The GISRS shares virological data via FluNet platform (15, 34). FluNet is a web-based tool for virological surveillance. The data at the country, regional and global levels are updated weekly and are publicly available. The data are collected by the GISRS's remote National Influenza Centres (NICs) and other national influenza reference laboratories collaborating with GISRS.

FluNet releases summaries of the latest influenza virus activities across the globe and weekly virological data by country, viral typing/subtyping and specified duration (see 'Further reading' section for more detail). The results are presented in tables, graphs and maps (15, 34, 35). Summarised in Figure 5.13, based on the FluNet web-based interactive data summary, we can see the changes in global influenza temporal trends overall.

Prior to the COVID-19 pandemic (up to the end of March 2020), influenza seasonality followed a regular annual spike pattern (consistent with the winter season in the northern hemisphere). Due to border closures and various COVID-19 restrictions, influenza activities were almost 'invisible' from April 2020 to late 2021. As influenza is also a respiratory infection, the implementation of public health interventions such as social distancing, mask wearing, working from home and lockdowns were effective measures in preventing the transmission of influenza. Following the removal of many restrictions in many countries in early 2022, we can see that influenza returned with two relatively small peaks in 2022 but a sharp epidemic in late 2022 and early 2023. Interestingly a secondary wave emerged from February 2023.

EXAMPLE 5.4 Continued

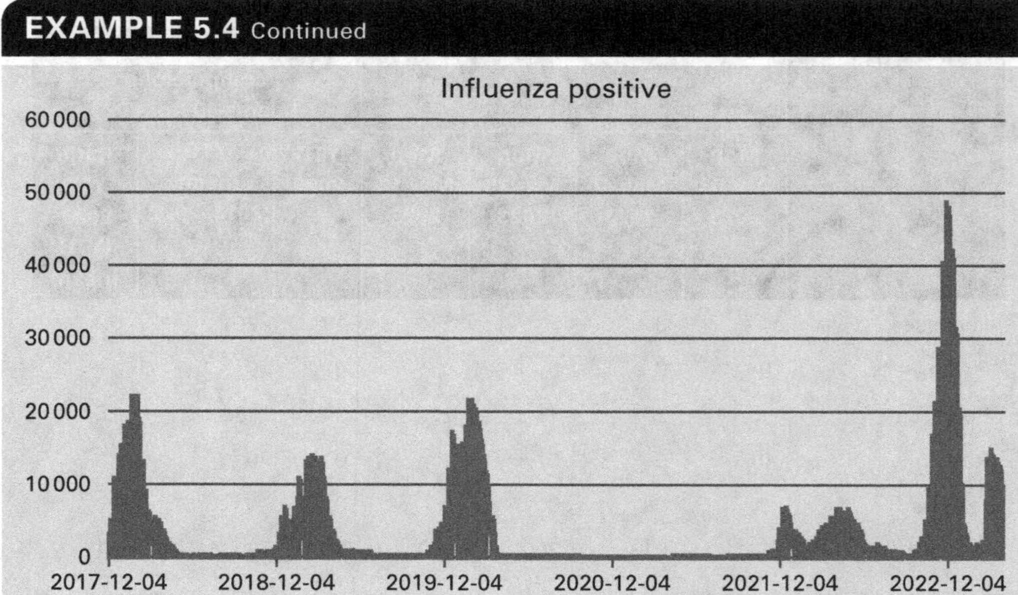

Figure 5.13 Influenza virus detections by viral subtype (all WHO member states) (34)

Global efforts on continuous monitoring of these changing and perhaps more unpredictable patterns of 'seasonal' influenza are required. Future research is also needed to investigate the factors (in addition to COVID-19 restrictions) contributing to these changes.

COVID-19 databases (global data)

As mentioned earlier, the WHO has been collating and updating COVID-19 cases and deaths since the PHEIC was declared in early 2020. All the updates with descriptive data visualisations (such as time trends and country distributions) are presented on the WHO COVID-19 Dashboard (34). For more details and data access, please see the link listed in the 'Further reading' section.

In addition, a group of interested researchers has been collecting COVID-19 related data from countries around the world and updates analysis results on 'Our World in Data' platform (https://ourworldindata.org/coronavirus). The group produces in-depth country profiles for 207 countries including interactive visualisations and sources of the data (36).

Cancer registry

A cancer registry is a database that collects information on people who have been newly diagnosed with cancer. The information is used to track the occurrence (incidence and prevalence) of various types of cancer, as well as to identify patterns of cancer distribution, long-term trends and projections. Cancer registries collect data on demographic information (such as age, sex and race), tumour characteristics (including diagnosis, site, stage and histology), and treatment information (such as surgery, radiation therapy and chemotherapy). They can be managed by cancer societies, governmental agencies or public health institutes (37). In Australia, cancer is a notifiable disease in all states and territories. Healthcare providers and pathology laboratories are required to notify all new cancer cases to the responsible jurisdiction's central cancer registry. The Australian Institute of Health and Welfare (AIHW) compiles the annual data supplied by states and territories and produces national cancer statistics. These enable a better understanding of how cancer might be detected and treated, as well as outcome monitoring and evaluation of cancer-prevention policies and interventions. The data can be made available on request (38). Cancer registries and associated data are of high quality in Nordic countries (37). The Association of the Nordic Cancer Registries (NORDCAN) compiles cancer data from member countries and updates comprehensive cancer statistics and data visualisation annually (39). A variety of interactive graphic and tabulation summaries with downloadable data are available on the 'Data visualization' page (https://nordcan.iarc.fr/en/dataviz). Globally, WHO's Global Cancer Observatory (GCO) is a web-based platform containing a wealth of population-based cancer statistics and cancer-prevention resources worldwide. The platform publishes visualisations of key cancer indicators using data from multiple organisations or projects. These summary graphs and tables are organised by sex, age group, indicator (incidence or mortality) and cancer site, and the related data can be accessed along with each visualisation item (40).

Australian national suicide and self-harm monitoring system

As suicide is the leading cause of death for Australians aged 15 to 49 years and the third leading cause of premature death from injury or disease, the Australian Government established the national suicide and self-harm surveillance system to collect information on suicide, intentional self-harm and suicidal behaviour to: (1) inform policies and services for suicide and self-harm prevention; (2) identify vulnerable at-risk groups; (3) understand emerging trends; and (4) address information gaps at the state and national levels (41). The AIWH collects the data on suicide and self-harm from multiple sources, and analyses and makes these data freely available online. The analysis results can be accessed through interactive visualisations and other relevant information on the demographics, trends and risk factors of these events. The datasets, organised by theme, are available on the 'data downloads' page (www.aihw.gov.au/suicide-self-harm-monitoring/data/data-downloads) (42).

Medical records

Medical or hospital records are official documents that contain information about a patient's medical history, diagnosis, treatment and outcomes. These are useful sources of morbidity data. Medical records can be accessed with patient consent or through a data-sharing agreement between health facilities. These data can be used to study the distribution of specific diseases or conditions within a healthcare system. All hospital admissions/discharges are recorded on a standard computerised system. The records contain diagnoses, procedures, lab tests and other relevant services. Analysing medical records allows us to examine patient characteristics, trends in the utilisation of healthcare services and the quality of care. For example, the US Electronic health records (EHR) are utilised for research purposes, such as evaluating the effectiveness of healthcare services and observing patients' responses to treatment. However, these records only relate to people who actually access medical care, so the data may not be representative (43). These data are not freely accessible but can be made available (e.g. for research purposes) upon request to the appropriate authorities. For ethical reasons, all identifiable personal information of individual patients will be removed prior to data release.

Other data sources

The Global Health Observatory (GHO) (44) is a large databank containing a wide range of data, analysed population health statistics, monitoring of health indicators and visualisations of data summary around the world. The platform compiles a comprehensive range of health-related data from various sources. The GHO statistics can be examined by theme/topic, health indicator and country. The GHO also encompasses many WHO data repositories such as Health SDGs, Global Health Estimates, mortality database and the COVID-19 Dashboard. The GHO also provides interactive data visualisations of trends and distributions of several non-communicable diseases and risk factors, including tobacco use, alcohol consumption, insufficient physical activity, prevalence of overweight and obesity, high blood pressure, blood glucose and nutrition. Many of the datasets are created for country comparisons over time. They are updated when more recent data become available from member states (44). These valuable resources allow countries, policy-makers, public health professionals and researchers to identify areas of needs, monitor progress toward health-related goals, inform policy formation and evaluate the impact of health.

Data linkage

Data linkage: A process of combining quantitative data from multiple sources based on the common identifiers.

There is a growing interest in **data linkage**, as it enables more comprehensive analyses through integrating data of different sources. Data linkage is a process of combining quantitative data from multiple sources based on the common identifiers. It allows researchers to explore broader and deeper insights beyond the scope of a single set of data collected for one study. It also has the benefit of reducing costs in conducting extensive surveys to collect data on additional variables within one study (especially when the study is facing time and financial constraints). For example, the data of individuals about behavioural risk factors such as smoking, alcohol consumption and physical activity collected in a prevalence survey can be linked to specific health outcomes using death records (e.g. death registry) in 20–30 years following the timing of the initial prevalence survey. The 'linkage' of different sources of data is normally done through the matching of unique individual identifiers such as citizen identification, Medicare number and social security number.

Rachael: I'm starting to think you can get information on anything!

Hugo: I guess the internet isn't just for funny videos about kittens …

Potential issues to be taken into consideration when using routine health data for descriptive studies

The above sections have presented a wide range of sources of routinely collected health data (many can be accessed online). They are used to monitor the health status of a country/community and assess variations in person, place and time. Since there is an abundant volume of routine health data available at various levels, it seems handy to make use of these data to design our descriptive studies. Routine sources of data are not collected for a particular research aim, but usually for management, planning and disease-prevention purposes. Caution needs to be taken when using routinely collected data to develop our own studies. Importantly, we need to consider the overall quality of data, including accuracy, completeness, timeliness and appropriateness. For example, if you are planning to use data from WHO Global Health Estimates to make multi-country comparisons in long-term trends of maternal mortality, you should be aware that the availability of long-term data may vary across the countries of your interest. In addition, the definitions used for diseases may vary in different jurisdictions. This would also impact the comparability of data. For instance, states and territories in Australia use different definitions and timeframes for notifications of COVID-19 infections, hospitalisations and deaths. These differences make data comparisons challenging even in the same country. The recently established Australian Centre for Disease Control (CDC) is expected to streamline the nationwide guidelines for disease surveillance to improve these issues.

As mentioned above, there is an urgent need to improve the availability and quality of population data (e.g. census data) in resource-poor countries. In addition, data about notifiable diseases tend to be under-reported, and the frequency of data collection may also differ, such as weekly or monthly collection. It is also important to ensure the data from different sources (e.g. countries or communities) are comparable, such as using the same definitions for key outcome variables. These issues need to be considered when undertaking data comparisons using routinely available data. A study (45) proposing a framework for conducting descriptive epidemiological studies can be used as guidance for designing a rigorous descriptive study (see 'Further reading' section for more details).

Importance of descriptive epidemiology

As discussed above, descriptive epidemiology allows us to identify sociodemographic and spatial patterns and long-term trends in the occurrence of diseases or health-related conditions and helps us to predict the trajectory of disease burden. It provides information for public health planning, policy decision-making and resource allocation, including funding, personnel and health services. For example, the incidence and mortality of infectious diseases remain major issues in many low-income countries, especially in the African region. Global funds can be directed towards the prevention and treatment of infectious diseases in that region. On the other hand, the burden of non-communicable diseases (NCDs) has been increasing and will continue to rise in developed countries, along with the challenges of population ageing and changing patterns of lifestyle factors. Global public health efforts can be made to generate strategies to tackle these challenges and proactively manage common risk factors to slow down the increasing burden of NCDs.

In addition, identifying the variations in disease patterns helps to establish the foundation for the development of hypotheses regarding what might have contributed to the increase in disease rates. In the hypotheses, we generate some *why* and *how* questions to search for underlying causes leading to the differences in disease rates. For instance, why was the incidence of COVID-19 higher in younger people (i.e. aged 20–29 years) than in older people at the early stage of the pandemic? A study based in the United States suggested that younger adults who were more likely to have mild or no symptoms of COVID-19 might have contributed to community transmission due to occupational and behavioural reasons (e.g. working in highly exposed industries, more socially active but less compliant with community mitigation measures) (46). The hypotheses generated through descriptive epidemiology can then be tested by analytical studies to assess associations between underlying 'determinants' and health outcomes. Although more recent surveillance data showed higher incidence of COVID-19 in older age groups (especially aged 90+), this change in age distribution may be reflecting healthcare-seeking behaviour in older populations concerning their higher risk of severe outcomes (47). Even though the hypotheses established in descriptive studies may need to be modified over time, they can inform further analytical studies to target specific determinants or investigate aetiology of disease. This is a process of searching for 'clues' or possible causes of disease. For example, if a particular group of people is more affected by a disease than others, researchers may investigate whether any sociodemographic, genetic, environmental or lifestyle factors have contributed to the disparity in disease rate between different groups of people. The findings of analytical studies can inform interventions or strategies for the prevention and control of the health issue of interest. Descriptive epidemiology is an important tool enabling you to take the first step of evidence-based practice in the health sciences.

Descriptive epidemiology is also crucial for detecting potential disease outbreaks. This function is particularly important for the monitoring of infectious diseases. Surveillance data help public health officials to quickly identify unusual patterns (such as a sharp increase in incident cases) and respond to outbreaks before they become widespread. Descriptive epidemiology is often the first step in an outbreak investigation. Descriptive data can be used to guide outbreak investigations in many ways. They can help investigators assess the demographic distribution, geographic clusters and type of epidemic curve of the event to determine the mode of transmission, which is urgently needed for timely control measures. The data collected from affected patients, such as clinical features, can also help investigators to establish a case definition at the early stage of the outbreak to identify more cases and prevent further transmission. These data also provide evidence to guide hypothesis formulation for the subsequent analytical study to identify the source of the outbreak. Finally, the continuous monitoring of the outbreak (e.g. changes in the number of cases over time or changes in the distribution of cases) can be utilised to evaluate the effectiveness of public health interventions in controlling the outbreak. Further reading of relevant content regarding outbreak investigation is recommended in *The CDC Field Epidemiology Manual* (1).

The following list presents the purposes of descriptive epidemiology adapted from the chapter 'Describing Epidemiologic Data' in *The CDC Field Epidemiology Manual* (1). These purposes highlight the importance of descriptive epidemiology in public health practice and summarise the key messages carried out in this chapter. Descriptive epidemiology:

- provides a systematic approach for breaking down a health problem into several component parts
- ensures that all basic dimensions of a health problem are addressed
- identifies specific populations at higher risk for the health problem being studied
- offers timely information to decision-makers, the public, the media and other stakeholders about ongoing investigations of a health issue
- supports the decision-making process for introducing or modifying disease-prevention and control measures
- assesses the progress of control and prevention programs targeting a specific health problem
- allows for the formation of hypotheses regarding aetiology, mode of exposure, effectiveness of control measures and other determinants of health problems
- aids in confirming the identification of causes or risk factors of a disease or health problem.

Conclusion

In this chapter, you have learnt how to use descriptive epidemiology to describe health-related problems, with specific patterns in relation to person, place and time. We have also explored descriptive studies used to collect various sources of data to compare the patterns of health issues and addressed the importance of descriptive epidemiology in developing evidence-based practice.

Learning objective 1: Examine the patterns of health-related issues by answering who, what, when and where questions

This chapter has demonstrated how we can unpack a health problem by asking a few 'W' questions – that is, who, what, when and where questions. In answering these questions, we are examining the 'patterns' of health issues in terms of personal, place and time characteristics. This chapter has also employed many real-world examples to compare the variations in disease frequency across different population groups and locations, and over time.

Learning objective 2: Be aware of the major sources of data and their uses for assessing the frequency and patterns of health events

You have also learnt various methods and sources to collect primary or secondary data to assess the mortality and morbidity of health-related events and compare the patterns of these events. By learning different sources of routine health data, we can use existing resources to describe a health problem and interpret the data in meaningful ways, enabling us to further explore underlying causes of the health problem.

Learning objective 3: Understand the importance and application of descriptive epidemiology to public health practice

Drawing on our understanding of the key concepts learnt in the first two sections, we have also learnt the areas of application of descriptive epidemiology, which reflect the importance of descriptive epidemiology in public health practice.

Further reading

Fontaine RE. Describing epidemiologic data. In: Rasmussen SA, Goodman, RA, eds. *The CDC Field Epidemiology Manual*. Oxford University Press; 2019. pp. 105–34.

Global Health Estimates. *Life Expectancy and Leading Causes of Death and Disability*. World Health Organization; 2020. www.who.int/data/gho/data/themes/mortality-and-global-health-estimates. To obtain the data of life expectancy, go to 'Life expectancy at birth (years)', then click the 'Data' tab to access the dataset of life expectancy at birth by sex, country (listed in alphabetic order) and year.

Lesko CR, Fox MP, Edwards JK. A framework for descriptive epidemiology. *American Journal of Epidemiology*, 2022;191(12):2063–70. https://academic.oup.com/aje/article/191/12/2063/6623869?login=false

World Health Organization (WHO). Data overview and visualizations. *WHO Coronavirus (COVID-19) Dashboard*. WHO; 2023. https://covid19.who.int/data. Downloadable country data from the beginning of the pandemic can be accessed by clicking the 'Data Download' tab.

World Health Organization (WHO). FluNet. *Global Influenza Programme*. WHO; 2023. www.who.int/tools/flunet. The datasets can be accessed on this page. Data of weekly reported influenza cases by country, influenza transmission zone, WHO region or hemisphere can be accessed.

Questions

Answers are available at the end of the book.

Multiple-choice questions

1. Which of the following is NOT a feature of descriptive epidemiology?
   A – Describing the long-term trend of cancer in a country
   B – Testing a hypothesis to determine whether or not an exposure is a risk factor of a disease
   C – Examining the difference in overall mortality between males and females in New South Wales, Australia
   D – Comparing the incidence rates of HIV between the United States and Nigeria.
2. The case series of high monkeypox incidence among gay, bisexual, and men who have sex with men in different countries/locations allow us to examine disease patterns in relation to:
   A – Person
   B – Place
   C – Time
   D – All of the above.
3. We can collect primary data to identify disease patterns using:
   A – Data from the WHO's Global Health Estimates
   B – Census data
   C – Cancer registry
   D – Case series.
4. By examining temporal changes in disease rate, we may be able to
   A – Determine population demographic changes
   B – Address health inequalities in country comparisons
   C – Evaluate the impact of a health intervention on disease prevention
   D – Identify the cause of the disease.
5. Figure 5.14 presents life expectancy at birth by sex and remoteness in Australia. Which of the following characteristics are we comparing?

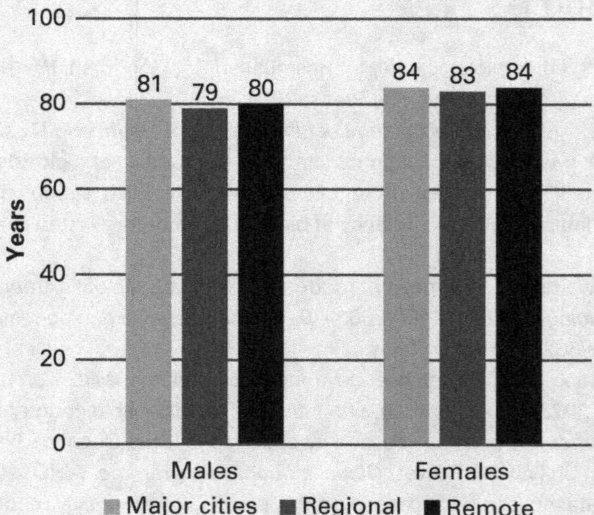

Figure 5.14 Life expectancy at birth by sex and remoteness in Australia's non-Indigenous population (8)

A – Person only
B – Place only
C – Time only
D – Person and place
E – Person and time.

Short-answer questions

1. What are the three characteristics of descriptive epidemiology?
2. Provide one example for each of the three characteristics listed in short-answer question 1.
3. Use the map in Figure 5.4 (produced by Dr John Snow) to explain why Snow suspected the Broad Street Pump as the source of the cholera outbreak.
4. How are the participants of a prevalence survey selected?
5. Describe the 'time lag' between the patterns of smoking prevalence and lung-cancer presented in Figure 5.9.
6. How can we use descriptive epidemiology to assess the effect of a population-based vaccination program on controlling a vaccine-preventable disease?
7. Figure 5.15 presents the comparisons of 'Under-5 mortality rate (per 1000 live births) in 1990, 2000 and 2020' across different WHO regions and a global average. What are the patterns of under-5 mortality being compared?

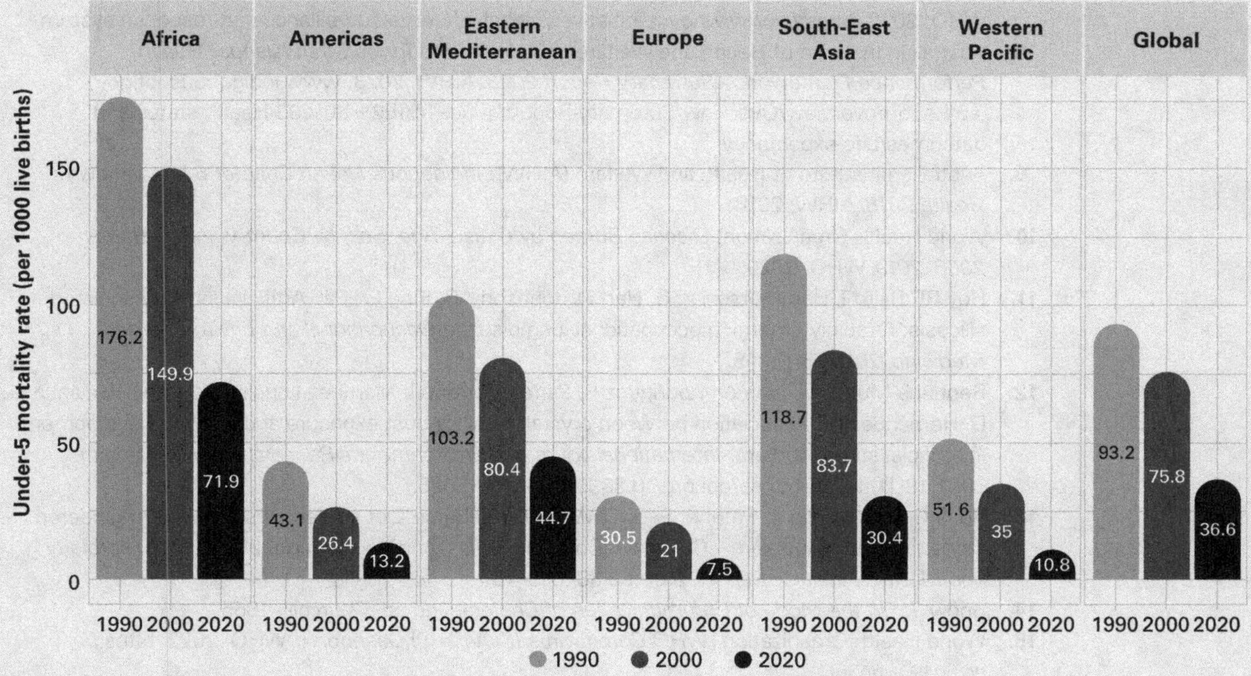

Figure 5.15 Under-5 mortality rate (per 1000 live births) in 1990, 2000 and 2020 across different WHO regions and global average (48)

8. Refer to Figure 5.15 in Question 7. Interpret the patterns of under-5 mortality in relation to the characteristics listed above.
9. Briefly describe how disability-adjusted life years (DALYs) is used as a health indicator to assess population health.

10. List two areas of application of descriptive epidemiology in public health/the health sciences.

References

1. Fontaine RE. Describing epidemiologic data. In: Rasmussen SA, Goodman, RA, eds. *The CDC Field Epidemiology Manual.* Oxford University Press; 2019. pp. 105–34.
2. Bots SH, Peters SAE, Woodward M. Sex differences in coronary heart disease and stroke mortality: A global assessment of the effect of ageing between 1980 and 2010. *BMJ Global Health.* 2017;2(2):e000298.
3. Glover JD, Hetzel DM, Tennant SK. The socioeconomic gradient and chronic illness and associated risk factors in Australia. *Australia and New Zealand Health Policy.* 2004;1(1):8.
4. Berkman LF, Kawachi I. A historical framework for social epidemiology: Social determinants of population health. In: Berkman LF, Kawachi I, eds. *Social Epidemiology*, 2nd ed. Oxford University Press; 2014: pp.1–16.
5. Queensland Health. *Influenza in Queensland Report.* Queensland Health; 2019. www.health.qld.gov.au/__data/assets/pdf_file/0029/713675/influenza-qld-ann=ual.pdf
6. World Health Organization (WHO). Monitoring health for the SDGs. In: *The Global Health Observatory – Explore a World of Health Data.* WHO; 2023. www.who.int/data/gho/data/themes/world-health-statistics
7. World Health Organization (WHO). *Global Influenza Surveillance and Response System (GISRS).* WHO; 2023. https://www.who.int/initiatives/global-influenza-surveillance-and-response-system
8. Australian Institute of Health and Welfare. *Aboriginal and Torres Strait Islander Health Performance Framework – Summary Report 2023.* AIHW; 2023. www.indigenoushpf.gov.au/Report-overview/Overview/Summary-Report/4-Tier-1-%E2%80%93-Health-status-and-outcomes/Life-expectancy
9. Australian Institute of Health and Welfare (AIHW). *Indigenous Health Chapter 6 in Australian's Health 2018.* AIHW; 2018.
10. World Health Organization. *Disease Burden by Cause, Age, Sex, by Country and by Region, 2000–2019.* WHO; 2020.
11. Hoy RF, Baird T, Hammerschlag G, Hart D, Johnson AR, King P et al. Artificial stone-associated silicosis: A rapidly emerging occupational lung disease. *Occupational and Environmental Medicine.* 2018;75(1):3–5.
12. Requena-Mullor M, Alarcón-Rodríguez R, Parrón-Carreño T, Martínez-López JJ, Lozano-Paniagua D, Hernández AF. Association between crystalline silica dust exposure and silicosis development in artificial stone workers. *International Journal of Environmental Research in Public Health.* 2021;18(11):5625. https://doi.org/10.3390/ijerph18115625.
13. Rose C, Heinzerling A, Patel K, Sack C, Wolff J, Zell-Baran L et al. Severe silicosis in engineered stone fabrication workers – California, Colorado, Texas, and Washington, 2017–2019. *Morbidity and Mortality Weekly Report.* 2019;68(38):813–18.
14. Snow J. *On the Mode of Communication of Cholera.* 2nd ed. Churchill; 1855.
15. World Health Organization. *WHO Coronavirus (COVID-19) Dashboard.* WHO; 2023. https://covid19.who.int
16. World Health Organization. *Maternal Mortality Ratio (per 100 000 Live Births) 2020.* WHO; 2024. www.who.int/data/gho/data/indicators/indicator-details/GHO/maternal-mortality-ratio-(per-100-000-live-births)
17. Australian Institute of Health and Welfare. The impact of a new disease: COVID-19 from 2020, 2021 and into 2022. In: *Australia's Health 2022: Data Insights.* AIHW; 2022: p. 1–60
18. Department of Health and Aged Care. Coronavirus (COVID-19) case numbers and statistics. Commonwealth of Australia; 2023. www.health.gov.au/health-alerts/covid-19/case-numbers-and-statistics#covid19-case-notifications

19. Australian Institute of Health and Welfare. Changing patterns of mortality in Australia since 1900. In: *Australia's Health 2022: Data Insights.* AIHW; 2022:153–96.

20. Greenhalgh EM, Bayly M, Jenkins S, Scollo MM. Prevalence of smoking – adults. In: *Tobacco in Australia: Facts & Figures.* Cancer Council Victoria; 2023. www.tobaccoinaustralia.org.au/chapter-1-prevalence/1-3-prevalence-of-smoking-adults

21. Patel A, Bilinska J, Tam JCH, Da Silva Fontoura D, Mason CY, Daunt A et al. Clinical features and novel presentations of human monkeypox in a central London centre during the 2022 outbreak: Descriptive case series. *British Medical Journal.* 2022;378:e072410.

22. Australian Bureau of Statistics. *National Health Survey: First Results Methodology 2020.* ABS; 2020. www.abs.gov.au/methodologies/national-health-survey-first-results-methodology/2020-21

23. Australian Institute of Health and Welfare. *Australia's Health 2022.* AIHW; 2022.

24. United Nations Population Fund. *Census.* UNFPA; 2023. www.unfpa.org/census

25. Australian Bureau of Statistics. *Snapshot of Australia: A Picture of the Economic, Social and Cultural Make-up of Australia on Census Night, 10 August 2021.* ABS; 2022. www.abs.gov.au/statistics/people/people-and-communities/snapshot-australia/latest-release

26. Office for National Statistics. England and Wales: Facts and figures about people living in England and Wales. 2021. www.ons.gov.uk/visualisations/areas/K04000001

27. United States Census Bureau. *Explore Census Data: Learn about America's People, Places, and Economy.* US Government; 2020. https://data.census.gov

28. United Nations Statistics Division. *Demographic and Social Statistics: Civil Registration and Vital Statistics.* United Nations; 2023. https://unstats.un.org/unsd/demographic-social/crvs

29. World Health Organization. *Global Health Estimates: Life Expectancy and Leading Causes of Death and Disability.* WHO; 2020. www.who.int/data/gho/data/themes/mortality-and-global-health-estimates

30. Institute for Health Metrics and Evaluation. *Global Burden of Disease (GBD).* Hans Rosling Center for Population Health; 2020. www.healthdata.org/research-analysis/gbd

31. Department of Health and Aged Care. *National Notifiable Diseases Surveillance System (NNDSS) Public Data Sets.* Australian Government; 2023. www.health.gov.au/resources/collections/nndss-public-datasets

32. Centers for Disease Control and Prevention. *Notifiable Infectious Disease Data Tables.* CDC; 2023. www.cdc.gov/nndss/data-statistics/infectious-tables/index.html

33. Queensland Health. Notifiable conditions weekly total Queensland. Queensland Government; 2023. www.health.qld.gov.au/clinical-practice/guidelines-procedures/diseases-infection/surveillance/reports/notifiable/weekly

34. World Health Organization. *FluNet: Global Influenza Programme.* WHO; 2023. www.who.int/tools/flunet

35. Hay AJ, McCauley JW. The WHO global influenza surveillance and response system (GISRS): A future perspective. *Influenza and Other Respiratory Viruses.* 2018;12(5):551–7.

36. Mathieu E, Ritchie H, Rodés-Guirao L, Appel C, Giattino C, Hasell J et al. Coronavirus Pandemic (COVID-19) United Kingdom. *Our World in Data*; 2020. https://ourworldindata.org/coronavirus

37. Wunsch G, Gourbin C. Mortality, morbidity and health in developed societies: A review of data sources. *Genus.* 2018;74(1):2.

38. Australian Institute of Health and Welfare. *Australian Cancer Database (ACD).* AIHW; 2023. www.aihw.gov.au/about-our-data/our-data-collections/australian-cancer-database

39. International Agency for Research on Cancer. Association of the Nordic Cancer Registries: NORDCAN. 2023. https://nordcan.iarc.fr/en

40. International Agency for Research on Cancer. *Global Cancer Observatory.* 2024. https://gco.iarc.fr/en

41. Department of Health and Aged Care. *National Suicide and Self-Harm Monitoring System.* 2021. www.health.gov.au/our-work/national-suicide-and-self-harm-monitoring-system

42. Australian Institute of Health and Welfare. Suicide and self-harm monitoring. AIHW; 2025. www.aihw.gov.au/suicide-self-harm-monitoring

43. National Library of Medicine. Health data sources: Medical records. 2023. www.nlm.nih.gov/oet/ed/stats/03-200.html

44. World Health Organization. The Global Health Observatory: Explore a world of health data. WHO; 2024. www.who.int/data/gho/data/major-themes/universal-health-coverage-major

45. Lesko CR, Fox MP, Edwards JK. A framework for descriptive epidemiology. American Journal of Epidemiology. 2022;191(12):2063–70.

46. Boehmer TK, DeVies J, Caruso E, van Santen KL, Tang S, Black CL et al. Changing age distribution of the COVID-19 pandemic – United States, May–August 2020. *Morbidity and Mortality Weekly Report.* 2020;69(39):1404–9.

47. New South Wales Health. *NSW Respiratory Surveillance Report – Fortnight Ending 6 January 2024.* NSW Government; 2024. www.health.nsw.gov.au/Infectious/covid-19/Documents/respiratory-surveillance-20240106.pdf

48. World Health Organization (WHO). *World Health Statistics 2022.* WHO; 2023. www.who.int/publications/i/item/9789240051157

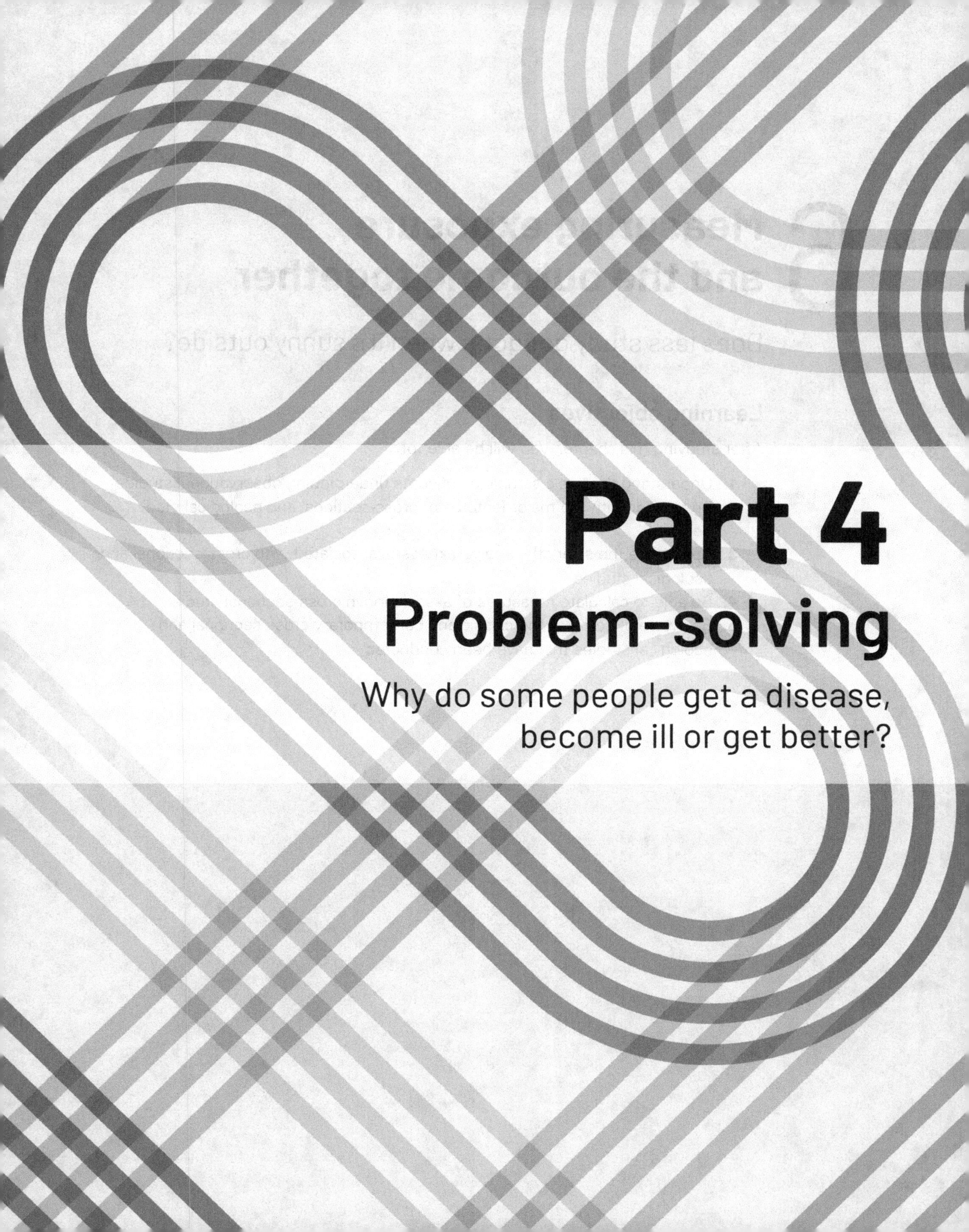

Part 4

Problem-solving

Why do some people get a disease, become ill or get better?

6 Measuring exposure and the outcome together

Does less study get done when it's sunny outside?

Learning objectives

After studying this chapter, you will be able to:

1. Understand the basic sampling concepts underpinning observational studies
2. Be familiar with the major features of cross-sectional and ecological study designs
3. Appreciate the strengths and weaknesses associated with cross-sectional and ecological studies
4. Be able to calculate measures of association in cross-sectional studies
5. Be aware of some of the classic and contemporary cross-sectional and ecological studies that have been conducted

Introduction

In epidemiology, we are interested in conducting studies to measure disease occurrence and to look for causes of disease. Such studies can be applied to public health, allowing us to modify the causes for disease prevention. In the previous chapters, we explored several commonly used public health measures and routinely collected health data. They form the basis of descriptive epidemiology and enable us to describe the frequency and patterns of health-related issues in relation to person, place and time characteristics. It is important to note that descriptive studies cannot be used to establish causal relationships, but they are useful for generating hypotheses. These need to be tested in analytical studies to determine whether the 'exposure' of interest is associated with the changes in disease morbidity or mortality to search for the possible causes of the disease. For instance, the COVID-19 pandemic had a negative impact on mental health, especially for younger people (1). We might want to identify the factors that caused the increase in mental health issues during the pandemic. It could be due to social isolation in lockdowns, lack of face-to-face contact with family and friends, fear of losing jobs or facing disruption of daily routines, and so on. Moreover, intrinsic characteristics of the individual, such as sex, age and ethnicity, could also be related to mental health issues. In this example, mental health issues are the outcome of interest, whereas any of the reasons or characteristics mentioned above could be the 'exposure' or study factor.

In epidemiology, the generic term 'exposure' is widely used to represent any determinant of interest. When we discuss analytical studies, we need to know that they are designed in the context of 'exposure' and 'disease'. There are several types of analytical study as outlined in Chapter 4. Following the logic of the hierarchy of analytical study designs (in the sequence of evidentiary strength), in this chapter we will start with the two common analytical designs at the bottom of the hierarchy: cross-sectional and ecological studies. These two designs provide the lowest level of evidence concerning a relationship between exposure and outcome among all analytical studies. Yet these types of studies are ideal when you are equally interested in looking at both sides of the relationship – exposures and outcomes together, not necessarily inferring a causal relationship. For example, we can design a cross-sectional study or an ecological study to answer a question like 'Does less study get done when it's sunny outside?'

Rachael: So, we can see disease patterns through descriptive studies that can help us to find the 'clues' or potential causes of a health issue, but how do we know what to look for in the first place?

Hugo: Yeah, do we need to find all the possible causes? That mental health example seemed to have lots of them!

Author (Patricia): These are important questions, Rachael and Hugo. When we identify differences in morbidity or mortality in descriptive studies, we can use a questionnaire survey to investigate a range of sociodemographic characteristics and other factors, such as health-related behaviours or environmental factors in an analytical study to find out which factors are associated with the outcome of our interest. We can consult with existing literature on similar topics to determine which factors to focus on in our study. It is important to understand the multicausal nature of disease. Most diseases are caused by multiple determinants. From a prevention point of view, if we address one or two key risk factors of a disease, we can prevent a large proportion of the disease in a population. It is not necessary to explore all possible causes in one study. In terms of assessing the association between exposure and outcome, we are normally interested in assessing a one-to-one relationship in analytical studies.

Quantitative methods: Those methods dealing with counting, measuring and comparing things.

Questionnaire surveys play a crucial role in analytical studies and are a common method used to collect data from our target population. They are used in conjunction with other **quantitative methods** to measure the 'exposure' and 'outcome' of our interest, as well as other relevant characteristics and factors known as *confounding factors*. In Part 4 of this book, on analytical studies, we will focus on establishing an association between exposure and outcome. The role and effect of confounding will be addressed in Part 6 (Chapter 11). As questionnaire surveys in analytical studies rely on the information collected from a study sample representing our target population, the next section will introduce the concepts of population, sample and sampling.

Population, sample and sampling

A population refers to the entire group of individuals, such as all people on the planet or in a country. It is an abstract concept: large in size and geographically broad. In the context of epidemiology, we need to clearly define the population of our interest – the target population for a specific study. As mentioned in Chapter 5, our target population in epidemiological studies can be defined in various ways, such as all residents in a geographic location, individuals of a particular age group or occupation, or people with a specific health condition. Directly collecting data from the entire population is often not feasible or practical unless abundant resources and funding are available for the study (such as using national census surveys to collect data). In most cases, we recruit a group of people or a *sample* from the population to conduct a study.

Sampling frame: A tangible source of material that provides individual identification, geographic locations, and contact information to allow researchers to access and select persons in a predetermined way for their studies.

Sampling unit: The minimum unit of observation. Ranges from an individual person, household, animal or specific microbe to an environmental hazard. In this book, the sampling unit refers to an individual person in the target population.

A sample is a smaller sub-set of people chosen from the target population to participate in a study. An ideal sample should exhibit similar sociodemographic characteristics, diversity and variability of the population. This means the sample is representative of the target population, so the results based on the study sample can be applied back to the population. If the sample perfectly represents our target population and the study is rigorously conducted, the study findings can be considered generalisable. However, achieving generalisability of findings within a study is not an easy task. Apart from sample representativeness, we also need to take into account other issues such as bias and confounding that emerge in the study. These issues will be discussed in more detail in Chapter 11.

Figure 6.1 illustrates the concept of drawing a *representative sample* from a study's target population. Assume that our target population is the entire population of a culturally diverse community (all people within the outer dashed line), from which the study sample is drawn. Prior to the sample selection procedures, we need to identify a **sampling frame** to allow us to access the study units within the population. A **sampling unit** can range from an individual person to a household, an animal, a specific microbe or an environmental hazard. In this book, our sampling unit refers to an individual person. A sampling frame is a tangible source

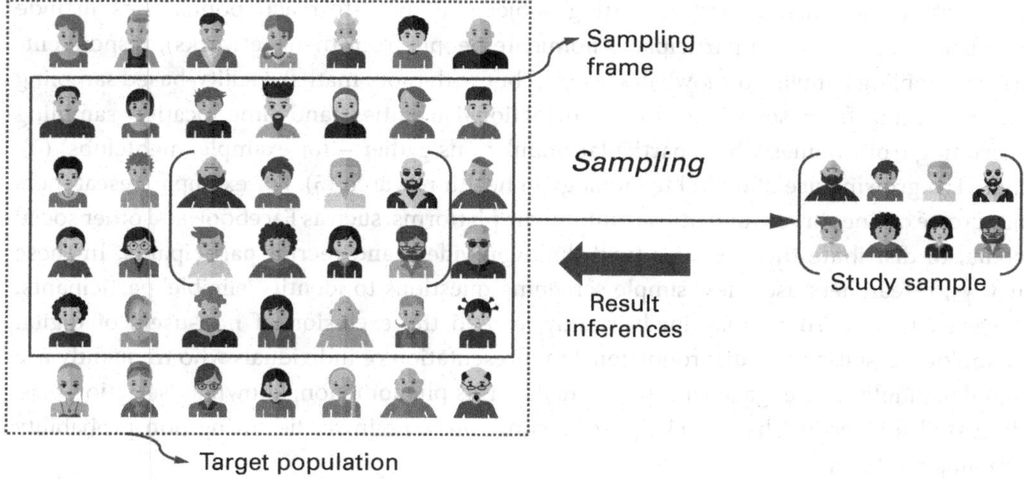

Figure 6.1 Population, sample and sampling

of material such as a list of individuals, households, streets, schools and so on. It provides individual identification, geographic locations and contact information to allow researchers to 'access' selected persons in a pre-determined way (such as through a particular random sampling method). A good sampling frame should be reasonably representative of the population of interest. For instance, a census, an electoral roll and a telephone directory are all common sampling frames for large population-based studies. If a study aims to investigate the quality of life among cancer patients, the researcher may contact the in-charge health authority to obtain cancer registry data for their sampling.

The different individuals in Figure 6.1 represent study units in our target population with a variety of demographic characteristics and a range of cultural diversity. To select a study sample, we need to obtain a sampling frame (all individuals within the solid line) to enable access to a list of people. The researcher can employ a sampling strategy to select a study sample – this is what we call 'sampling'. To ensure the representativeness of our study sample, a probability sampling technique (or any form of random sampling in which everyone in a sampling frame has an equal chance or a pre-determined probability of being selected into the sample) is usually applied in epidemiological studies. The commonly used random sampling methods are simple random, systematic, stratified and cluster sampling techniques. The details of these sampling techniques can be found in most methodology or statistics textbooks. (You will learn a little more about this in Chapter 9.) Some relevant resources are listed in the 'Further reading' section (2, 3). It is important to acknowledge potential **sampling errors** *and selection errors* that may arise during sample selection and recruitment processes. These issues of error/bias will be detailed in Part 6. While it may be impossible to completely eliminate these issues, we should always make every effort to minimise errors in the sampling process and the conduct of research.

Sampling error: A type of random error that occurs when the characteristics of the selected study sample differ from those of the target population. As such, the data collected from this sample does not truly represent the population data. It arises at random as the people we select into each sample may be slightly different (e.g. with slightly different sociodemographic distributions).

In some situations, using random sampling may not be achievable or suitable due to the nature of the target population or resource constraints. For example, identifying a sampling frame would be very challenging when studying hard-to-reach populations such as people living with HIV, people who use drugs or homeless people. In such cases, a non-probability sampling alternative is often used to overcome the difficulties. The non-probability sampling strategies for identifying and recruiting subjects in hard-to-reach populations include snowball sampling (when participants nominate people from their networks), respondent-driven sampling (similar to snowball sampling but with more maths), facility-based sampling (e.g. recruiting from sexual health or correctional facilities) and time-location sampling (recruiting from venues where particular populations gather – for example, nightclubs) (4). There is a growing use of digital technology in health research (5). For example, researchers may create online surveys and utilise multimedia platforms, such as Facebook and other social media, to distribute their surveys (with links provided) and recruit participants. In these surveys, researchers use a few simple screening questions to identify 'eligible' participants. However, this approach may inadvertently lead to the exclusion of non-users of digital technology, resulting in a disproportionate representation of individuals who frequently use digital technology or engage with social media. This phenomenon, known as 'selection bias' (discussed further in Chapter 11), poses a common issue in studies using non-probability sampling methods.

Hugo: So, if I wanted to see if less studying got done on sunny days and wanted a sample of students in our university, what sampling frame would I need? Should I use a non-probability sampling method?

Rachael: Yeah, right! As students, we don't have access to lists of students in other programs.

Author (Patricia): This is a challenging issue for all researchers. Identifying a representative sampling frame is not easy and obtaining it can be even harder. If selecting a probability sample is not achievable, we would have to go for a non-probability option. Please bear in mind that the sample selected using a non-probability method is not representative, so the generalisability of results is limited. Having said that, in educational settings, random sampling can be done in different ways. The easiest sampling technique is cluster sampling (details can be found in the 'Further reading' section), as students or different groups of personnel can be found in natural clusters (e.g. first year, second year, health sciences major, business major, etc.). In this sense, we can identify a sampling frame in a more accessible way such as at higher levels of cluster. For example, we can find the lists of all programs under each study group (such as health, business and sciences) presented on the university website. The next step is to randomly select programs in each study group. We can then contact the program directors to request dissemination of our survey link to their students.

As most research teams have limited time and resources to develop their studies, a minimum sample size is often determined prior to the sampling process. The calculation of sample size is beyond the scope of this text, although we will learn a bit more about this later in the book. Further details about sample size calculation with examples and useful links are covered in Chapter 10. Once sufficient study subjects have been recruited, we can then proceed to collect data (such as survey data) from them according to the study design, and analyse the data based on this 'study sample'. The findings derived from the sample data are used to draw inferences (i.e. statistical inferences) for the target population.

Cross-sectional studies: Their features, strengths and limitations

As discussed in Chapter 5, the variations in disease patterns identified in descriptive studies help us to establish hypotheses regarding what might have contributed to the increase in disease rates. The hypotheses need to be tested by analytical studies to *assess associations* between underlying 'determinants' and health outcomes. This is a process of searching for possible causes of disease. The determinants of a health event can be demographic characteristics, socioeconomic status, genetic factors, immunological status, environmental exposures and other behavioural risk factors. Once again, we normally focus on determining a one-to-one relationship between exposure and outcome in an analytical study. The exposure may be a *risk factor*, a **protective factor** or a treatment or intervention, depending on the nature of the exposure and the study design.

Protective factor: A factor/variable that decreases the chance of having a particular disease or health condition among the people who are exposed to this factor.

In Chapter 4, we learned that all experimental studies and many observational designs can be categorised as analytical studies. Under each of these categories are several study designs that guide our plan to collect data from the study sample. When it comes to establishing causation, in Chapter 4 we also learnt that study designs can be ranked in a hierarchy according the strength of the evidence they can provide. In ascending order of evidence, the hierarchy goes from ecological and cross-sectional studies, to case-control studies, on to cohort studies, with experimental study designs at the top. As opposed to experimental studies involving an intervention, we observe the effect of an exposure on the occurrence of a health event in natural settings in observational studies. In this section, we will begin with cross-sectional studies and discuss their key features, strengths and limitations.

Features of cross-sectional studies

Cross-sectional studies are also known as prevalence studies. They are, as the name suggests, investigations of a cross-section of the population. The central feature of these studies is that the data on exposure and outcome are both collected and measured at a given point in time. The second key feature of cross-sectional studies is that study subjects are selected according to a pre-determined sampling method (normally a type of random sampling technique), without specifying their exposure or outcome status in the sample selection process. In addition, data on multiple exposures and health outcomes can be collected in a survey.

Figure 6.2 illustrates the design of a cross-sectional study. Following the idea of sample selection explained earlier, we draw a study sample from our target population. The initial sample of a cross-sectional study involves only one group, ideally a good representative of the population. The shaded individuals represent people with the exposure of our interest and those with a triangle symbol are people with a specific health condition. However, the researcher does not know each individual's exposure or outcome status when selecting the study sample.

The study subjects can further be categorised according to the status of exposure or outcome. As shown in Figure 6.3, the study sample is split into two groups according to exposure status: subjects with and without exposure. At the same point in time, we also investigate the subjects' outcome status. The shaded individuals in the exposed and unexposed groups represent those who have the disease. Conversely, the study sample can

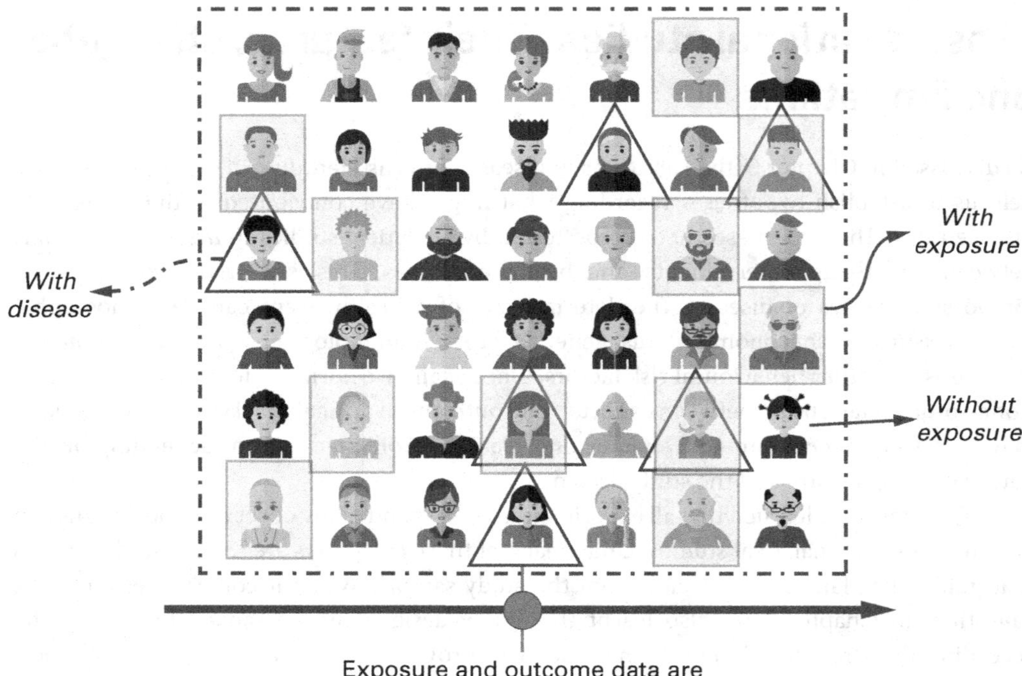

Figure 6.2 A cross-sectional study design: initial sample

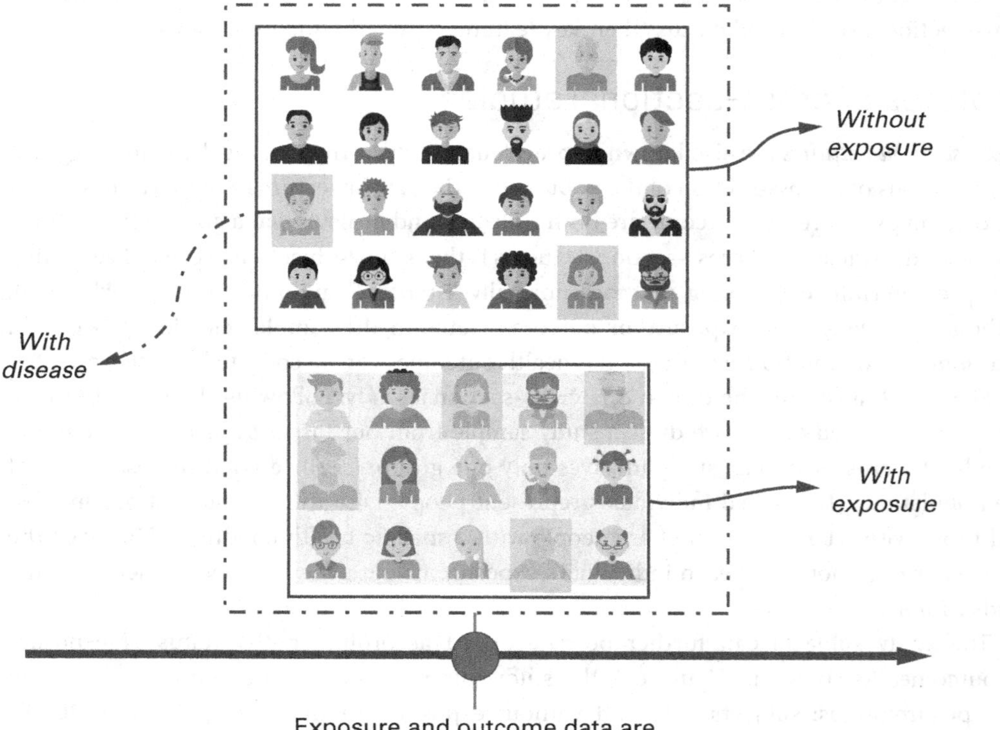

Figure 6.3 A cross-sectional study design: study samples for analysis

also be split into groups based on outcome status. This joint collection of data on both disease and exposure allows analysis of their association, and thus it is analytical in nature. Cross-sectional studies can be particularly useful for examining exposures that do not change over time for everyone included in the study. These exposures include personal characteristics such as sex, race/ethnicity, blood type and family history of disease.

Cross-sectional studies can be used to identify prevalent cases of disease (prevalence of disease). Likewise, we can also calculate the prevalence of exposure in these studies. For example, we can assess the prevalence of physical inactivity in a cross-sectional study if it is the exposure in which we are interested. As mentioned above, questionnaire surveys are commonly used to collect data in analytical studies. In cross-sectional studies, we can use surveys to collect data on multiple factors and various outcomes.

We have learned in Chapter 5 that prevalence surveys are conducted to collect data on the overall health and well-being of a population, including the prevalence of specific health conditions, social determinants of health and common health risk factors. These studies involving surveys are categorised as cross-sectional studies. Prevalence surveys are classified as descriptive studies if they are conducted to examine the patterns of disease occurrence in relation to person, place and time characteristics as detailed in Chapter 5. For example, population surveys (such as National Health Surveys) are carried out by health or statistical agencies to collect data from a population sample. These surveys focus on assessing the prevalence of specific health conditions such as chronic diseases and common health risk factors within a defined population, as well as exploring the distributions of these health conditions in subpopulations (e.g. different age, sex and ethnic groups) and geographic locations. On the other hand, a survey study is classified as an analytical cross-sectional study when the study goes beyond simply describing the prevalence and distribution of diseases/health conditions in a population and aims to determine the relationship between an exposure or risk factor and the presence of a health outcome. In other words, a cross-sectional survey study is designed not only to estimate the prevalence of a health outcome but also to quantify an association between a specific exposure and the health outcome.

The information collected on various exposure and outcome factors in a survey is based on participants' self-reported data. A typical survey questionnaire often includes sociodemographic characteristics, specific health outcomes, an exposure of interest and other health risk factors. Many standardised questionnaires or validated measurement tools have been developed for the assessment of exposure and outcome status. For example, some psychometric scales can be used to identify potential mental health issues such as stress, anxiety and depression. A wide range of assessment tools are also available for measuring abstract constructs such as knowledge, attitudes and behaviours (e.g. KAP scales). We can also apply other data-collection methods in addition to surveys. For instance, we may use hospital records or clinical/diagnostic testing results to determine the presence of certain diseases to determine 'outcome status' in more objective and reliable ways. Similarly, biological samples may be taken from study participants to measure exposure/outcome status such as levels of serum cholesterol, triglycerides, lipoproteins and micronutrients (e.g. vitamin D, iron, folic acid). For example, we can investigate whether people have uncontrolled diabetes mellitus through a questionnaire survey (using self-reported data). However, the data are more objective if we check glycated haemoglobin (HbA1c) levels in the blood. Of course, additional costs and potential ethical issues (as taking blood samples is minimally invasive) should be taken into consideration when choosing data-collection methods.

An example of a population-based cross-sectional study was reported in 2021 which aimed to assess how migration was associated with small gestational age (SGA, <10th percentile of all babies of the same age) in Victoria, Australia (6). The study made use of routinely collected population data on all singleton births in Victoria between 2009 and 2018. The study found that the prevalence of the overall SGA among babies born in Victoria during the study period was 8.7 per cent. However, the prevalence of SGA was higher among infants born to migrant mothers (11.3 per cent) compared with those born to Australian-born mothers (7.3 per cent). This study also suggested that migrant women from Southern Central Asia, South-East Asia and sub-Saharan Africa were at particularly higher risk of birthing an SGA child than Australian women. As being born small for gestational age is a strong predictor of the short- and long-term health of an individual (from infancy to adulthood), the findings of the study provided crucial evidence for SGA prevention, particularly addressing health inequality and improving the health and well-being of migrant women and their children.

Rachael: In the example you just described, the population data was collected over a long period of time (2009–18). Why didn't the study collect data at a specific time point if this is a cross-sectional study?

Hugo: Yeah, right – that was 10 years!

Author (Patricia): That is a brilliant question, Rachael. Although the data were collected over a long period of time, the prevalence of the health event (SGA) and other characteristics was still measured cross-sectionally (at various time points). In this example, period prevalence (instead of point prevalence) was used because it is obviously not possible to expect all babies to be born at the same point in time! This is like needing a lot of sunny days to effectively measure whether they are associated with reduced study.

EXPLANATION 6.1: What is period prevalence? When can it be used?

Unlike point prevalence assessing the proportion of existing cases of a disease/health condition in a defined population *at a given time point* (e.g. at a cross-sectional survey), period prevalence measures the proportion of a health condition in a population *during a period of time*. Period prevalence is a useful measure in public health practice, especially when the health event of interest is rare or uncommon, and using a cross-sectional survey to capture cases would be impractical.

Following the SGA example, the prevalence of SGA in each calendar year is determined by the proportion of SGA newborns in the total live births in the same year. It is important to note that the numerator (SGA newborns) is included in the denominator (total babies born live). In other words, the denominator includes SGA babies and non-SGA babies. The annual period prevalence accounted for all SGA cases at various time points throughout each year. Similarly, we can also use period prevalence to determine the proportion of babies born with a birth defect such as Down Syndrome in all newborns during a year.

The population denominator in period prevalence is different from that in incidence. It is not practical to use incidence to assess the 'risk' of developing Down Syndrome in the newborn population, because in those babies with Down Syndrome, the condition already exists at birth. Therefore, the outcome (existing cases of Down Syndrome) is assessed cross-sectionally. It does not make sense to follow up a group of babies without Down Syndrome over a period of time to see whether they will develop this condition later in their lives. However, if we follow up a cohort of babies to compare the rates of a particular childhood disease between babies born with Down Syndrome and those without Down Syndrome, incidence would be the most appropriate measure in this case.

Strengths and weaknesses of cross-sectional studies

Since data on all variables (including exposure and outcome) in cross-sectional studies are collected at once and do not require follow-ups, they are less expensive and relatively easy to do compared with other forms of analytical studies (these will be detailed in Chapters 7–9). It is also important to note that cross-sectional studies have the features of both descriptive and analytical studies, as such, they can be used to generate and test hypotheses important to identifying the aetiology of disease (causal pathway). We can study multiple outcomes and exposures: measuring the prevalence of a specific disease or other outcomes and various health-related factors. This information can be used to assess the burden of disease and provide information for health planning and resource allocation. Additionally, cross-sectional studies allow researchers to establish a basic association between the outcome and exposure in which they are interested. The findings of these studies form a basis to guide further analytical studies investigating the potential causal relationship between exposure and outcome. For example, cross-sectional studies provide baseline data for cohort and experimental studies, helping researchers evaluate the effect of exposure over time.

On the other hand, cross-sectional studies also have several limitations. First, due to the simultaneous measurement of outcome and exposures, these studies do not capture the temporal sequence of exposure and outcome events, making it difficult to determine causality. Since we don't know whether exposure preceded or resulted from the outcome, reverse causality may occur (which came first, the chicken or the egg?). Second, cross-sectional studies are not suitable for studying rare diseases or health conditions. To capture sufficient cases of a rare outcome event for analysis, the study requires a large sample size at any given point in time. It makes the design impractical and inefficient. Third, we need to be aware that incidence cannot be measured in cross-sectional studies, so we are unable to assess the 'risk' of developing a disease in these studies. Lastly, cross-sectional studies are prone to various types of bias (selection bias and information bias) and confounding. We will learn more about these issues later in this book.

The strengths and weaknesses of cross-sectional studies should be considered carefully in comparison with other forms of analytical studies (Chapters 7–9) in order to choose the most appropriate study design with the time and resources available in various circumstances. Example 6.1 presents a cross-sectional study designed to investigate the impact of COVID-19-related stress on the changes in alcohol consumption habits among American adults. It also highlights the major limitations of the study in reflection on the major issues discussed previously.

EXAMPLE 6.1

A cross-sectional study was developed to determine the impact of the COVID-19 pandemic on adult alcohol consumption in the United States. A questionnaire was used to assess alcohol consumption and COVID-19 related stress. Convenience sampling was used to recruit participants through social media posts and emails (sent via listservs of selected consumer groups and the American Public Health Association). Snowball sampling was also utilised to further distribute the survey link.

The study found that 34.1 per cent and 7.0 per cent of participants reported binge drinking and extreme binge drinking, respectively, since the pandemic began. Those who experienced COVID-19-related stress were more likely to drink a greater amount of alcohol and engage in alcohol consumption on more days than those who did not perceive stress. It was concerning that 60 per cent of the study participants increased alcohol drinking compared with their pre-COVID-19 habits. The study also revealed that increased stress (45.7 per cent), greater alcohol availability (34.4 per cent) and boredom (30.1 per cent) were the main reasons for increasing alcohol consumption during the pandemic.

As the participants were recruited through convenience sampling, the sample was not representative (e.g. the majority of participants were female, white, aged <50 and middle- or higher-income) and had limited generalisability. Due to its cross-sectional design, it was difficult to determine the temporal sequence of binge-drinking behaviours and COVID-19-related stress among all the participants. The researchers were unable to determine whether stress occurred before binge drinking behaviours among the participants. As such, a causal relationship between alcohol drinking and COVID-19 related stress could not be established through this research. Despite these limitations, this study provided valuable information on the changes in unhealthy behaviours under the influences of the COVID-19 restrictions and lockdowns.

Source: (7).

Establishing associations in cross-sectional studies

In the previous chapters, we learned that the differences in disease occurrence identified in descriptive studies help us generate hypotheses in order to search for the possible causes of the disease. An analytical study can be developed to test the hypotheses, determining whether an association between exposure and disease exists. Measures of association in analytical studies are calculated differently depending on the type of study design. To assess an association in analytical studies, we often start by constructing a contingency (2 × 2) table to display the numbers of subjects according to their exposure and outcome status.

Table 6.1 presents a standard format of 2 × 2 tabulation. The denoted values a, b, c and d indicate the quantities of subjects in relation to four different combinations of exposure and outcome status. Unlike other analytical studies that select two or more study samples based on exposure status (such as cohort studies) or outcome status (such as case-control studies), in cross-sectional studies, only one study sample is selected. The researchers can split the sample into groups according to a specific exposure or outcome of their interest.

Table 6.1 Standard format of a 2 x 2 table in analytical studies

Exposure	Disease		Total
	Presence (+)	Absence (–)	
Presence (+)	a	b	a + b
Absence (–)	c	d	c + d
Total	a + c	b + d	a + b + c + d

Measures of association in cross-sectional studies: Prevalence ratio and prevalence odds ratio

Measures of association allow researchers to quantify the strength and direction of an effect of a specific exposure on a health outcome and are fundamental to assessing causality. The choice of measure of association depends on the study design. In cross-sectional studies, measures of association can be estimated in different ways, depending on how study subjects are grouped (based on exposure or outcome status). A measure of association based on exposure status is more frequently used in practice. To avoid confusion, we only focus on this way of subject grouping for the measure of association in cross-sectional studies. Using the standard 2 x 2 table shown in Table 6.1, the prevalence of the disease in the two exposure groups can be measured as follows:

Exposure (+) group: a/(a + b)
Exposure (–) group: c/(c + d)

Prevalence ratio (PR): A quantitative measure used to determine the strength and direction of association between exposure and outcome in cross-sectional studies. It is computed by dividing the prevalence of disease in the exposed group by that of the unexposed group.

We can calculate the **prevalence ratio (PR)** of disease as the measure of association by simply dividing the prevalence of disease in the exposed group by that of the unexposed group:

$$\text{Prevalence ratio (PR) of disease} = \frac{a/(a+b)}{c/(c+d)}$$

Hugo: That looks like a calculation!!

Rachael: We may need a bit of help sorting this out ...

Author (Patricia): No worries, Hugo and Rachael. You are not alone in feeling that way. Many students find calculations intimidating at first, but with practice and patience you can certainly master them. We can use some basic worked examples (let's start with Worked Example 6.1) and familiar calculations to build your understanding and confidence step by step. We can work through this together!

WORKED EXAMPLE 6.1

Table 6.2 demonstrates a 2 x 2 table of a hypothetical cross-sectional study on the relationship between physical inactivity and cardiovascular disease (CVD). Assume that the study participants (10 000 in total) are categorised according to their exposure status (physically inactive group vs physically active group). Given that the total number of CVD cases is 500, the overall prevalence of CVD in this example is 5 per cent (500 ÷ 10 000 = 0.05 = 5%). The numbers of subjects in a and b grids represent people with and without CVD respectively among those who are physically inactive. Similarly, values c and d are people with and without CVD among physically active people.

(A) Prevalence ratio (PR)

We can calculate the measure of association using the prevalence ratio formula above. In this scenario, we calculate the prevalence ratio of CVD to estimate the 'association' between physical activity and CVD. It is calculated by dividing the prevalence of CVD in the exposed (Exposure (+), physical inactivity) by the prevalence of CVD in the unexposed (Exposure (–), physical activity).

Table 6.2 Physical inactivity and CVD

Exposure	CVD		Total
	Presence (+)	Absence (–)	
Physically inactive (+)	260 (a)	3200 (b)	3460
Physically active (–)	240 (c)	6300 (d)	6540
Total	500	9500	10000

Prevalence of CVD in physical inactivity group = 260/3460 = 0.075 = 7.5%
Prevalence of CVD in physical activity group = 240/6540 = 0.037 = 3.7%
Prevalence ratio (PR) of CVD between exposure (+) and (–) is:

$$PR = \frac{a/(a+b)}{c(c+d)} = \frac{260/3460}{240/6540} \cong 2.05$$

This result of the prevalence ratio tells us that the odds of CVD prevalence among physically inactive people are around two times (PR = 2.05) as likely to be suffering from CVD *as those who are physically active*. As a measure of association is a relative measure, it needs to be interpreted in comparison with a 'reference' group (physically active group in this case).

Please note that, as the data of both exposure and outcome are collected at the same point in time, we can only assess the association between the presence of an exposure factor (physical inactivity) and the prevalence of an outcome (CVD). In this example, the cases of CVD are already present (they are survivors of CVD) in the population at the time of the study. As discussed above, we cannot determine the temporal sequence of participants' physical activity habits and their incidence of CVD.

Also, incidence cannot be assessed in a cross-sectional study. Therefore, we are unable to determine whether physically inactive subjects are at a higher 'risk' of developing CVD than those physically active individuals. For instance, some participants might have to adjust their levels of physical activity due to the conditions of CVD. As physical activity/inactivity and CVD are measured at the same point in time, we are not certain which one came first. This shortcoming makes the interpretation of measures of association in cross-sectional studies challenging with respect to disease aetiology.

(B) Prevalence odds ratio (POR)

Another commonly used measure of association in cross-sectional studies is the **prevalence odds ratio (POR)**. It is calculated by using the odds of disease in the exposed group divided by the odds of disease in the unexposed group. Using the standard format of 2 x 2 table as shown in Table 6.1, the odds of disease in these groups are expressed as follows:

Exposure (+) group: a/b
Exposure (–) group: c/d

$$\text{Prevalence odds ratio (POR) of disease} = \frac{a/b}{c/d} = \frac{a \times d}{b \times c}$$

Let's use the example in Table 6.2 to calculate the POR to assess the association between physical inactivity and CVD.

Odds of CVD in physical inactivity group = a/b = 260/3200 = 0.081
Odds of CVD in physical activity group = c/d = 240/6300 = 0.038

$$\text{Prevalence odds ratio (POR) of CVD} = \frac{a \times d}{b \times c} = \frac{260 \times 6300}{3200 \times 240} \cong 2.13$$

The result indicates that the odds of CVD prevalence are 2.13 times higher among people who are physically inactive than those who are physically active.

Both PR and POR show consistent results that those people who identify themselves as physically inactive at the survey have around a twofold higher chance to be living with CVD than those who are active.

Prevalence odds ratio (POR): Another measure of association commonly used in cross-sectional studies. It can be measured in two different ways: (1) by dividing the odds of outcome in the exposed group by that of the unexposed group; and (2) by dividing the odds of exposure in the diseased group by that of the non-diseased group.

Rachael: I guess the calculations weren't too difficult after all!

Hugo: The PR and POR results look pretty similar, though – how do we know which ones to use?

Author (Patricia): Thanks for your question, Hugo. You are right. As you can see in Worked Example 6.1 (A) and (B), the value of POR shows a slightly stronger association than that of PR. Existing studies suggest a tendency to over-estimate the strength of association by POR in comparison with PR. Some researchers prefer PR over POR when the prevalence of the target outcome is high (e.g. >20%) (8, 9). Nevertheless, they are both valid measures of association in cross-sectional studies (10–12). One systematic review found that the prevalence odds ratio is the most commonly used measure of association in cross-sectional studies (13).

Strength and direction of an association

As mentioned earlier, measures of association allow us to assess the strength and direction of the effect of an exposure on a health outcome. In analytical studies, these measures are calculated using divisions known as ratios (see Chapter 2). In the CVD example, the 'strength' of association is comparing the prevalence or odds of CVD in the 'exposed' (physically inactive group) relative to the odds in the 'unexposed' (physically active group).

If the result of the measure of association shows PR or POR = 1, it means that the numerator and denominator are equal in quantity. In an epidemiological context, the result indicates 'no association' between exposure and outcome — that is, the prevalence or odds of the outcome are the same in both exposed and unexposed groups. Table 6.3 summarises the interpretation of a measured association in different directions.

EXPLANATION 6.2A: How do we determine the strength of association in different directions?

Table 6.3 Strength and direction of a measure of association

Value of estimate	Strength of association	Direction	Type of exposure
PR/POR = 1	No association	No association	Not a contributing factor
PR/POR >1	Stronger when away from 1	A positive association	A risk factor
PR/POR <1	Stronger towards 0 or away from 1	A negative association	A protective factor

Note: The estimates of association measures are PR or POR in cross-sectional studies.

If the calculated PR or POR is a value greater than 1, the result shows a positive association, such as the PR/POR >2 in Worked Example 6.1. Based on the value of PR/POR (if >1), the exposure factor (e.g. physical inactivity) in the study is defined as a 'risk factor' – that is, people who are physically inactive have an increased odds of having CVD. We use the value 1 as the base value to determine the strength of an association. The further away from 1 (in both directions) the estimated PR/POR is, the stronger association. Conversely, if our measured association is <1, it is a negative association. The exposure factor is defined as a protective factor, meaning that the exposure is likely to lower the chance of disease prevalence. Once again, if the PR/POR is closer to 0 but away from 1, the magnitude of association is considered stronger as opposed to a value closer to 1.

Rachael: I am a bit confused with the interpretation of a PR/POR <1. Why does the association become stronger when the value is closer to 0? Could you please explain this again?

Hugo: I think how we determine the strength of a negative association must have something to do with the ratio concept. It would be great if you could give us a specific example.

Author (Patricia): No worries, Rachael and Hugo. I am happy to explain the concept of a 'negative association' using Figure 6.4 and revisit the example in Table 6.2 (physical inactivity and CVD) to help you understand it.

EXPLANATION 6.2B: How do we determine the strength of association in different directions?

Figure 6.4 illustrates the strength and direction of an association depending on the calculated value. This concept can be applied to all analytical studies. As mentioned before, measures of association in analytical studies are ratios, simply using one number divided by another number. The value of a ratio is ranging from 0 to infinity. In terms of a measure of association, 1 is the null value (no association) where the two study groups have equal prevalence (or odds) of outcome. Interpreting the strength and direction of a positive association is quite straightforward. As indicated in Figure 6.4, an estimated association near 1 (the value of no association) is relatively weak, whereas an association is considered stronger when the value is further away from 1. This is how we quantify the 'strength' of a positive association.

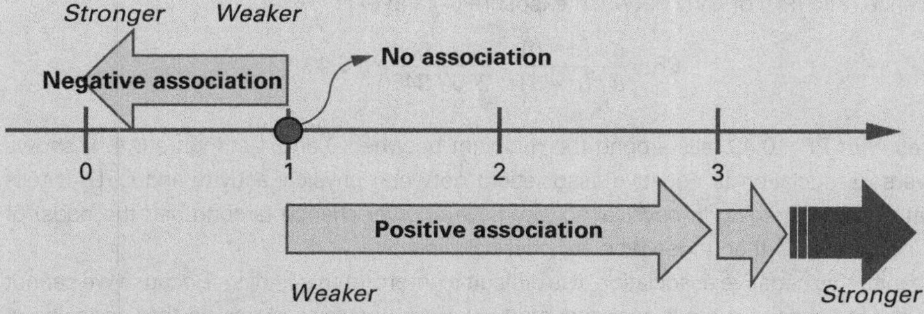

Figure 6.4 Strength and direction of an association

Unlike a positive association with a value ranging from >1 to infinity, the value of a negative association is limited from 0 to 1 (when the quantity of the numerator is less than the quantity of the denominator). As 1 is the base value, an association of 0.98 (very close to 1) shows very little difference in the prevalence of outcome between the exposed and unexposed groups (e.g. assuming the prevalence in each group is numerator (exposed) = 0.04; denominator (unexposed) = 0.041; the association = 0.98), indicating a weak association. On the other hand, an association closer to 0 (but away from 1) reflects a greater difference in the prevalence between the two groups (e.g. exposed = 0.04; unexposed = 0.25). This 'large difference' in prevalence implies that exposure to this 'protective factor' is associated with a lower chance of having the disease compared with the unexposed group.

Let's use the example presented in Table 6.2 to elaborate on this concept. Instead of considering 'physical inactivity' as the risk factor of our interest, we now make 'physical activity' the exposure factor and see how the association changes.

WORKED EXAMPLE 6.2

Table 6.4 demonstrates the reversed exposure status and the updated 2 x 2 table according to the outcome status in relation to the new 'exposed' and 'unexposed' groups. (Physically active people are assigned as exposure (+) in this new table.) In this example, we still want to measure the association of physical activity with CVD, but the direction of the association is completely opposite. Remember, we have only swapped the 'exposure' status between the groups. All the values according to the exposure and outcome status in the 2 x 2 table remain unchanged.

Table 6.4 Physical activity and CVD

Exposure	CVD		Total
	Presence (+)	Absence (–)	
Physically active (+)	240 (a)	6300 (b)	6540
Physically inactive (–)	260 (c)	3200 (d)	3460
Total	500	9500	10 000

Prevalence of CVD in physical activity group = 240/6540 = 0.037 = 3.7%
Prevalence of CVD in physical inactivity group = 260/3460 = 0.075 = 7.5%
Prevalence ratio (PR) of CVD between exposure (+) and (-) is:

$$PR = \frac{a/(a+b)}{c/(c+d)} = \frac{240/6540}{260/3460} \cong 0.49$$

This result of PR= 0.49 falls around the midpoint between 0 and 1 in Figure 6.4. It shows an inverse association (a negative association) between physical activity and CVD. It tells us that people engaging in physical activity have a lower chance (around half the odds) of suffering from CVD than those who are physically inactive.

Despite this negative association, it is difficult to interpret this finding. Because we cannot measure incidence in a cross-sectional study, we are unable to conclude that engaging in physical activity protects people from developing CVD or reduces the 'risk' of developing CVD. In addition, this new PR' = 0.49 is equivalent to an inverse value of the previous PR in relation to Table 6.2 (see calculation below).

$PR' = 1 \div PR = 1 \div 2.05 = 0.487 \cong 0.49$

Likewise, if we use the new values in Table 6.4, the POR can be calculated as follows:

$$\text{Prevalence odds ratio (POR) of CVD} = \frac{a \times d}{b \times c} = \frac{240 \times 3200}{6300 \times 260} \cong 0.47$$

Once again, this new POR' equals the inverse value of the previous POR:

$POR' = 1 \div POR = 1 \div 2.13 = 0.469 \cong 0.47$

This result means that people who are physically active have a reduced odds (reduced by 53%, 1 – 0.47 = 0.53) of having CVD than those who are physically inactive.

As suggested above, prevalence odds ratios tend to estimate stronger associations compared with prevalence ratios. In relation to the two examples, we can see that the calculated PORs are slightly away from the null value of 1 than the PRs.

Ecological studies: Their features, strengths and limitations

'Longitudinal' cross-sectional studies

In Chapter 5, we learned that many countries routinely conduct repeated cross-sectional population studies, using questionnaire surveys to collect information on the prevalence of specific health conditions, health-related issues, utilisation of health services, nutrition and lifestyle factors. For instance, the New Zealand Health Survey has been carried out on a yearly basis since 2011 (14). In Australia, the National Health Survey is conducted by the ABS every three to four years to collect population data for long-term health conditions, mental well-being, sociodemographic characteristics and health risk factors (15, 16). Another typical example of this kind is the Global Burden of Disease (GBD) study. As mentioned in Chapter 5, the GBD study is the most comprehensive observational study in the world, regularly collecting global data on mortality, morbidity and risk factors (17). Please find the link to the *Lancet* GBD Study in the 'Further reading' section for more information. These cross-sectional surveys, which are carried out on multiple occasions, are sometimes called 'longitudinal' studies because they collect information at various time points to monitor long-term trends of diseases and health issues. It is important to note that the results of these cross-sectional surveys are only comparable if the sampling method remains consistent over time.

We need to recognise that these repeated cross-sectional surveys differ from follow-up studies – including cohort and experimental studies (these designs will be detailed in Chapters 8 and 9), which are sometimes also called longitudinal studies. Follow-up studies track the same individuals over time to examine the effect of exposure on the incidence of a disease, while routine cross-sectional surveys do not monitor the same group of people at different time points. Instead, they recruit a different sample of people for each survey and then study the changes in prevalence of specific health conditions, mental well-being and health risks.

Features of ecological studies

Ecological studies are also known as *correlational studies.* Building upon our understanding of 'longitudinal' cross-sectional surveys, ecological studies analyse existing data at the group or population level. These existing data can be obtained from the results of repeated cross-sectional surveys, records of long-term monitoring of specific health conditions and disease surveillance. These group- or population-level data include the occurrence of health outcomes (such as incidence, prevalence and mortality), aggregate measures of risk factors, environmental variables or other determinants.

Ecological studies are a special type of observational study. Some researchers (2, 11) consider ecological studies as a type of descriptive study (or consider them as both descriptive and analytical studies) because they cannot be used to directly measure associations between exposure and outcome among study subjects (at the individual level). In other words, individual data on exposures, outcomes and other variables (such as personal characteristics) are not available in these studies.

Similar to cross-sectional studies, ecological studies can also be used to describe the patterns (time, place and personal characteristics) of health-related issues or factors as discussed in Chapter 5. For example, Figure 5.10 presents the long-term patterns of the prevalence of daily smoking and mortality of lung cancer in Australia. The graph demonstrates the effect of smoking prevalence on the changes in lung cancer mortality in male and female populations. The data are presented at the 'population level', including annual data on smoking prevalence and lung cancer-specific mortality (deaths per 100 000). The data cannot tell us whether or not individual smokers in the population were more likely to die from lung cancer than non-smokers. Individual data are not available to enable us to draw up a 2 x 2 table according to all study subjects' exposure and outcome status. Therefore, we are unable to directly measure an association relating an exposure to a specific outcome at the individual level.

Correlation: A relationship between variables in which the values of the variables change in relationship with each other.

In terms of its analytical feature, we can assess a **correlation** at the population level as an alternative way of measuring a relationship between exposure and outcome in an ecological study. For example, a study utilised the vital statistics and the National Nutritional Survey in Japan from 1955 to 1993 to evaluate the relationship between food/nutrient intake and cancer mortality (18). The results of this study suggested correlations between westernised dietary habits and the mortality of colon, breast, ovary and prostate cancers; and the correlation between traditional Japanese dietary habits and stomach cancer mortality. To make the concept of 'correlation' easier to understand, we can revisit Figure 5.10. This helps us visualise the relationship between smoking prevalence and lung cancer mortality. It is clear that lung cancer mortality increased with an increasing trend of smoking prevalence over time (with a time lag of 20 to 30 years). Following the logic of positive and negative associations (Table 6.3), the directions of correlation can be understood in a similar way. In contrast, like the example in Figure 5.9, the continuous decrease in the COVID-19 case-fatality rate seemed to correspond with the rollout of the vaccination program in Australia (correlating with the increasing uptake of vaccination).

Gross domestic product (GDP) per capita: A global indicator used to measure and compare the economic growth of countries around the world. It is calculated by dividing the GDP of a country by its mid-year population (World Bank Metadata Glossary: https://databank.worldbank.org/metadataglossary/world-development-indicators/series/NY.GDP.PCAP.KN). Developed countries tend to have a higher GDP per capita than developing countries.

EXAMPLE 6.2

Figure 6.5 demonstrates another example of using ecological data to examine the relationship between life expectancy and **gross domestic product (GDP) per capita**. We can see that most of the countries are scattered around the diagonal line, a positive gradient. It seems that more developed or rich nations (the countries around the top-right corner of the graph) have longer life expectancy. This example shows a 'positive' correlation between GDP per capita and life expectancy.

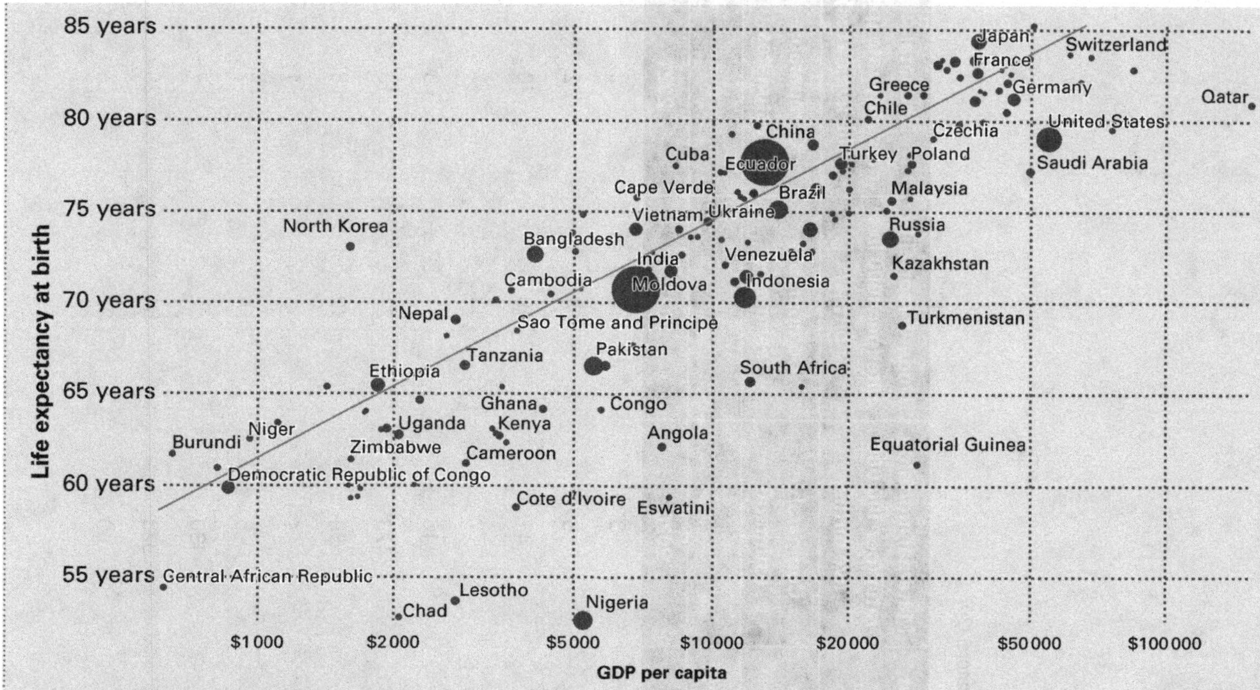

Figure 6.5 Life expectancy vs GDP per capita, 2018 (19)

Note: GDP per capita is adjusted for inflation and differences in the cost of living between countries. Larger dots represent countries with bigger populations.

Hugo: I noticed that the data of different countries compared in Figure 6.5 were based on the data of 2018. Is this a cross-sectional study?

Author (Patricia): No, Hugo, this is an ecological study because the data used to determine the relationship between GDP and life expectancy are aggregate data at the country level. In a cross-sectional study, we need to have the data of individual subjects. In the next section, I will show you the differences in datasets between ecological and cross-sectional studies.

Table 6.5 shows an extracted section of the WHO Health Statistics database. This type of data is a typical source of ecological studies. The data present each country's average life expectancy (in males and females separately and both sexes combined) in 2019 and the levels of several key health indicators. For example, the life expectancy of both sexes in 2019 may contribute to the y-axis value for each country dot similar to Figure 6.5. We also need to collect the data of overall GDP per capita (e.g. collecting from the World Bank data) for all the compared countries. These data were aggregated at the country/population level. The unit of analysis is the entire country. We don't have detailed data from individual residents of each country.

Table 6.5 Example of ecological data (aggregate data on life expectancy by sex and selected health indicators) (20)

Countries and areas	Life expectancy at birth (years)			Healthy life expectancy at birth (years)			Maternal mortality ratio (per 100 000 live births)	Under-5 mortality rate (per 1000 live births)	Neonatal mortality rate (per 1000 live births)
	Comparable estimates			Comparable estimates			Comparable estimates	Comparable estimates	Comparable estimates
	Male	Female	Both sexes	Male	Female	Both sexes			
	2019			2019			2020	2021	2021
Australia	81.3	84.8	83.0	70.2	71.7	70.9	3	4	2
Austria	79.4	83.8	81.6	69.9	71.9	70.9	5	4	2
Azerbaijan	68.8	74.1	71.4	62.1	65.2	63.6	41	19	10
Bahamas	69.9	76.6	73.2	62.3	66.5	64.4	77	13	7
Bahrain	75.0	77.0	75.8	66.0	65.5	65.9	16	7	3
Bangladesh	73.0	75.6	74.3	64.2	64.4	64.3	123	27	16
Barbados	74.3	77.7	76.0	66.2	67.7	67.0	39	12	8
Belarus	69.7	79.6	74.8	62.3	69.4	66.0	1	3	1
Belgium	79.3	83.5	81.4	69.8	71.3	70.6	5	4	2
Belize	71.4	77.8	74.4	63.5	67.3	65.3	130	11	7
Benin	61.2	65.7	63.4	54.5	56.6	55.5	523	84	29
Bhutan	72.0	74.4	73.1	63.2	63.5	63.4	60	27	15

Countries and areas	Life expectancy at birth (years)			Healthy life expectancy at birth (years)			Maternal mortality ratio (per 100 000 live births)	Under-5 mortality rate (per 1000 live births)	Neonatal mortality rate (per 1000 live births)
	Comparable estimates			Comparable estimates			Comparable estimates	Comparable estimates	Comparable estimates
	Male	Female	Both sexes	Male	Female	Both sexes			
	2019			2019			2020	2021	2021
Bolivia (Plurinational State of)	71.1	73.1	72.1	63.2	63.3	63.3	161	25	13
Bosnia and Herzegovina	74.4	79.1	76.8	65.7	68.7	67.2	6	6	4
Botswana	58.9	65.5	62.2	51.9	55.8	53.9	186	35	18
Brazil	72.4	79.4	75.9	63.4	67.4	65.4	72	14	8
Brunei Darussalam	73.4	75.4	74.3	65.2	66.1	65.6	44	11	6
Bulgaria	71.6	78.6	75.1	63.9	68.7	66.3	7	6	3
Burkina Faso	60.1	65.2	62.7	53.4	56.3	54.9	264	83	25
Burundi	61.5	66.1	63.8	54.0	57.2	55.6	494	53	20
Cabo Verde	69.9	77.9	74.0	62.2	67.2	64.8	42	14	8
Cambodia	67.2	72.7	70.1	59.8	63.0	61.5	218	25	13

Table 6.6 presents a partial dataset of a cross-sectional study. The study participants were university students (21). We can see that each line of the data contains information from a participant. The unit of analysis in this example is individual participants. The data enables us to relate one variable to the other at the individual level. For instance, if we are interested in investigating the relationship between exercise and stress, we can draw up a table to classify the subjects according to different levels of exercise and the presence/absence of stress, then calculate a measure of association (PR or POR). This dataset also includes information on participants' demographic characteristics and other variables, which may also be related to stress. As mentioned in the previous chapters of this book, most diseases and health issues are caused by the interplay of multiple factors. The additional variables in the dataset could

Table 6.6 Example of a dataset of a cross-sectional study. Adapted from (21)

ID	Age	Gender	Marital_ status	Hours_ work	Hours_ exercise	Weight_ in_kg	Height_ in_cm	Current_ smoker	Stress
1	20	1	1	3.00	5.00	80	176	2	1
2	19	1	1	2.00	4.00	90	183	2	1
3	23	1	1	2.00	5.00	78	188	2	1
8	19	1	2	1.00	4.00	110	190	2	2
9	22	2	1	3.00	4.00	55	163	2	2
10	20	2	2	1.00	4.00	60	168	2	1
11	19	1	1	2.00	5.00	75	191	2	2
12	21	1	1	3.00	4.00	91	178	2	2
13	22	1	1	1.00	5.00	65	171	2	1
14	22	1	1	3.00	4.00	78	180	2	1
15	22	1	2	3.00	4.00	81	186	2	1
16	20	1	2	3.00	5.00	87	178	2	1
17	18	1	1	3.00	4.00	66	180	2	1
18	21	1	1	2.00	4.00	75	175	2	2
19	21	1	1	3.00	5.00	65	170	2	1
20	28	2	1	3.00	2.00	53	160	2	2
21	22	2	1	1.00	4.00	45	160	2	2
24	22	1	1	1.00	5.00	77	174	2	2
25	20	1	1	1.00	2.00	65	175	2	2
26	22	1	1	2.00	4.00	68	175	2	2
27	22	1	1	1.00	5.00	70	165	1	1
28	23	1	1	1.00	4.00	83	181	2	2
29	20	1	2	2.00	5.00	87	190	2	1
31	19	2	1	1.00	2.00	65	163	2	1

be potential *confounding factors* in the relationship between exercise and stress. Collecting data on such factors enables researchers to further control for their effects on the measured association. The concepts of confounding factors and strategies for adjusting for confounding will be addressed in more detail in Chapter 11.

Ecological studies are typically used to examine the effects of climate change on human health. Researchers collect data on long-term patterns of meteorological variables such as temperature, humidity, rainfall and extreme weather events to explore how changes in these climate variables correspond to changes in the occurrence of a specific disease or health issue within a given population or a geographic area. Example 6.3 presents an example of an ecological study used to link the changes in daily temperature and renal disease.

EXAMPLE 6.3

A study was developed to investigate the relationship between daily temperature and kidney disease, in consideration of more frequent, intensified and long-lasting heatwaves due to climate change. The study obtained daily data on maximum, minimum and average temperatures from July 2003 to March 2014, with a focus on the warm season (October to March) in Adelaide, South Australia. In addition, hospital admission data (including emergency department admissions and inpatient admissions) for renal disease (the incidence of eight temperature-prone renal disease categories) in the same period was collected.

The research findings showed that the rising daily temperature per 1°C was correlated with an increased incidence of all renal disease categories except for pyelonephritis. The study also suggested that an increased frequency of renal disease (including urolithiasis, acute kidney injury and urinary tract infections) is predicted with increasing temperatures due to climate change. The results of this research provided useful information regarding the management of renal diseases in the context of climate change.

The authors also acknowledge the limitations of their findings based on an ecological study. They suggest that future studies can collect data on targeted renal diseases from hospital records during heat events, taking into account other clinical, social and behavioural risk factors.

Source: (22).

Hugo: It's cool that ecological studies let you see how changes in one factor works with changes in another!

Rachael: We could use an ecological design to see whether studying is negatively correlated with sunny days!

Strengths and weaknesses of ecological studies

Ecological studies are usually attractive because they are relatively easy to conduct if the routine data for the exposure and outcome of interest are available. One advantage of ecological studies is that they are relatively cost-effective to conduct by using existing databases or resources such as the data of the National Health Survey, Global Burden of Disease and

WHO Global Health Estimates. Accessing many of these data is free of charge and collection of existing data can be conducted relatively quickly compared with other forms of analytical studies. Ecological studies enable researchers to identify the patterns of health-related issues and risk factors. They are useful for generating hypotheses and informing health policies and interventions (as per features of descriptive studies). They also provide information about population-level relationships (correlations) between exposures and health outcomes (when designed as analytical studies) to guide further analytical studies to explore disease aetiology. Moreover, ecological studies are more practical and efficient for studying rare diseases/outcomes than cross-sectional studies because collecting individual-level data for a rare outcome in a cross-sectional study would require a very large sample size.

Ecological studies also have several weaknesses. A major concern is *ecological fallacy*. This occurs when correlations observed at the group/population level are incorrectly assumed to apply at the individual level. Applying inferences drawn from ecological studies (using aggregate data or population average) to individuals can be misleading since we don't have the details of individual information. We don't know whether the people who develop the disease (included as part of the population-level disease rate) are the same as those who are exposed to the factor of interest (those individuals contributing to the population percentage of exposure). For example, as mentioned in the Japanese study above, we cannot determine whether those people who died of colon, breast, ovary and prostate cancers had truly established westernised dietary habits for a long period of time (18). Furthermore, ecological studies are often prone to confounding. The relationship between exposure and outcome being observed could actually be influenced by something else, such as individual-level differences (e.g. variations in sociodemographic characteristics and/or behaviours). Another major limitation of ecological studies is their inability to establish an association or causation. Additionally, it is challenging to generalise the findings of ecological studies to other populations due to variations in the context of the measured correlation and factors affecting this relationship. Overall, ecological studies are relatively easy to do and they can be valuable for generating hypotheses for further analytical studies and informing public health planning and policies. However, their limitations should be considered carefully when interpreting the findings about relationships between exposures and outcomes.

Conclusion

In this chapter, we have moved from descriptive epidemiology to analytical epidemiology, focusing on two specific designs: cross-sectional and ecological studies. These two study designs provide basic evidence for assessing the effect of an exposure on a specific outcome quantitatively, which is the central purpose of all analytical studies. We have learned the details of these two study designs and the quantitative measures used to determine the relationship between exposure and outcome in these studies.

Learning objective 1: Understand the basic sampling concepts underpinning observational studies

This chapter has explained the concepts of sampling fundamental to epidemiological studies, especially observational studies, to select a representative sample to draw study inferences for our target population. It has also briefly introduced the principles and the common methods of probability (random) and non-probability sampling.

Learning objective 2: Be familiar with the major features of cross-sectional and ecological study designs

In this chapter, we have learned the features of cross-sectional and ecological studies, and how they are conducted. The category of 'cross-sectional study' includes descriptive studies and prevalence surveys involving only one study sample (individuals selected from the target population). They are classified as a type of analytical study when the study subjects are split into groups for measures of association. Ecological studies make use of routinely collected/existing data to examine the relationship between exposure and outcome at the population/group level.

Learning objective 3: Appreciate the strengths and weaknesses associated with cross-sectional and ecological studies

This chapter has also highlighted the advantages and disadvantages of cross-sectional and ecological studies. The strengths and weaknesses of these studies should be understood in comparison with other forms of analytical studies in order to choose the most appropriate study design for our research with the time and resources available in various circumstances.

Learning objective 4: Be able to calculate measures of association in cross-sectional studies

We have learned how to calculate prevalence ratio and prevalence odds ratio as the common measures of association in cross-sectional studies. Although measures of association at the individual level cannot be calculated in ecological studies, we have learned that 'correlations' are often used in these studies to explore the relationship between exposure and the outcome in which we are interested.

Learning objective 5: Be aware of some of the classic and contemporary cross-sectional and ecological studies that have been conducted

In addition to the basic concepts relevant to cross-sectional and ecological studies, this chapter has illustrated several real-world examples to enhance the learning of the key concepts.

Further reading

Büttner P, Muller R. Sampling strategy and sample size calculation. In: Büttner P, Muller R. eds. *Epidemiology*. 2nd ed. Oxford University Press; 2015. pp. 385–408.

Neuman WL. Qualitative and quantitative sampling. In *Social Research Methods: Qualitative and Quantitative Approaches*. 7th ed. Pearson Education; 2011: p. 240–74.

The Lancet. Global burden of disease. 2020. https://www.thelancet.com/gbd

Questions

Answers are available at the end of the book.

Multiple-choice questions

1. Why is sampling used in a cross-sectional study?

A – To study the entire population

B – To eliminate the need for data analysis

C – To make data collection easier and more manageable
D – To ensure good data accuracy.

2. What is main characteristic of a cross-sectional study?
A – Intervention design
B – Follow-up of disease outcome
C – Measuring incidence of disease
D – Exposure and outcome data collected at the same point in time.
3. Which of the following is a limitation of cross-sectional studies?
A – Temporal relationships between exposure and outcome cannot be established.
B – They can provide insights into potential causal relationships.
C – They are relatively expensive and time-consuming compared with follow-up studies.
D – They cannot be used to measure an association at the individual level.
4. What is the ecological fallacy in an ecological study?
A – A situation where the study's findings are applicable to all individuals in the target population
B – An error that arises when the exposure and outcome factors are not correlated
C – A mistake that occurs when the data of exposure and outcome are collected from different populations
D – An error that occurs in interpreting a relationship at the population level as if it applies to individuals in the population.
5. Which of the following is a limitation of ecological studies?
A – They are costly and time-consuming.
B – They cannot be used to establish an association at the individual level.
C – They are not suitable for studying rare outcomes.
D – They can be used to generate hypotheses and inform health policies.

Short-answer questions

1. Describe three key features of cross-sectional studies.
2. What are the strengths of cross-sectional studies?
3. What are the limitations of cross-sectional studies?
4. Why are cross-sectional (prevalence) studies considered both descriptive and analytical studies?
5. A cross-sectional study is developed to explore the association between the use of electronic vaping products and mental health among high school students. Table 6.7 summarises the study results. Compare the prevalence of mental health issues between the students who use vaping products and those who do not use such products.

Table 6.7 Vaping and mental health issues

Exposure	Mental health issues		Total
	Yes (+)	No (–)	
Vaping (+)	230 (a)	670 (b)	900
No vaping (–)	615 (c)	3485 (d)	4100
Total	845	4155	5000

6. Use Table 6.7 in Question 5 to calculate the prevalence ratio (PR) to determine the relationship between vaping and mental health issues. Interpret your result.

7. Use Table 6.7 in Question 5 to calculate the prevalence odds ratio (POR) and interpret your result.
8. How does the ecological fallacy occur?
9. What are the advantages of using ecological studies?
10. How is probability sampling typically conducted in a cross-sectional study?

References

1. Australian Institute of Health and Welfare (AIHW). The impact of a new disease: COVID-19 from 2020, 2021 and into 2022. In: *Australia's Health 2022.* AIHW; 2022. www.aihw.gov.au/reports-data/australias-health
2. Büttner P, Muller R. *Epidemiology*. 2nd ed. Oxford University Press; 2015.
3. Neuman WL. *Social Research Methods: Qualitative and Quantitative Approaches*. 7th ed. Pearson Education; 2011.
4. Shaghaghi A, Bhopal RS, Sheikh A. Approaches to recruiting hard-to-reach populations into research: A review of the literature. *Health Promotion Perspectives*. 2011;1(2):86–94.
5. Belt RV, Rahimi K, Cai S. Reaching the hard-to-reach: A scoping review protocol of digital health research in hidden, marginal and excluded populations. *BMJ Open*. 2022;12(9):e061361.
6. Grundy S, Lee P, Small KFA. Maternal region of origin and small for gestational age: A cross-sectional analysis of Victorian perinatal data. *BMC Pregnancy and Childbirth*. 2021;21(1):1–12.
7. Grossman ER, Benjamin-Neelon SE, Sonnenschein S. Alcohol consumption during the COVID-19 pandemic: A cross-sectional survey of US Adults. *International Journal of Environmental Research and Public Health*. 2020;17:9189.
8. Behren T, Taeger D, Wellmann J, Keil U. Different methods to calculate effect estimates in cross-sectional studies: A comparison between prevalence odds ratio and prevalence ratio. *Methods of Information in Medicine*. 2004;43(5):505–9.
9. Schiaffino A, Rodríguez M, Pasarín MI, Regidor E, Borrell C, Fernández E. (2003). Odds ratio or prevalence ratio? Their use in cross-sectional studies. *Gaceta Sanitaria*. 2003;17(1):70–4.
10. Tamhane AR, Westfall AO, Burkholder GA, Cutter GR. Prevalence odds ratio versus prevalence ratio: Choice comes with consequences. *Statistics in Medicine*. 2016;35(30):5730–5.
11. Webb P, Bain C, Page A. *Essential Epidemiology: An Introduction for Students and Health Professionals*. 4th ed. Cambridge University Press; 2020.
12. Zocchetti C, Consonni D, Bertazzi PA. Relationship between prevalence rate ratios and odds ratios in cross-sectional studies. *International Journal of Epidemiology*. 1997;26(1):220–3.
13. Martinez BAF, Leotti VB, Silva GSE, Nunes LN, Machado G, Corbellini LG. Odds ratio or prevalence ratio? An overview of reported statistical methods and appropriateness of interpretations in cross-sectional studies with dichotomous outcomes in veterinary medicine. *Frontiers in Veterinary Science*. 2017;4:193.
14. Ministry of Health New Zealand. *New Zealand Health Survey*. 2023. www.health.govt.nz/nz-health-statistics/surveys/new-zealand-health-survey
15. Australian Bureau of Statistics (ABS). National Health Survey: First Results. ABS; 2018. www.abs.gov.au/statistics/health/health-conditions-and-risks/national-health-survey-first-results/latest-release#about-the-national-health-survey.
16. Australian Institute of Health and Welfare. *Australian Bureau of Statistics – National Health Survey (NHS)*. AIHW; 2023. www.aihw.gov.au/australias-disability-strategy/technical-resources/data-sources/australian-bureau-of-statistics-nhs
17. *The Lancet*. Global burden of disease. 2020. https://www.thelancet.com/gbd
18. Tominaga S, Kuroishi T. An ecological study on diet/nutrition and cancer in Japan. *Internal Journal of Cancer*. 1997;71:2–6.
19. Our World in Data. Life expectancy vs. GDP per capita. 2022. https://ourworldindata.org/grapher/life-expectancy-vs-gdp-per-capita

20. World Health Organization. Country, area, WHO region and global health statistics (Annex 1-1). *World Health Statistics 2023*. WHO; 2023. www.who.int/data/gho/publications/world-health-statistics

21. Papier K, Ahmed F, Lee P, Wiseman J. Stress and dietary behaviour among first-year university students in Australia: Sex differences. *Nutrition*. 2014;31(2):324–30.

22. Borg M, Bi P, Nitschke M, Williams S, McDonald S. The impact of daily temperature on renal disease incidence: An ecological study. *Environmental Health*. 2017;16(1):114.

7

Starting with the outcome

What do you think might cause headaches in health science students?

Learning objectives

After studying this chapter, you will be able to:

1. Describe the main features and uses of case-control studies
2. Understand the importance of case definition and selection of controls
3. Describe the main types of potential sources of bias in case-control studies and understand some of the methods to address these
4. Appreciate the strengths and limitations of case-control designs

Introduction

In Chapter 6 we heard about how we can identify and quantify associations between exposures and health outcomes within populations, and even between countries. We learnt how useful cross-sectional studies were for looking at a range of risk factors and outcomes as they exist in a defined population at a particular point in time. While they have a great number of advantages, it can sometimes be difficult to sort out the direction of the relationships identified using cross-sectional approaches – that is, current risk factors or exposures may not necessarily have caused current outcomes or diseases. If we want to move towards thinking about potential causal relationships, we need an approach that allows us to determine the relative strength of relationships between exposures and outcomes and provide some hints about temporality – that is, to give us a start on determining whether the exposure preceded the health event. We will need this type of study to address question posed for this chapter: What might be causing all those headaches that health science students seem to complain about?

Hugo: I think they are caused by all that calculating you make us do!

Rachael: But wouldn't non-health science students who don't get as many headaches have to do calculations too?

Author (Emma): I'm not sure that we have been asking you to do that many calculations! It is possible that calculations may be responsible, of course, but it could also be lots of other things. We need an epidemiological study design that will allow us to investigate the role of lots of potential exposures, including making you do too many calculations. We also need a design that would let us find out whether students who don't get as many headaches have the same exposure history.

Background rate: The rate of disease occurring in a population without direct exposure to a risk factor of interest.

We previously heard a little bit about surveillance (see Chapter 1), through which new cases of disease are notified to health authorities so that changes in disease occurrence can be monitored. One thing that might be noticed by authorities is an 'outbreak' (synonym 'epidemic'), which is an increase in the number of cases beyond what is normally expected for a particular region at a particular period of time (with the normal situation often referred to as the **background rate**). The number of cases at which an outbreak is declared varies from disease to disease and from area to area. For instance, a single case of locally acquired dengue (a mosquito-borne viral infection) is deemed an 'outbreak' in Queensland, Australia (1). In Kenya, where malaria (another disease involving mosquitos) is *endemic* (the persistent presence of a given disease in a specified population), authorities are required to regularly update specific regional thresholds based on the numbers of malaria cases notified in the previous five years. An outbreak will be declared once case numbers are notified above these regional thresholds, often set at above 50 cases per week, which will then trigger an appropriate response from health authorities (2).

For diseases such as dengue and malaria, which we know are transmitted by mosquitos and for which we have a good understanding of mitigation strategies, there are very well-established protocols for responding to outbreaks when they occur. However, the situation commonly arises that a defined case of disease, or other health event, is identified without a clear understanding of its cause or risk factors – similar to the case of headaches in health science students.

In this chapter, we will look at a type of study that is suitable when you are pretty sure about the outcome but want to find out more about the exposures or risk factors that are associated with that outcome: a case-control study.

Case-control studies

Case-control studies are observational (non-experimental) studies that start with the identification of 'cases', who are people experiencing the condition or event of interest. Then appropriate 'controls' are identified, which are people with similar characteristics to the cases who do not have the condition (glossing very lightly over the difficulties associated with selecting controls for now). Then both cases and controls are classified according to their exposure status and those histories are compared. The direction of investigation for case-control studies is presented in Figure 7.1.

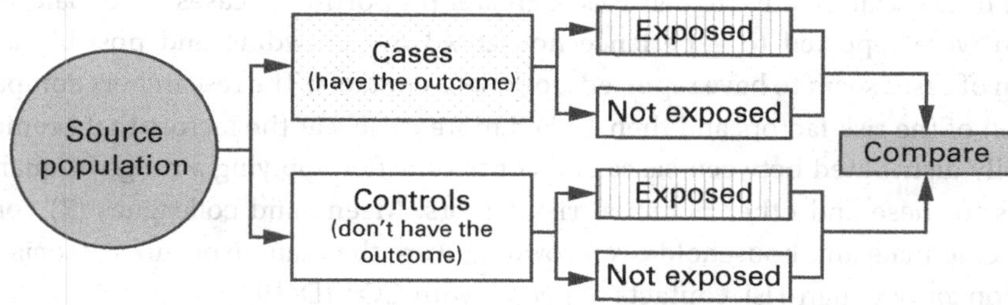

Figure 7.1 Direction of investigation for case-control studies

Case-control studies are also called 'case-referent' studies and, because the design looks back towards exposures that may have led to the current situation, are also known as 'retrospective' studies (not to be confused with a type of cohort study that we will hear about in Chapter 8). Because case-control designs allow for the investigation of multiple potential exposures that could be associated with a specified outcome, they provide the perfect design to quickly investigate things that have might have led to disease outbreaks. Investigations of outbreaks of gastrointestinal disease frequently undertake rapid case-control studies to identify potential contaminated food types, shared venues, caterers or food producers that might be associated with the cases. Case-control studies can also be used to identify risky practices that may have occurred in the past. Following an outbreak of COVID-19 in a district of India called Madurai, for instance, researchers were interested in knowing what characteristics and behavioural factors led to greater transmission of COVID-19 (3). During the period from March to May 2020, the researchers selected 139 people who were newly diagnosed with COVID-19 infection and identified those who could be described as 'high-risk contacts' due to the level of exposure they had to the infected person. The 'cases' were 50 high-risk contacts who subsequently tested positive to COVID-19 and the 'controls' were 551 high-risk contacts who tested negative to COVID-19. Table 7.1 presents how cases and controls are classified according to their exposure to selected risk factors for COVID-19 transmission.

Table 7.1 Distribution of risk factors among 601 cases and controls in Madurai, 2020. Adapted from (3).

Factor	Cases % (n = 51)	Controls % (n = 501)
Male	66	46
Female	34	54
Other health condition	14	7
No other health condition	8	93
Household overcrowding	90	65
No household overcrowding	10	35
Type of contact		
Household	84	87
Friends	8	7
Workplace	8	4
Healthcare	0	2

While these are by no means all the factors investigated in their study, can you see any differences between the exposure histories of cases and controls as presented in Table 7.1? You might notice that, relative to controls, a greater proportion of cases were male, a greater proportion were reported to experience household overcrowding and possibly a greater proportion of cases seem to have reported workplace contacts. The researchers compared the distribution of the risk factors and then looked more closely at the factors that seemed to be differentially distributed between cases and controls. After applying a range of quantitative techniques to these and other potential risk factors, Meena and colleagues (3) confirmed that that being male and household overcrowding were the main exposures associated with transmission among high-risk contacts of people with COVID-19.

Hugo: Great! Let's start looking at things that might be causing those headaches for health science students!

Rachael: But how do we know what to look for?

Author (Emma): This is an important point – deciding on potential exposures to look at isn't simply a fishing expedition …

Potential exposures

Deciding on potential exposures to investigate in case-control studies is not a random process, but is in fact based on a great deal of critical thinking. Investigators know a bit about the outcome of interest but must undertake some research to gain a good understanding of the types of exposures and risk factors that could be associated with that outcome. Analysis and evaluation of the available information helps the development of a list of potential exposures that might include what I like to call the 'usual suspects' because they nearly always play at least some part – things like age, sex, comorbidities (additional coexisting health conditions) and socioeconomic factors. Reviewing existing information will also help to develop a list of what I like to call the 'likely suspects' – factors that have played a part in similar conditions, or that informed reasoning suggests might be implicated.

If we were looking at the headache situation in health science students, for instance, we couldn't simply pull potential exposures out of a hat, but would need to carefully evaluate the evidence for potential risk factors and undertake some logical reasoning in order to develop a tight list of usual and likely suspects to investigate. It is possible that the excess calculations allegedly required of health science students might make the list of exposures, but looking at the relationship between headaches and, say, shoe colour might throw up some intriguing but probably misleading avenues of investigation. Applying critical thinking here will not only help to determine the exposures to look at but also help to explain any relationships identified and help to shape potential strategies for intervention.

Once we have developed our evidence-based list of exposures to investigate, we need to make sure that information on these exposures is available in relation to both cases and controls. Where possible, the exposure information should be derived from the same source for each group. When cases and controls are actively recruited for participation in a case-control study, exposure information may be collected directly from the participants via interviews or questionnaires. In non-clinical studies, this may actually be the only way such information can be collected. In investigating a food-borne disease outbreak, for instance, participants are directly interviewed to get a complete recent history of their food intake and sources of food to make sure all potential risk factors are identified (4), although sometimes data about the types of food eaten by healthy 'controls' are actually obtained from large-scale population surveys (5). Where available, objective measurements might provide high-quality exposure data. For instance, existing medical records might provide all that is needed to provide exposure data on COVID-19 outcomes in hospitalised patients (6) with no interviewing required. Many countries have established human tissue banks, or 'biobanks', which are essentially large repositories of human tissue specimens linked to demographic, genetic and health information that can be used by researchers to obtain high-quality exposure information (7). Finally, if active participants in a case-control study are too young, too ill or deceased, exposure information can be obtained from 'proxy' respondents such as a spouse, parent or other family member. For example, in a case-control study of hip fracture risks in elderly Australians, 27 per cent of the exposure information was derived from proxy respondents due to the health and cognition status of the elderly participants (8).

Each method of deriving exposure information introduces the potential for various types of bias. This, along with some of the complexities of selecting cases and controls in the first place, will be discussed in a little more detail later in this chapter. For now, let's assume that we have managed to recruit suitable participants to our study, about whom we now proudly possess high-quality exposure information. We now need a way to compare this information between our cases and controls so that we can easily quantify any differences in the distribution of exposures. The most common way is to do this is to develop a measure that describes the probability (or odds) of exposure in cases relative to the odds of exposure in the controls – the odds ratio (OR). A lot more detail about OR and other measures of association will be discussed in Chapter 10, but an introduction to OR is provided below.

Odds ratios

The OR (also known as a 'cross-product ratio' and 'relative odds') is essentially a ratio of the odds of an event occurring in one group relative to the odds of the same event occurring in another group. The OR can tell us a lot about the size and strength of a particular relationship between an exposure and outcome as well as how much the odds of exposure differ between groups, such as cases and controls. ORs are calculated by dividing the odds of exposure in cases by the odds of exposure in controls. If you had the same odds of exposure in both groups, dividing one number by another would equal 1. So, we interpret OR by how much it differs from 1 (known as the 'null' value). The null value of 1 means there is no difference in exposure between the two groups. If OR exceeds 1 (OR >1), it indicates that the odds of exposure are higher in cases. If OR is less than 1 (OR <1), the odds of exposure are lower in cases. Note that the OR relates to the odds of the *exposure* and not the risk of disease, as the disease has already developed.

EXAMPLE 7.1

One case-control study investigated factors associated with mortality in patients with severe COVID-19 infection admitted to a hospital in China (6).

A total of 124 patients were hospitalised with severe COVID-19 in early 2020, of whom 89 ultimately died and were classified as 'cases' and 35 recovered and were classified as 'controls'. The researchers then compared demographic details, clinical findings, and laboratory and radiographic changes occurring during the course of the infection in cases and controls.

Relative to controls (those who recovered), the researchers found that the most important risk factors associated with cases (those who died of COVID-19) were having lower oxygen saturation (OR 3); having differences in immune response to infection as measured by lower white blood cells called lymphocytes (OR 4) but higher liver proteins called C-reactive protein (OR 3); developing a blood infection (sepsis) measured by procalcitonin (OR 3); and having higher markers of disease or tissue damage as measured by the enzyme lactate dehydrogenase (OR 3). Neither time of admission after onset of symptoms (OR 1) nor body temperature at admission (OR 1) was associated with case status.

The researchers recommended using oxygen levels, immune markers, serum markers for sepsis and tissue damage to predict increased mortality risk when COVID-19 patients are admitted to hospital (6).

In Example 7.1, the researchers presented ORs to demonstrate the strength of the relationship between the different sorts of exposures and patients who died from COVID-19 (cases) relative to patients who recovered from COVID-19 (controls). The OR of 3 for lower oxygen at admission to hospital can be interpreted to mean that the odds of low oxygen were three times higher in cases than in controls. The OR of 4 for lower lymphocytes can be interpreted to mean that the odds of low lymphocytes was four times higher in cases compared with controls. The OR of 1 for both time of admission and appearance of symptoms means there was no difference in odds of this between cases and controls. Sometimes, you might read about an OR that is less than 1 – this could happen if you were looking at a protective exposure such as vaccines. For instance, one study estimated that people with symptomatic COVID-19 had an OR of 0.3 after having had three doses of vaccine (9). The OR of 0.3 can be interpreted as meaning that, relative to controls, cases had 70 per cent greater odds of being unvaccinated than vaccinated.

The way ORs are calculated is described in Explanation 7.1.

EXPLANATION 7.1: Calculating odds ratios

Construct a 2 x 2 table that cross-references the exposure status of cases and controls – disease status in the columns and exposure status in the rows (see Figure 7.2).

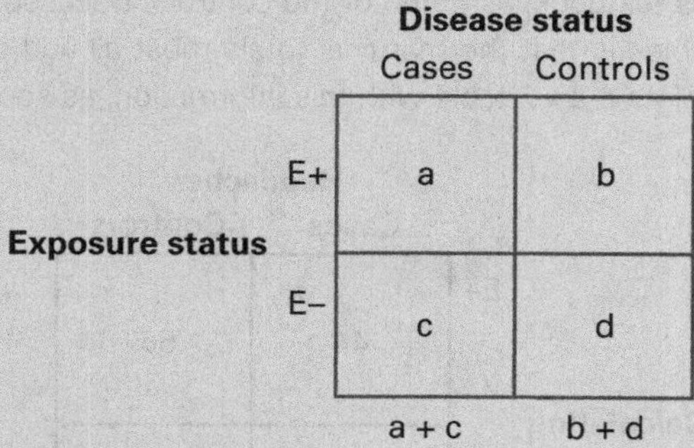

Figure 7.2 Cross-tabulation of case and exposure status to calculate OR.

Cells:

a = number of cases exposed to a particular risk factor
b = number of controls exposed to a particular risk factor
c = number of cases not exposed to a particular risk factor
d = number of controls not exposed to a particular factor
a + c = number of cases
b + d = number of controls
Odds of exposure in cases = a divided by c (a/c)
Odds of exposure in controls = b divided by d (b/d)

$$\text{OR} = \text{a/c divided by b/d} \left(\frac{a/c}{b/d}\right)$$

OR can also be calculated by ad/cb, which is why OR is also sometimes called a 'cross product ratio'.

Rachael: Okay … that all looks a bit headache producing …

Hugo: Can you show us how this works, Emma?

Author (Emma): I would love to – 2 x 2 tables are just about my most favourite thing in epidemiology!

Let us briefly return to the *hypothetical* example concerning headaches in health science students.

WORKED EXAMPLE 7.1

We will first identify health science students who have reported headaches in the past week; these students will be our cases. We will use students who haven't had headaches in the past week as our controls. Let's say we find 115 cases and select 200 controls (they don't have to be the same number in each group) and classify them by their exposure to epidemiological calculations. Say 44 of cases insist they have been diligently doing all the calculations described in this textbook, as do 56 of the controls. Because one of the many great properties of 2 x 2 tables is that the marginal totals must all add up, we now have enough information to complete a 2 x 2 table with this information, as seen in Figure 7.3

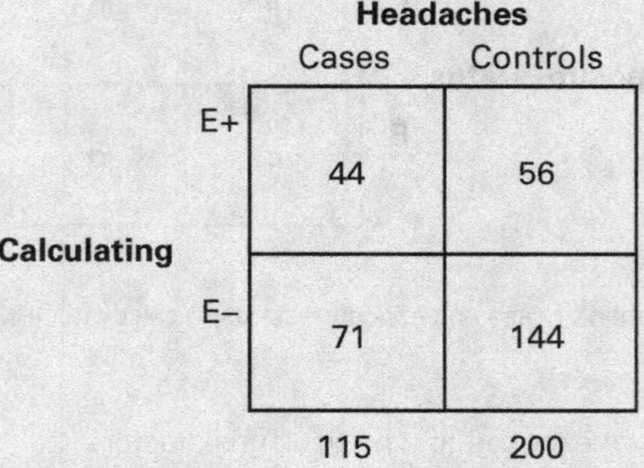

Figure 7.3 Headache status in health science students cross-tabulated by exposure to epidemiological calculations – set up to calculate an odds ratio (OR)

The OR is calculated by dividing the odds of exposure in the cases by the odds of exposure in the controls:

$$
\begin{aligned}
OR &= \frac{(a / c)}{(b / d)} \\
&= \frac{(44 / 71)}{(56 / 144)} \\
&= 0.62 / 0.39 \\
&= 1.59
\end{aligned}
$$

In Worked Example 7.1, we calculated an OR of around 1.6. This is a bigger number than 1, so the odds of calculating was higher in those experiencing headaches in the past week. The odds of doing calculations were more than one and a half times higher (or increased by 60 per cent) in cases compared with controls.

Rachael: That was a bit tricky, but I think I worked it out.

Hugo: I think I have a headache coming on.

Author (Emma): You do realise that this was a hypothetical example that in no way provides real evidence to support the calculating-headache relationship?

A little about *p* values and confidence intervals

In a real investigation using a case-control design, researchers will calculate odds ratios for all of the exposures and risk factors that interest them. They will usually do some statistical testing to assure themselves that the odds ratios are not just visually different from 1, but are what they call 'statistically' different from 1 (or the difference is 'statistically significant'). That is, researchers want to know that any differences they see are likely to be real differences and haven't just arisen by chance.

Researchers usually quantify the level of significance of odds ratios with what is known as a ***p* value** – the long-run probability that a result of the value they have calculated would have arisen by chance in a world where the OR would really be 1 (with 1 meaning that there is no difference between groups). We do not need to trouble ourselves with the actual statistical acrobatics here, but deriving the *p* value takes into account a number of things including the numbers of cases and controls in the study. The important thing to remember is that the *p* value is a measure of probability. *p* values have a maximum value of 1.0, which would indicate that the probability of the result arising by chance was 100 per cent (an unlikely claim in the world of science) ranging down to very tiny numbers, sometimes with multiple decimal points.

***p* value:** The long-run probability that a statistical finding of a particular value would have arisen by chance in a world defined by the null value.

The smaller the *p* value is, the less likely it is that the result would have arisen by chance and most researchers will decide to accept that their results are exciting, that they may have found a real difference, at a *p* value of 0.05. A *p* value of 0.05 essentially means that if I were to repeat this same measurement in study after study, having conducted those studies exactly as I have conducted this one, a result of this magnitude would arise on fewer than 5 per cent of occasions in a world defined by the null hypothesis. That is pretty unlikely, so if I had derived a *p* value that was small– or smaller – in relation to my OR of 1.6 for epidemiological calculations and headaches, I might start to think about accepting that this was a true difference (which, of course, we know is only hypothetical!).

There is some controversy about relying on *p* values to make decisions about the meaningfulness of findings, much of which centres on their misinterpretation and of the assumptions underpinning them (10, 11). Most researchers therefore also (and increasingly instead) report a range of values around their estimates, called a **confidence interval.** Like *p* values, confidence intervals are a statement of probability, but they also have other useful functions. They consist of a lower number and a higher number forming a range around the odds ratio or other outcome measure calculated in the study. Again, we do not have to consider the complex inner workings here, but both of the numbers in the confidence interval are based around various parameters including the size of the study – that is, the number of participants – and the statistically derived estimate of error in the measurement (a mystery for another day). They may be constructed around a single estimate of prevalence, a ratio, an estimate of a difference in means or any other statistic that might be developed from study results. Confidence intervals can also be set at any probability level, but typically they are set at the 95 per cent level. Essentially, the researcher is saying is that if we were to repeat this study over and over and obtain this measure again and again, in the long run, 95 per cent of those measures would lie between the upper and lower numbers of this confidence interval.

Confidence interval: A range of values constructed around an estimate arising from an analysis (e.g. odds ratios, prevalence, incidence rate) that represents the specified probability (typically, 95 per cent) that, on repeated measurements in the same circumstances, the true value will lie between the lower and upper bounds of the interval.

As well, confidence intervals can provide an idea of how precise a measurement is. Because of the factors that go into calculating confidence intervals, things such as sample size can make a big difference in how tightly the interval clusters around the study finding. For example, an estimate derived from a bigger study will have a narrower interval, while a small study will lead to a larger interval. Thus, a wide confidence interval indicates low precision (e.g. inaccuracy about the exact value of the measure) and a narrow confidence interval indicates higher precision. What actually constitutes a 'narrow' or 'wide' confidence interval has never been exactly specified. The main thing to understand is that confidence intervals clustering tightly around an estimate place limits on alternative values, while a certain amount of vagueness remains about the true value (along a range) associated with wider confidences.

A further useful property of confidence intervals is they can, like *p* values, tell us whether the finding that is presented is statistically different from the 'null' value. If the confidence interval includes the null value (which is a 1 for ORs), the result is not considered statistically significant. A 95 per cent confidence interval that includes the null value is essentially saying that the true value of the measure of interest could vary in either direction (e.g. the true OR could be anywhere from <1 to >1). Like *p* values, using confidence intervals alone to determine significance can lead to misinterpretation due to the influence of the statistical models underpinning them (10). Used cautiously, however, both *p* values and confidence intervals provide the best available guide to interpreting research findings. See Explanation 7.2 for examples of how to interpret *p* values and confidence intervals.

EXPLANATION 7.2: Interpreting *p* values

In our hypothetical example of headaches in health science students, depending on how we conducted the case-control study, we might hypothetically find:

'The OR for calculations was 1.6 ($p < 0.04$).'

- We can be pretty sure that the odds of calculations in cases was increased relative to controls and we can accept that this was a significant difference on the basis that there is less than 4 per cent probability that an OR of 1.6 could occur by chance if there wasn't real difference in exposure.

'The OR for calculations was 1.6 ($p = 0.23$).'

- We are not that sure about the difference in exposure between the cases and controls and cannot rule out that there is no difference at all. This is on the basis that there is up to a 23 per cent probability that an OR of 1.6 could have occurred by chance alone.

Interpreting 95 per cent confidence intervals

In our hypothetical example of headaches in health science students, depending on how we conducted the case-control study, we might hypothetically find:

'The OR for calculations was 1.6 (95% CI: 1.3, 1.9).'

- The confidence interval does not include 1, which is the null value, so this estimate of OR is statistically significant and denotes a real difference in risk between the cases and controls. The relative narrowness of the confidence interval also gives us some confidence in the precision of the estimate.

'The OR for calculations was 1.6 (95% CI: 1.1, 67.3).'

- The confidence interval does not include 1, so this sample estimate is also statistically significant and denotes a real difference in risk between cases and controls. However, the difference could be anything from very tiny (only 10 per cent higher odds of calculations) to very substantial (more than 67 times higher odds of calculations). The width of the confidence interval makes us a little uncertain about the precision of the estimate.

'The OR for calculations was 1.6 (95% CI: 0.9, 2.6).'

- The confidence interval includes 1, so this sample estimate is not statistically significant and an OR of 1.6 may have occurred completely by chance.

Some more information about interpreting *p* values and confidence intervals will come up throughout this book, and you will have lots of opportunity to become more familiar with these concepts via the review questions and through your reading of the scientific literature. For those who would like more detail, a useful open access student resource (12) is listed in the 'Further reading' section.

Rachael: I always wondered what those *p* things were that people reported in journal articles!

Hugo: As long as we don't have to calculate them, but I guess I get it ...

Author (Emma): If you want to get more into it, there is plenty more to know! But for the time being, it is really very useful to think about what they mean when you see them in the scientific literature.

Selecting cases and controls

In the discussions so far, I have hinted that the selection of cases and controls might not be quite as simple as it first appears to be. Here we will be looking at some of the complexities around defining cases and selecting controls.

Suitable cases

In case-control studies, we start by assembling a group of people who are known to be affected by a condition of interest. But herein lies the rub – what makes a case? The accurate definition of cases is actually a tricky business for both research and surveillance efforts when dealing with morbidity (illness) as opposed to mortality (death), with the latter being much easier to characterise. For just about all surveillance purposes, concise and (often) internationally agreed-upon case definitions are crucial. For instance, the WHO regularly prescribes expert-informed and agreed case definitions that include the circumstances for identifying suspected, probable and confirmed cases of a vast number of conditions. In relation to infectious disease, cases are usually defined using epidemiological and clinical evidence, probable cases are defined using the criteria for suspected cases plus evidence of direct links to other cases and confirmed cases are those that test positive using specified diagnostic or screening tests (sometimes in conjunction with other compelling epidemiologic or clinical evidence, depending on test accuracy). You might wish to view the WHO COVID-19 case definition in the 'Further reading' section (13).

Having a clear and tight case definition is important to ensure that we are measuring what we think we are. For surveillance purposes, cases may be defined in two ways:

- *Syndromic:* the case is defined by the pattern of clinical signs and symptoms with which they present (e.g. the simultaneous occurrence of fever, cough and fatigue is the agreed syndromic case definition for influenza).
- *Laboratory confirmed:* the case is defined by returning a specific laboratory test for the condition (e.g. a positive HIV virological or antigen test).

The importance of having consistent, reliable and valid case definitions to various areas of health science is described in Table 7.2.

Table 7.2 Importance of case definitions in health-related activities. Adapted from (14)

Surveillance	• Basis of case identification • Consistency and comparability in reporting • Tracking the presence and distribution of cases
Research	• Measure morbidity and mortality accurately • Detect biological markers • Ideally, depend on whether gold-standard tests available/accessible
Clinical care	• Early case finding • Isolation of infectious diseases cases • Allows timely initiation treatment and infection control
Service provision	• Crucial to effective outbreak investigation • Standardisation of the cases during epidemic investigations • Allows comparisons between outbreaks at different times and places

In case-control studies, validly identifying cases of the condition of interest is a critical first step, requiring some sort of operational and standardised definition that can be applied consistently. Ideally, cases will be incident cases (newly diagnosed), as this will aid in the accurate recollection of potential exposures and the identification of contemporary information from medical records. In the investigation of an active outbreak, it can be easier to select incident cases of acute disease. Cases are typically defined by clusters of symptoms and can be confirmed by laboratory testing, and contain elements of person, time and place. For example, in relation to an outbreak of food-borne disease (15), a case definition might include the following elements:

- *Clinical symptoms:* gastrointestinal illness (e.g. vomiting and x number of loose stools over a defined period)
- *Laboratory results:* pathogen (e.g. bacteria, serotype)
- *Person:* age group, sex, occupation, exclusion criteria (e.g. aged 5 to 10 years, females, primary school teacher, chronic gastrointestinal conditions excluded)
- *Time:* onset of illness (e.g. symptoms appeared on or after 17 March)
- *Place:* specified location, specified source (e.g. school sports event, catering company).

In contexts other than the investigation of active outbreaks of infectious disease, it can be a little harder to identify incident cases. In reality, investigators usually have to compromise, particularly when the condition of interest is rare. Investigating rare diseases is actually one of the greatest benefits of a case-control study design, as we don't have to wait for cases to occur but can select a group of existing cases that are usually sourced from medical records and disease registries. This means the cases selected for study are most often prevalent rather than incident cases. For instance, you might want to conduct a case-control study on a rare type of cancer, and decide to approach a cancer registry to identify your cases. Since many jurisdictions have mandatory notification of new cancer cases to state registries, this would make a great source of confirmed incident cases of the cancer that interests you (subject to appropriate approvals, of course). However, the data are generally subject to substantial delays in notification, registering, cross-checking, governance and privacy protocols before they might finally be made available, sometimes years after their initial diagnosis. In a well-established cancer registry of one Australian jurisdiction, for instance, data are only available following up to a three-year time lag (16). In the United States, the 'standard delay' even to report new cases to the registry after diagnosis is two years, with incidence data then only reported publicly the following year (17). Further, considerable time might elapse before sufficient numbers of cases of rare cancers are notified to be part of a case-control study in the first place.

Using prevalent cases may end up being an unavoidable compromise; however, in case-control studies that actively recruit participants, this can make it difficult to untangle whether exposures are associated with case status or with surviving the condition in the first place. Clearly, being dead would preclude recruitment opportunities! Indeed, the same issues could arise when actively recruiting incident cases affected by conditions of short duration but with high mortality. In case-control studies using only medical and/or registry data – that is, that do not involve active participation of cases – survival-related issues can be less problematic, but at the cost of being restricted solely to the information that has been documented.

Whether investigating diseases of short or long duration, rare or common, infectious or non-communicable, it is important that case definitions be reliable, valid and applied consistently within the study to avoid misclassification of cases and controls, and misleading conclusions. Tight and specific case definitions also allow comparability with other research on the same health condition and ultimately contribute to appropriate intervention strategies.

Suitable controls

If there are complexities surrounding defining cases, the problem of identifying suitable controls can be even more fraught.

Rachael: Oh no! Why is it always so complicated?

Hugo: Seriously, what is it with epidemiology?

Author (Emma): I would argue that overcoming the complexities is like solving a puzzle (which is right up my alley!) as well as contributing to the methodological rigour of epidemiological studies.

If we are going to make comparisons between the exposure histories of cases and controls, we would want to select controls that are as similar to the cases as possible. This is so we can have a little more confidence that it is the exposures, not characteristics of the participants themselves, that are most likely to be associated with case or control status. If we are interested in looking at arthritis, say, we might recruit cases from a clinic population. We could be very clear about our case definition and so make sure that we can exclude arthritis in our potential controls. Clearly, a group of children recruited from the local school would not make a great comparison group. We already know that advancing age and obesity are strongly associated with arthritis and both of these characteristics are far less likely to be found in school children. Further, all sorts of potential exposures that we might want to investigate are also more likely to occur in older people than school-aged people. We wouldn't know if potential exposures such as smoking, alcohol consumption or sedentary activity patterns were associated with arthritis or with the relative age of the cases and controls.

We need to source the controls from a population that is similar to the population in which the cases were identified, but which is likely to represent 'normal' exposure levels to provide a basis of valid comparison.

Sources of controls

Generally, controls are best drawn from a population at risk for the condition of interest. The population may be the same population that gave rise to the cases or one that is comparable to that population. Controls may be completely disease free or have other diseases, depending on what specific exposures and their relationships are being investigated. The other important principles for controls is that they must be selected independently of their exposure status and must not be eligible to be a case themselves.

Community or *population-based* controls might be identified from random samples of the whole population or of neighbourhoods, potentially also randomly selected samples of those with demographic similarities to the cases. Telephone number listings, electoral registers or rolls of registered voters – for example, in the United States – can be used to identify potential controls. For our arthritis study, we might randomly identify only older age groups in the population. We could also identify potential controls from aged-related community groupings, such as church or social groups. We could even go knocking door to door in a particular location or use random telephone dialling methods. Poor response rates, however, are a serious and increasing issue for population-based recruitment, especially when participants are required to complete a survey or provide a sample (18).

Clinic- or hospital-based patients can be a good source of controls that are easy to identify and tend to have higher response rates than population-based controls. In our hypothetical arthritis investigation, we might recruit controls from the same primary healthcare practice attended by the cases. If our cases were hospitalised, we could recruit controls from a different ward in the same hospital. The important selection criteria for controls would be that they are not presenting to the primary healthcare practice/clinic or hospitalised with a condition that has similar risk factors. For instance, cardiovascular patients might not make a good comparison for lung cancer patients, since both conditions are associated with smoking. Due to this, we might be tempted to select controls from hospitalised or clinic-based patients with a disease that differs substantially from the condition affecting cases. However, a consideration here might be that the controls start to be quite unrepresentative of the population that gave rise to the cases.

Relatives or *friends* of cases have also been used as controls and can be quite representative of the population from which the cases arose. Using friends and family for controls can produce good response rates, but such people have far more similarities in genetics, social pastimes and behavioural factors than randomly selected controls and so also share many of the same exposure histories with the cases to which they are related (19).

While there are issues with all types of control selection, both methodological and statistical steps can be taken to minimise some of these issues. One of these is the idea of not using actual controls at all. As discussed earlier in this chapter, comparison exposure data might sometimes be obtained from large-scale population nutrition history surveys (5), from medical records (6) or from human tissue repositories or 'biobanks' (7).

Addressing the control problem

I mentioned earlier that we don't have to have the same number of cases and controls. I also mentioned that more precision was associated with larger studies. So, we can increase the likelihood that our controls will be representative of the population giving rise to the cases by increasing the number of controls. More controls per case, who can be sourced from the same or multiple population groups, will also increase the ability of our study to find any differences between the exposure histories of cases and controls (known as the statistical 'power' of the study – more on this in later chapters).

Another method used to increase the similarities of cases and controls is to consider 'matching', which can be done either on an individual or group level. In individual matching, for every case a control is selected that is matched for characteristics that might otherwise confuse the relationship between exposures of interest and case status. For instance, if we were looking at exposures that might be associated with arthritis, we could match each of our cases (those with arthritis) with a control person. A female case aged 74 years could be matched with a female control aged 74 years, a male case aged 81 years could be matched with a male control of the same age, and so on. If we then found associations between a risk factor or exposure, we would know that age and sex were not involved in the relationship.

In group matching, we would match our controls on the proportion of the cases with certain characteristics. For example, if 63 per cent of our cases were female and 57 per cent were assessed as having low socioeconomic status, 63 per cent of our controls would also be female and 57 per cent would have low socioeconomic status. Group matching allows us to create a control group with identical proportions of whatever characteristics are deemed important.

Matching does allow us to 'control' for variables that might confuse relationships between exposures and case status, but there are consequences. Once you have matched on a characteristic, it is no longer possible to investigate that characteristic as a potential exposure. Over-matching (matching on the basis of multiple characteristics) can make it very difficult to find suitable controls that meet all the matching variables required. The other (not insurmountable) consequence is that different statistical methods are required for analysing data from matched relative to unmatched case-control studies, as well as for individual versus group matching. While it is important to be aware of this, we will not trouble ourselves further with these statistical hijinks.

A real-life example of a case-control study is presented in Example 7.2. Take a look and see how many of the epidemiological concepts you now recognise.

EXAMPLE 7.2

Researchers in London investigated why people from minority ethnic backgrounds seemed to be getting far sicker with COVID-19 and have worse outcomes than other COVID-19 patients (20).

Part of their investigation involved undertaking a case-control study of hospitalised COVID-19 patients (cases), matched to non-hospitalised COVID-19 patients (controls) from the same inner-city area who were identified in a primary healthcare clinical database. Four controls were individually matched to each case on the characteristics of age and sex. There were 872 cases and 3488 matched controls.

Using complex statistical methods (on account of the matching and other reasons), the researchers found higher odds of being Black among hospitalised patients than in controls (OR 3.1, 95% CI: 2.6, 3.7) as well as higher odds for mixed ethnicity (OR 3.0, 95% CI: 2.3, 3.9). Further statistical acrobatics revealed that adjusting for additional illnesses (comorbidities) and low socioeconomic status only slightly reduced these associations (OR 2.2, 95% CI: 1.8, 2.7 for being Black; OR 2.7, 95% CI: 2.0–3.6 for mixed ethnicity). Asian ethnicity was not associated with higher admission risk (OR 1.0, 95% CI: 0.7, 1.5).

The researchers concluded that being admitted to hospital with COVID-19 was associated with higher odds of being Black or of mixed ethnicity (but not Asian), and this was only partially explained by comorbidities and socioeconomic status (20).

Rachael: I can see that the study design is a matched case-control study, and they would have matched and used more controls per cases to increase the similarities between them!

Hugo: And the ORs for Black or mixed ethnicity were greater than 1 and had significant confidence intervals!

Author (Emma): That is exactly right! Perhaps someone should do a case-control study to see whether understanding epidemiological concepts is associated with higher odds of having read this book!

Bias in case-control studies

Measurement bias: (synonym 'information bias') Systematic error introduced by inaccurate and/or inconsistent measurement of study variables or misclassification of participants according to exposure or disease status.

One of the main things about case-control studies is that, despite being classified as observational studies, they involve artificial groupings of people. We are not just watching to see what happens to people, but are actively selecting them based on their case or control status. Case-control studies usually collect data about exposure retrospectively, sometimes long after the actual exposure occurred. Now this situation introduces a whole world of woe in terms of the potential for bias of both major types – selection and **measurement bias.** Selection bias occurs when participants are selected for a study (or the information about them is included) but have different characteristics from those who are not selected for study. Measurement bias can occur when measurements taken or other information collected are inconsistently accurate. Both selection and measurement bias will lead to misleading findings from which valid inferences cannot be made about the real world – the major point of most quantitative studies. There are actually multiple sub-categories of selection and measurement bias that will be discussed in detail in Chapter 11, but here we will outline those most associated with case-control studies.

Selection bias

As described earlier, cases are often selected from registry or surveillance system notifications, hospitals, community clinics and elsewhere. If we were looking at a social phenomenon, such as homelessness or those experiencing poverty, we might try to select cases accessing community-based organisations or charities. Then we would attempt to select appropriate controls using similar contact points. If we want to have something to say about all people with the condition, or all those experiencing the social phenomenon, we want both of our comparison groups to look as much like the true population as possible. Because study participants do not tend to be random samples of the population but are usually samples of convenience (although some designs do incorporate some level of randomness, particularly in relation to selection of controls), extreme care should be taken to recognise and minimise the impact of selection bias if we want to investigate the true relationship between exposures and case status.

In our earlier discussion of the issues involved in identifying suitable cases and controls, I mentioned that prevalent rather than incident cases are often recruited to case-control studies. I touched on the possibility that our sample of cases might end up excluding people who had already died of the condition of interest, which is actually a situation that could be described by epidemiologists as **survivor bias**. This might result in the selection of a sample of cases that doesn't represent the range of cases and their exposures that would occur in the real world, because those with particular disease and/or physiological characteristics did not survive to be selected (21). Another type of survivor bias known to investigators of workplace-related conditions is called the **healthy worker effect**. In this situation, unwell workers leave the workplace due to their health status, leaving those who are least affected by both the condition and the workplace exposure to be recruited (22). Thus, both types of survivor bias run the risk of reducing the study's ability to identify potentially important exposures, since those with high exposure would have been systematically excluded from being selected as cases.

Survivor bias: (synonym 'survivorship bias') Occurs when a sample of participants (or their data) includes only those who still exist (are alive, or are still in the setting of interest) and omits those who are no longer alive or available. This is a particular problem when their absence is related to the phenomenon of interest (a form of selection bias).

Healthy worker effect: A problem for studies looking at occupational exposures that results in lower incidence of disease in workers relative to the general population due to sicker persons having already left the workforce (a form of selection bias).

The problem of introducing selection bias doesn't stop at recruitment but continues to exert an influence at various points until data collection is complete. Depending on what sampling method is used to identify our cases and controls, we then will need to apply our inclusion and exclusion criteria. These will include our case definitions (described above) and any other specifications that are important to our investigation – for example, duration of illness, age groups, sex, and so on. Such attributes might be important to answer our specified scientific question but, again, start to move our cases and controls away from representing the real-world picture. The picture becomes even more distorted when people deemed eligible to be in our study decline to participate. As we have already seen, poor response rates during control selection can impact their representativeness and lead to bias (18).

Once we have successfully recruited our cases and controls, we then face the problem of non-response and missing information. Selection bias also includes the actual data included in the analysis (21). So, if your participants are unwilling or unable to provide the information your investigation requires, or this information is not available from medical records or elsewhere, those participants will not feature in your analysis.

Figure 7.4 shows how study groups can eventually come to look completely different from the populations from which they were sampled, and also come to have unrepresentative exposure histories. Selection bias can be introduced at any stage through the sampling method, via the inclusion criteria, in the recruitment process and through to non-response and incomplete information.

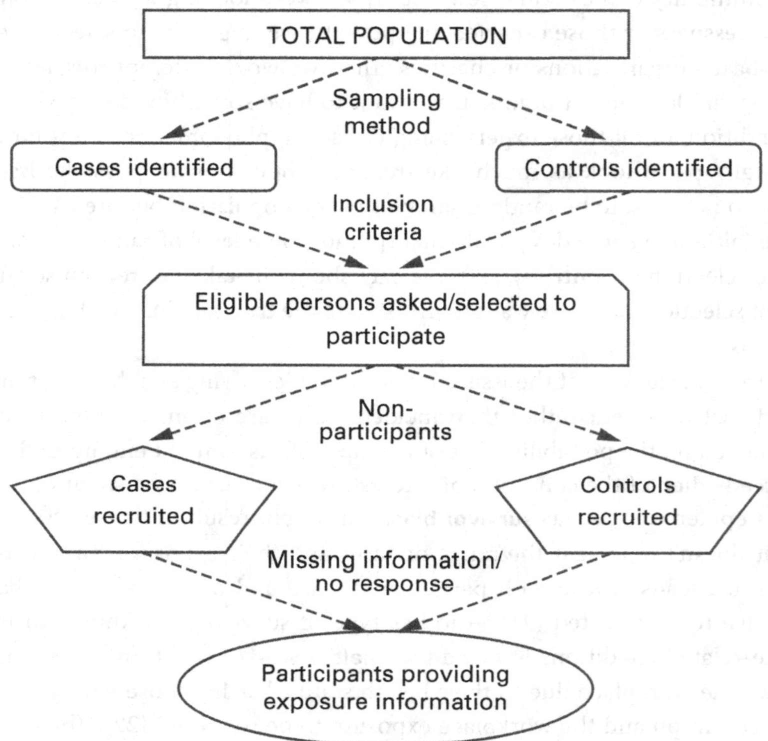

Figure 7.4 Potential for introducing bias during the process of sample selection

The potential for selection bias can never be eliminated, but steps can be taken to minimise, or at least measure, its potential impact. The first thing to do is to consider all the places where selection bias can occur (see Figure 7.4) and take active steps to minimise the potential at the time. This means potential sources of bias should be anticipated from the outset and steps to minimise these sources should be specifically described in the study protocol (the written guide for how a study is to proceed). In published studies, you should find a full account of all the steps taken to minimise bias in the methods section. The conclusions of any study should take into account the near-certainty of persistent sources of bias (usually written in the limitations section). Any confident assertions you might read to the contrary, or omission of discussion on potential bias noted, should be a red flag to all critical thinkers to question the quality of the study being read.

The steps to minimise selection bias include paying attention to much of what has already been discussed in this chapter. Precise case and exposure definitions should be used by all investigators and those in the control group should be selected independently of their exposure status while reflecting the population that gave rise to the cases. As well, strategies that improve participation can reduce the problem of incomplete data through achieving higher response rates. Things that make it easier to contribute information will help here. For instance, careful attention to designing surveys so they only include questions to collect information that is absolutely required will take less time to complete and reduce the overall burden on participants. Sending reminders to participants – for example, by email or SMS – to complete their surveys can sometimes be helpful in increasing response rates, as can including digital links to online surveys rather than relying on paper-based surveys. In case-control studies that don't involve active participants, careful planning ahead of time will ensure it is actually possible to obtain any health record information required, and that these data are routinely and consistently recorded and readily accessible. In such cases, a data collection form or database interface that reflects the order in which data are stored in medical records can greatly improve both the efficiency and completeness of data collection.

Measurement bias

Measurement bias is a systematic error introduced by inaccurate and/or inconsistent measurement of study variables, leading to the misclassification of exposures attributed to cases or controls. Because they rely on exploring exposure histories, the major type of measurement bias to which case-control studies are most prone is known as 'recall bias'. Many studies types involving interviewing participants can be affected by problems of recall, as the ability to remember facts about anything varies from person to person and tends to worsen as time passes. This is a particular problem in case-control studies, as much of the exposure information is obtained from interviewing cases and controls. As well as simply forgetting experiences, there are some exposures that people might be reluctant to disclose, particularly where the behaviour involved might be frowned upon, illegal or stigmatised (behaviours with respect to substance misuse, for instance). Now, as long as the level of forgetting or reluctance to disclose is roughly the same for both cases and controls, we still have the problem of inaccurate measurement, but we haven't really introduced a bias. Actual recall bias is when there is differential recollection between cases and controls.

Recall bias is thought to be a serious problem in case-control studies that rely on participants for exposure information because the risk of differential recollection of exposures among cases and controls is almost always present. For example, if you have developed a strange rash that keeps you up itching at night, you will probably spend your hours of torture thinking about all the things you have eaten, touched or otherwise come into contact with that may have caused the rash. If I selected you as a case of 'mysterious rash disease', even many weeks later you would likely be able to provide far greater detailed information about your exposure history than would, say, one of your friends, selected as a control because they didn't have a rash.

A fairly well-known Australian example of potential recall bias pertains to white-tail spider bites and the development of ulcerative and necrotic skin lesions. Despite strong evidence against the relationship, the fear of white-tail spider-induced necrosis persists across the population, with the creatures blamed for many chronic ulcerative skin conditions even when no evidence of spider bites exists (23). Results from a hypothetical example of a case-control study of the relationship between white-tail spider bites and the development of ulcerative and necrotic skin conditions is presented in Table 7.3. Cases are people who have newly developed ulcerative skin lesions, and controls are those who did not develop a skin lesion. Since white-tail spiders are frequently suspected, even when patients do not remember having been bitten by one (24), the exposure is defined as having seen a white-tail spider nearby in the previous six months. For the sake of the exercise, let's assume we have the amazing ability to know with certainty the true exposure history (reality) so that we can compare it with what is reported by our participants.

Table 7.3 Hypothetical example of recall bias in the development of skin ulcers and presumed white-tail spider bites – 80 cases, 100 controls

	Cases	Controls	OR
Reality			
Saw a white-tail spider	12	15	1.0
Did not see a white-tail spider	68	85	
Perceived reality			
Saw a white-tail spider	38	10	10.8
Did not see a white-tail spider	42	90	

Rachael: Eeeew! Spiders and necrosis in the same sentence!

Hugo: First, necrotising ulcers, yuck! Second, why would people think they saw spiders if they didn't?

Author (Emma): As I mentioned, people with a condition of some type tend to spend time thinking about possible causes and these people may have even heard the myth about white-tail spiders. Perhaps the interviewer had heard the myth too, and interviewed the cases slightly differently to controls. In comparison, the controls may have seen just as many spiders but forgot about it because nothing jogged their memory over the past six months. (Also – hopefully you have attempted the calculations yourself and came up with the same ORs as in Table 7.3.)

Incidentally, I have used a hypothetical example in Table 7.3 as there are actually very few demonstrated instances of recall bias in case-control studies published in scientific journals. It may well be that the peer-review process for journal submissions is working (see Chapter 1), or perhaps studies clearly affected by recall bias are not even submitted to journals in the first place. Nonetheless, there remains a strong potential for recall bias in case-control studies that could vastly influence conclusions, as demonstrated by the large difference in the ORs calculated for our hypothetical example (Table 7.3). So, it remains crucial to take steps to minimise the potential for recall bias in case-control studies.

As with selection bias, the best ways to address measurement bias is to recognise the potential from the outset and attempt to minimise this potential as much as possible in the study design. If we were taking actual physical measurements, such as body temperature or blood glucose levels, we would make sure we were using the most accurate technology, that the technology was properly calibrated and that it was used consistently for each test and by everyone conducting the tests. If we were collecting exposure information using a survey, we could ensure that the questions were unambiguous and collected the actual information we were expecting. We might 'pilot' the survey by getting a representative group to test it ahead of the real study or get a group of people to complete it again after a period of time and then test the level of agreement between their responses. We would keep the survey as brief as possible to prevent participant fatigue and, where possible, use questions that had previously been 'validated' (tested for accuracy) by other researchers.

Improving recall for both cases and controls can be achieved by minimising as much as possible the time period that participants are required to remember. Strategies such as providing participants with a list of possible exposures can help by acting as cues to memory. Providing contextual information in brief examples can facilitate participant recall of long past events and using non-judgemental language can help to reduce reluctance to disclose information about stigmatised risk behaviours. Strategies that address recall bias (differential recall) could include selecting cases and controls that have both had reason to consider the possible causes of their condition. If you recruited cancer patients for cases, you might consider recruiting controls who have been diagnosed with a different type of cancer. To address both differential and non-differential recall errors, we might consider using more than one source for the same information, such as using medical records or secondary interviewees in addition to primary surveys and interviews.

Strengths and limitations of case-control studies

Given all you have heard so far, it probably won't surprise you to hear that there are advantages and disadvantages associated with case-control research designs. There are certainly occasions when only a case-control study will do. For instance, if we have a good understanding of a particular condition, but don't know what might be causing it, case-control designs allow us to investigate a range of exposures and provide the first evidence of causal relationships. In fact, strong evidence from case-control studies can inform swift public health action in outbreak situations. For instance, a 2015 outbreak of hepatitis A cases in Australia was so strongly epidemiologically linked to imported frozen berries that the product was removed from supermarket shelves before the organism was even isolated in the product (25).

Although an almost endless (well, within reason) variety of exposures can be investigated in a case-control study, we are stuck with the outcome that defines the cases – that is, we have selected our participants on the basis of their case status and so have lost the freedom to explore the relationships between exposures and other conditions. The other consequence of having selected the cases (rather than waiting for the condition of interest to occur in a group of people) is that it is not possible to generate incidence data from a case-control study. This means we can't provide an estimate of the risk of developing a particular condition in a given population. If the condition is a rare one, however, we can happily use a case-control design to look at causes and contributing factors in a way than runs rings around other epidemiological designs. We don't have to sit around waiting for cases to occur but can spread our net wide and identify as many cases as we need to, and find out exposure information right away without going through the trouble of following-up a large number of people over time (and, for rare conditions, this can be a very large population followed up for a very long time) and losing contact with many of them along the way. Because case-control studies tend to be small and the exposure information is already existing and waiting to be collected, findings can be very quickly generated at relatively low cost. What's not to love about case-control studies?

Well, we have already discussed the difficulties in finding suitable controls and have heard quite a bit about how prone case-control studies can be to bias – particularly that form of measurement bias known as recall bias. Because of this, case-control studies are considered less 'rigorous' (scientifically sound and unbiased) than some other epidemiological designs, such as cohort studies or randomised controlled trials, although they do improve on case reports and other cross-sectional designs that do not include controls. Finally, with precise case definitions and exposure criteria, case-control studies can be designed to provide some hints about temporality (that the exposure preceded the outcome); however, the precise order of events can get muddled – particularly when dealing with chronic conditions. For instance, does consuming diet drinks lead to obesity or is consuming diet drinks a response to obesity (26)? To truly explore the sequence of events, a cohort study would work better, and this is the focus of Chapter 8.

Some of the advantages and disadvantages of case-control studies are presented in Table 7.4.

Table 7.4 Advantages and disadvantages of case-control studies. Adapted from (27).

Advantages	Disadvantages
Can investigate a wide range of potential exposures and risk factors	Cannot be used to generate incidence data
Useful for investigating rare diseases	Not suitable for the investigation of rare study factors or exposures
No losses to follow up	Difficulty in sourcing appropriate controls
Can generate findings quickly and (relatively) cheaply	Subject to selection and measurement bias (particularly prone to recall bias)
	Problems in sorting out sequence of events

Rachael: We should go and do a case-control study now and finally find out what's causing headaches in health science students!

Hugo: I guess we could look at lots of headache-provoking exposures, but my money is still on all the calculating.

Author (Emma): I agree, a case-control study is the best design for investigating potential causes of rare conditions!

Conclusion

In this chapter, we have learnt about the main features and uses of case-control studies, how they can be used to measure exposures and how we can calculate the odds of exposure in cases relative to controls. We also introduced the concept of statistical significance, including a brief look at interpreting *p* values and confidence intervals. Below are summaries of the ways we addressed each of the learning objectives.

Learning objective 1: Describe the main features and uses of case-control studies

We learnt that case-control studies start with the identification of cases of the condition of interest, and we compare their exposure histories with those of a comparison group without the condition, called controls. We also had a go at calculating odds ratios (OR), which are the main method of measuring the strength of the association between exposures and cases in case-control studies.

Learning objective 2: Understand the importance of case definition and selection of controls

We learnt how developing precise and clear case definitions assists in the identification of cases, decreases the potential for misclassification and misleading findings and increases the capacity for comparing findings with other studies. We also discussed the pros and cons of using incident and prevalent cases. We learnt how controls should, as much as possible, resemble the population that gave rise to the cases and the various strategies for achieving this.

Learning objective 3: Describe the main types of potential sources of bias in case-control studies and understand some of the methods to address these

We learnt that selection bias and measurement bias were the main broad categories of bias that apply in studies. We discussed how selection bias can be introduced at all stages throughout the conduction of the study, from recruitment to data analysis. We identified the main type of measurement bias associated with case-control studies as recall bias because exposure data are collected retrospectively. We also had a brief look at strategies for minimising the potential for selection and measurement bias in case-control studies.

Learning objective 4: Appreciate the strengths and limitations of case-control designs

We finished the chapter by looking at the advantages and disadvantages of case-control studies. We learned that case-control studies were really good at examining a range of exposures that could guide rapid public health action in outbreaks and were great at looking at rare diseases but not rare exposures. While case-control studies are a good first step, we learnt that to fully explore the temporality of exposures and outcomes, we would need other designs, which will be explored in the next few chapters.

Further reading

Fein, EC, Gilmour, J, Machin, T, Hendry, L. *Statistics for Research Students: An Open Access Resource with Self-Tests and Illustrative Examples*. University of Southern Queensland; 2022. https://usq.pressbooks.pub/statisticsforresearchstudents

World Health Organization (WHO). WHO COVID-19 case definition. 2022. www.who.int/publications/i/item/WHO-2019-nCoV-Surveillance_Case_Definition-2022.1

Questions

Answers are available at the end of the book.

Multiple-choice questions

1. Which of the following scientific questions can be answered using a case-control study design?
   A – What is the incidence of breast cancer in low socioeconomic areas of Pakistan?
   B – What is the risk of cardiovascular disease in smokers relative to non-smokers?
   C – What risk factors are associated with the development of Alzheimer's disease?
   D – What is the experience of single parents living in metropolitan areas?
2. Epidemiologists were investigating an outbreak of hepatitis A in a small village in India. They asked everyone in the village to provide a comprehensive history of their food preparation and consumption practices, then waited to see whether more cases of hepatitis arose during a two-week study period. Is this an example of a case-control study? Why or why not?
   A – Yes. The investigators compared exposure histories among those with hepatitis and those without hepatitis.
   B – No. The direction of study was from exposure to outcome, with the proportion affected by hepatitis unknown at the outset.
   C – Yes. All the villagers had an equal chance of being in the study, which was a strategy to reduce the potential for selection bias.
   D – No. Case-control studies are not appropriate for studying outbreaks of infectious diseases.
3. How does having clear and precise case definitions assist in the surveillance of disease across populations?
   A – Ensures consistency of reporting across time and place
   B – Allows accurate measurement of morbidity and mortality
   C – Facilitates early case finding and isolation of infectious cases
   D – All of the above.
4. What among the following is an important principle for selecting controls in case-control studies?
   A – Controls must be completely disease free.
   B – The controls should not have been exposed to the same risk factors as the cases.
   C – The controls should come from a population that is as comparable as possible to that in which the cases arose.
   D – Controls must be from the same population as the cases.
5. A case-control study was conducted on risk factors associated with cardiovascular disease. Cases were hospitalised patients with diagnoses of coronary heart disease and controls were randomly selected from the neighbourhood serviced by the hospital. What main sort of bias might be introduced by this design?
   A – Survivor bias
   B – Measurement bias
   C – Selection bias
   D – Recall bias.

Short-answer questions

1. A researcher is planning to undertake an investigation on chronic asthma in adults. Specifically, they want to look at the relationship between childhood exposures and risk factors and chronic asthma in adults. Would a case-control study be the best study design to investigate this relationship? If so, why? If not, why not?
2. An investigation was undertaken in high school students to see whether academic success was associated with extra reading and writing support during primary school. At the end of the academic year, Year 10 high school students with average grades that were above those achieved by 75 per cent of their classmates were interviewed about their participation in volunteer-led reading and writing support programs in primary school, engagement in homework activities and any family support for academic activities provided at home. The same information was obtained from their classmates whose grades were, on average, at the 75 per cent or lower range of academic achievement. What sort of study design is this and what are the features that make you think so?
3. Having clear and consistent case definitions is very important for all sorts of purposes in the health sciences. After conducting a brief search on the internet, develop a case definition that might apply to one of the conditions on the following list and explain your reasoning:
   - asthma
   - diabetes (either type 1 or 2)
   - obesity
   - influenza.
4. If you were to undertake a case-control study on the condition defined in Question 3, where would you source your cases and what controls would you use?
5. Table 7.5 shows the association of sociodemographic factors and multi-drug resistant tuberculosis among cases and controls in India. Comment on the distribution of the characteristics in cases and controls. *Hint: look at the differences in percentages that are presented.*

Table 7.5 Characteristic of study participants with multi-drug resistant TB at a TB-specialised hospital in India, 2011 – 90 cases and 90 controls. Adapted from (28).

	Cases – n (%)	Controls – n (%)
Age in years		
≤30	66 (73.3)	38 (42.2)
>30	24 (26.7)	52 (57.8)
Sex		
Male	41 (45.6)	52 (57.8)
Female	49 (54.4)	38 (42.2)
Literacy		
Able to read	11 (12.2)	22 (24.4)
Unable to read	79 (87.8)	68 (75.6)
Relationship status		
Partnered	62 (68.9)	43 (47.8)
Single	28 (31.1)	47 (52.2)

6. Complete Table 7.5 by calculating the odds ratios for each of the four exposure categories. Remember that OR is calculated by dividing the odds of exposure in cases by the odds of exposure in controls: OR = (a/c)/(b/d). *Hint: in your calculations, use either only the counts in each cell or only the percentages in each cell.*
7. How do you interpret the ORs that you calculated for Question 6 and added to Table 7.5?
8. The authors of the findings in Table 7.4 (28) also calculated confidence intervals for each of their odds ratios (hopefully you calculated the same results!). If I were to tell you just one of these confidence intervals, how would it change your interpretation of the findings? The 95 per cent confidence interval associated with the OR for literacy is 0.19 to 1.95.
9. Marouf et al. (29) conducted a case-control study looking at the relationship of dental health and outcomes for hospitalised COVID-19 patients in Qatar. They used national data from health records in Qatar for the period February to July 2020. Patients who developed severe COVID-19 complications (such as ICU admissions and death) were cases. Controls were COVID-19 patients who recovered and were discharged without major complications. They used dental x-rays to identify the main exposures of interest, which were periodontal conditions (inflammatory gum disease). They used a range of fancy statistical techniques to examine the links between periodontitis and COVID 19 complications while controlling for demographic, medical and behavioural factors. They included 568 patients, 40 cases and 528 controls in their analysis. Among the cases, there were 14 deaths, 36 ICU admissions and 20 people who required assisted ventilation. The ORs associated with periodontitis and the complications suffered by the 40 cases were: death (OR = 8.8, 95% CI 1.0, 77.7); ICU admission OR = 3.5, 95% CI 1.4, 9.1); assisted ventilation (OR = 4.6, 95% CI 1.2–17.3). Take a careful look at the above information, comment on the findings and form a conclusion.
10. Researchers want to investigate the relationships between childhood exposure to asbestos and the development of mesothelioma (a type of cancer that is specific to asbestos exposure). Due to the known dangers of exposure to asbestos and disease, asbestos is no longer mined or used in building products in Australia and mesothelioma has pretty much stopped occurring as a result of workplace exposure (30). However, mesothelioma continues to develop as asbestos was used everywhere in Australia and most buildings built prior to the ban (1983) contain asbestos. The incidence of disease is higher in Australia than just about any other country, but still amounts to only 2.7 cases of mesothelioma per 100 000 people, and it can take 20 to 60 years for mesothelioma to develop after exposure to asbestos (31). With lots of home renovations occurring over the past few decades in Australia, the researchers want to know if childhood exposures via home renovations, school renovations and duration of exposure are related to the development of mesothelioma in later life. Do you think a case-control study design would be appropriate for this investigation and what is your reasoning?

References

1. Queensland Health. *Queensland Dengue Management Plan 2015–2020.* Queensland Health; 2015.
2. Ministry of Health. *Guidelines for Malaria Epidemic Preparedness and Response in Kenya.* 2nd ed. Ministry of Health; 2020.
3. Meena MS, Priya S, Thirukumaran R, Gowrilakshmi M, Essakiraja K, Madhumitha MS. Factors influencing the acquisition of COVID infection among high-risk contacts of COVID-19 patients in Madurai district: A case control study. *Journal of Family Medical Primary Care.* 2022;11(1):182–9.

4. Centers for Disease Control and Prevention. Types of data collected in foodborne outbreak investigations. CDC; 2022. www.cdc.gov/foodborne-outbreaks/about-data/?CDC_AAref_Val=https://www.cdc.gov/foodsafety/outbreaks/basics/data-types-collected.html
5. Centers for Disease Control and Prevention. *Foodborne Diseases Active Surveillance Network (FoodNet) Population Survey*. Centers for Disease Control and Prevention; 2022 www.cdc.gov/foodnet/surveys/population.html
6. Pan F, Yang L, Li Y, Liang B, Li L, Ye T et al. Factors associated with death outcome in patients with severe coronavirus disease-19 (COVID-19): A case-control study. *International Journal of Medical Sciences*. 2020;17(9):1281–92.
7. National Health and Medical Research Council (NHMRC). *Biobanks Information Paper 2010*. NHMRC; 2010.
8. Cumming RG, Klineberg RJ. Case-control study of risk factors for hip fractures in the elderly. *American Journal of Epidemiology*. 1994;139(5):493–503.
9. Accorsi EK, Britton A, Fleming-Dutra KE, Smith ZR, Shang N, Derado G et al. Association Between 3 doses of mRNA COVID-19 vaccine and symptomatic infection caused by the SARS-CoV-2 Omicron and Delta variants. *JAMA*. 2022;327(7):639–51.
10. Greenland S, Senn SJ, Rothman KJ, Carlin JB, Poole C, Goodman SN et al. Statistical tests, P values, confidence intervals, and power: A guide to misinterpretations. *European Journal of Epidemiology*. 2016;31(4):337–50.
11. Wasserstein RL, Lazar NA. The ASA statement on *p*-values: Context, process, and purpose. *The American Statistician*. 2016;70(2):129–33.
12. Fein, EC, Gilmour, J, Machin, T, Hendry, L. *Statistics for Research Students: An Open Access Resource with Self-Tests and Illustrative Examples*. University of Southern Queensland; 2022. https://usq.pressbooks.pub/statisticsforresearchstudents
13. World Health Organization (WHO). WHO COVID-19 case definition. WHO; 2022. www.who.int/publications/i/item/WHO-2019-nCoV-Surveillance_Case_Definition-2022
14. El-Gilany AH. COVID-19 caseness: An epidemiologic perspective. *Journal of Infection and Public Health*. 2021;14(1):61–5.
15. Public Health Agency of Canada. *Outbreak Toolkit: Enteric Outbreak Investigations*. National Collaborating Centre for Infectious Diseases; 2023. https://outbreaktools.ca
16. Cancer Institute NSW. Cancer incidence and mortality New South Wales, Australia. 2022. www.cancer.nsw.gov.au/research-and-data/cancer-data-and-statistics/cancer-statistics-nsw/cancer-incidence-and-mortality
17. National Cancer Institute. Cancer incidence rates adjusted for reporting delay. 2022. https://surveillance.cancer.gov/delay
18. Sneyd MJ, Cox B. Commentary: Decreasing response rates require investigators to quantify and report the impact of selection bias in case-control studies. *International Journal of Epidemiology*. 2011;40(5):1355–7.
19. Bunin GR, Vardhanabhuti S, Lin A, Anschuetz GL, Mitra N. Practical and analytical aspects of using friend controls in case-control studies: experience from a case-control study of childhood cancer. *Paediatric and Perinatal Epidemiology*. 2011;25(5):402–12.
20. Zakeria R, Bendayanb R, Ashworth M, Bean DM, Dodhiad H, Durbabad S et al. A case-control and cohort study to determine the relationship between ethnic background and severe COVID-19. *eClinical Medicine*. 2020;28:100574.
21. Delgado-Rodríguez M, Llorca J. Bias. *Journal of Epidemiology and Community Health*. 2004;58(8):635–41.
22. Li C-Y, Sung F-C. A review of the healthy worker effect in occupational epidemiology. *Occupational Medicine*. 1999;49(4):225–9.
23. Isbister GK, Gray MR. White-tail spider bite: A prospective study of 130 definite bites by *Lampona* species. *Medical Journal of Australia*. 2003;179(4):199–202.
24. Isbister GK, Whyte IM. Suspected white-tail spider bite and necrotic ulcers. *Internal Medicine Journal*. 2004;34(1–2):38–44.

25. Victorian Government. Hepatitis A outbreak associated with frozen berries (update). Media release. 24 February 2015.

26. Apovian CM. Sugar-sweetened soft drinks, obesity, and type 2 diabetes. *JAMA*. 2004;292(8):978–9.

27. Lewallen S, Courtright P. Epidemiology in practice: Case-control studies. *Community Eye Health*. 1998;11(28):57–8.

28. Workicho A, Kassahun W, Alemseged F. Risk factors for multidrug-resistant tuberculosis among tuberculosis patients: A case-control study. *Infection and Drug Resistance*. 2017;10:91–6.

29. Marouf N, Cai W, Said KN, Daas H, Diab H, Chinta VR et al. Association between periodontitis and severity of COVID-19 infection: A case–control study. *Journal of Clinical Periodontology*. 2021;48(4):483–91.

30. Asbestos Safety and Eradication Agency. *National Asbestos Profile for Australia*. Asbestos Safety and Eradication Agency; 2017.

31. Cancer Council Australia. *Mesothelioma.* 2023. www.cancer.org.au/cancer-information/types-of-cancer/mesothelioma

8

Starting with exposure

What happens if you eat pizza and potato chips every day?

Learning objectives

After studying this chapter, you will be able to:

1. Describe the main features, types and uses of cohort studies
2. Interpret the common outcome measures of cohort studies
3. Identify the main types of potential sources of bias in cohort studies and understand some of the methods used to address these
4. Discuss the strengths and limitations of cohort studies

Introduction

In Chapter 7, we found out all about case-control studies and how they are great for exploring multiple potential exposures. For a case-control study to be a suitable design, we need a good idea about the outcome of interest (or condition) described by a strong case definition. But what if we know quite a bit about the exposures that interest us, but we are a little hazy on the potential outcomes associated with those exposures? If we consider a scientific question like the one posed in this chapter – 'What happens if you eat pizza and chips every day?' – we have specifically identified the exposures of interest but can only guess about what the outcomes might be. Okay, we could probably make fairly educated guesses about some of the potential outcomes (weight gain being chief among them), but there remains a level of uncertainty about their timing, magnitude and variety. What is really needed to answer a question like this is a 'cohort study', a type of observational study in which 'cohorts' of people (population groups who share certain characteristics, such as being in the same work environment, or who are born in the same year) are sorted into groups on the basis of whether they have or have not been exposed to specific health-related factors. Health outcomes for exposed and not-exposed groups are then compared over time. Like the pizza and potato chip thing, we usually would have an idea of what sort of outcomes to expect (based on scientific evidence and/or experience), so we would have to plan a study with a sufficiently long follow-up period for the expected outcomes to emerge; however, the design also provides the freedom to explore any number of outcomes linked to the identified exposures, as well as providing precise measures of incidence and mortality.

Hugo: Let's go – bring me the pizza and chips!

Rachael: I would love to eat them every day but I am pretty sure it wouldn't take long to know what would happen!

Author (Emma): If we did do a cohort study on this, we might not have to use a very long follow-up period to see quantifiable outcomes like weight changes, fluid retention and changes in blood pressure (from all the salt). But you would have to maintain your daily pizza and potato chip habit for quite a bit longer if we wanted to look at longer range outcomes, such as obesity, chronic hypertension and cardiovascular disease (and did you notice the word 'mortality' above?).

Compared with other observational study designs, a cohort study provides a lot more certainty about the temporality of things. This is because the study always starts with people who are free of disease in the first place (but at risk of it) who we know have been exposed to a particular risk factor prior to them developing any disease – that is, the design does much to assure us that the presumed cause preceded the effect.

In this chapter, we are going to have a close look at the cohort study – the best type of observational study for when you know what exposures or risk factors are at play but want to know more about the outcomes that might be associated with those exposures or risk factors.

Cohort studies

In a cohort study, those in a population without the conditions of interest are sorted into groups based on their exposure to a specified factor and then followed up over time to measure outcomes that develop in each group. Because this allows for the identification of new events when they occur, cohort studies are great for generating and comparing incidence and mortality rates. When the study population (or cohort) is recruited in the present and followed up into the future – that is, the investigators age with the project and its participants – this is called a 'prospective cohort study' (also known as a 'concurrent study'). The cohort can also be identified from historical records, then data about them are chased up through registries and other databases to find out what has happened to them later on (or in the present). This is known as a 'retrospective cohort study'. There are differences in the data-collection methods, but the direction of the investigation is exactly the same, starting with identifying a population prior to the development of disease, determining their status with respect to specified risk factors (exposure status), then comparing the occurrence of disease in the two groups. The basic direction of inquiry in cohort studies is presented in Figure 8.1.

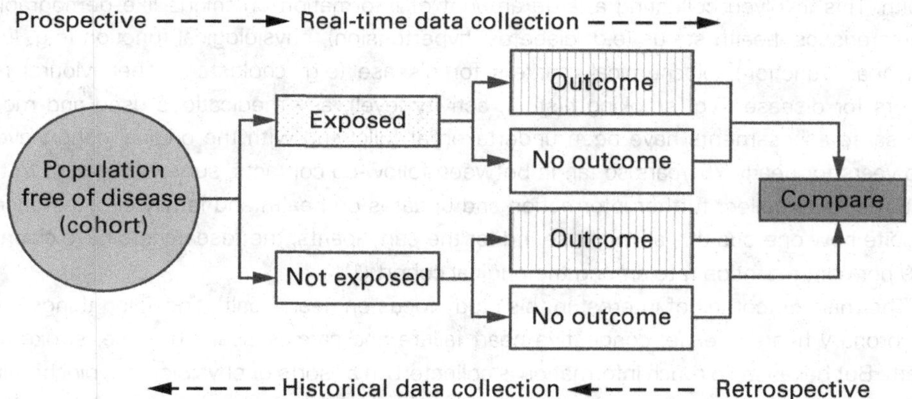

Figure 8.1 Cohort direction of inquiry for prospective and retrospective cohort studies

Rachael: Okay, so I might need to think about this a little bit ...

Hugo: Yep, this is bending my mind a little ... So, what is the difference between a retrospective cohort study and a case-control study then?

Author (Emma): They are both retrospective study designs, but the similarity pretty much ends there. You might remember that case-control studies are made up of participants who are purposely selected on the basis of either having or not having a defined condition, and the thing that is being investigated is what *exposures* might be associated with a known condition. In a retrospective cohort study, we are looking to see what *outcomes* might have occurred after exposure to a well-defined risk factor. So, the whole focus of the investigation differs and, as we will see later, the outcome measures that can be estimated from them also vary considerably between the two study designs.

Prospective cohort studies

Cohort studies are famous for their ability to precisely estimate incidence and mortality rates, and prospective cohort studies are particularly good for this. Their ability to establish the direction of the relationship between exposure and outcomes also moves the cohort study far closer to establishing causality than other observational designs. Because they start with a healthy population and then have to wait for conditions of interest to develop, prospective studies can take a really long time to complete and some have been going for generations. One very famous prospective cohort study, the ongoing Framingham Heart Study, is summarised in Example 8.1.

EXAMPLE 8.1

In the context of rising morbidity and mortality due to cardiovascular disease, the US Public Health Service established a cohort study in 1948, in the hope of better understanding the condition that had consistently ranked as the number one health threat (1). In Framingham, a city in Massachusetts, a cohort of 5209 male and female participants were recruited and underwent baseline measurements of factors thought to be associated with cardiovascular health. This involved collecting a large amount of information on things like demographic characteristics, health status (e.g. diabetes, hypertension), physiological function (e.g. lung and heart function), biochemical markers for disease (e.g. cholesterol), behavioural risk factors for disease (e.g. smoking history, activity level), any medications used and more. The same assessments have been undertaken at follow-up with the original cohort every two years for nearly 75 years so far. In between follow-up contacts, surveys are sent to the participants to collect further information and updates on health and family circumstances. Despite how onerous this all might sound for the participants, the researchers have claimed a 99 per cent retention rate among the original cohort (1).

The main outcomes of interest in this study focus on heart health, including things such as coronary heart disease, congestive heart failure and cardiovascular disease, stroke and death. But because so much information is collected on all sorts of physiological, biochemical and behavioural characteristics, this now vast longitudinal dataset has been used to study all sorts of exposures and outcomes related to health, such as smoking behaviour (2), obesity (3), diabetes (4) and oral contraception use (5), among many other health topics.

A lot of the routine stuff now undertaken in primary healthcare is actually based on the evidence first discovered in the Framingham Heart Study, including checking blood pressures, testing for serum cholesterol and providing counselling about healthy diets, smoking, physical activity and weight control (6).

The Framingham Heart Study now has a number of offshoot cohort studies, such as the 'Offspring Cohort' that was established in 1971 (7), and has continued to follow up the children of spouses from the original Framingham cohort ever since. Framingham Heart Study data are available for researchers to undertake their own research, and so far there have been almost 4000 publications based on these analyses (8). You can find out more about the Framingham Heart Study by visiting their website listed in the 'Further reading' section.

Prospective cohort studies are often conducted over a long period of time, but most do not go on to outlive their original research teams, subject as they are to the availability of funding and the ongoing commitment of research staff. More commonly, prospective cohort studies occur over a defined period of time. The main thing is that the follow-up period should be long enough for the outcome of interest to occur. A much shorter prospective cohort study about COVID-19 transmission in healthcare workers is described in Example 8.2.

EXAMPLE 8.2

A prospective cohort study was undertaken to estimate the risk of contracting COVID-19 in front-line healthcare workers (defined as those with direct patient contact) relative to the general community (9). The researchers recruited people using a COVID-19 symptom app in the United Kingdom and the United States in early 2020. Participants first provided a range of baseline information on demographic factors (age, sex, ethnicity, occupation) and medical history. Front-line healthcare workers were further questioned on their main place of work and use of personal protective equipment (PPE). Participants reported their COVID-19 symptoms on a daily basis (using the app) and follow-up continued for up to 30 days or until the participant reported a COVID-19 positive test.

Nearly 100 000 front-line healthcare workers and more than two million members of the general community were enrolled in the study and the median length of follow-up was 19 days. During follow-up, 5545 COVID-19 incident cases (new cases) were reported and the incidence per 30 person-days of follow-up was calculated as 3.96 per cent for front-line healthcare workers compared with 0.33 per cent for the general community, or 12 times the risk for front-line healthcare workers. The COVID-19 risk among front-line healthcare workers varied according to the intensity of patient contact, ranging from 1.99 per cent per 30 person-days for clinical settings to 9.18 per cent per 30 person-days for inpatient settings. Greatly increased risk for all settings was associated with inadequate use of personal protective equipment (such as reuse and unavailability of PPE).

The researchers concluded that there was increased risk for COVID-19 in front-line healthcare workers relative to the general community in the United Kingdom and the United States, and they recommended that health systems ensure the adequate availability of PPE (9).

I think we can all agree that one month of follow-up is much shorter than 75 years! Unlike the Framingham Heart Study, Nguyen's team (9) was mainly interested in just one outcome: infection with SARS-CoV-2. In the context of a highly infectious pandemic, the researchers knew it would not take very long for the cases to arise, especially in a very large cohort. And did you notice that follow-up of individuals stopped as soon a positive test was recorded? This is because cohort studies are essentially interested in movement from the denominator to the numerator – that is, people moving from the at-risk group to being identified as an incident case. This movement is often expressed in cohort studies as 'person time', which we will find out more about later in this chapter.

Retrospective cohort studies

In prospective cohort studies, the exposure status of a people within a defined cohort is classified and then the cohort is followed up in real time by investigators who age along with the research project. In the case of studies such as the Framingham Heart Study, the original investigators can grow very old indeed! Although the direction of study is exactly the same as prospective studies (moving from exposure to outcome), retrospective studies use historical data to identify cohorts and exposure histories rather than collecting the data in real time. This means they can be a lot cheaper and take far less time to complete, even when we are interested in outcomes that typically take a really long time to develop. The trade-off is that we will be stuck with the records as they were documented yesterday. Unlike starting off fresh with a prospective cohort study, we can only identify the baseline, exposure and (frequently) outcome information that was recorded in the past. Data might be missing or inaccurate, and some people from the defined cohort may prove to be impossible to trace (they could leave the country, change their names, or go 'off grid'). Still, assuming good access to complete-*ish* data, it is certainly possible to conduct retrospective studies of high quality. A retrospective cohort study is summarised in Example 8.3. This study looked at the relationship between exposure to computerised tomography (CT) scans in earlier life and the subsequent development of cancer (10).

EXAMPLE 8.3

A retrospective cohort study was undertaken in the United Kingdom to assess the cancer risks that might be associated with exposure to CT scans in children and young adults – that is, those younger than 22 years of age (10).

The participants all had CT scans in the UK healthcare system (the National Health Service (NHS)) at some time between 1985 and 2002, when no evidence of cancer was apparent. The researchers defined the cohort from radiological records kept at 81 health centres in the United Kingdom. The data in the radiology records were then linked to cancer notifications made to the NHS Central Registry between 1985 and 2008. The NHS Central Registry has records of everyone in the United Kingdom who is registered with a general practitioner and is updated with all births, deaths, marriages, cancer notifications and more on a continuous basis. The outcomes of interest in the cohort study were leukaemia (diagnosed at least two years after the first CT) and brain tumours (diagnosed at least five years after the first CT), which they also compared with the radiation dosage received from the earlier CT scan.

Among approximately 180 000 individuals forming the cohort, 74 cases of leukemia and 185 brain cancer cases were diagnosed. The researchers undertook some complex techniques to statistically correlate the data to show an excess risk of leukaemia and brain tumours that increased along with the dose of radiation received during their CT scans. The leukaemia risk for those receiving 30 milligray (mGy) of radiation was more than three times that of those receiving 5 mGy (RR = 3.2; 95% CI: 1.5, 6.9) and the brain cancer risk for young people receiving 50–74 mGy was nearly three times that of those receiving 5 mGy (RR = 2.8; 95% CI: 1.3, 6.0).

Although the relative risks associated with higher radiation doses were high, leukemia and brain tumours are quite rare, so the total number of excess cases was small (only one excess leukemia case and one excess brain cancer case during the decade following the first scan undertaken in patients younger than 10 years of age). Nonetheless, the authors recommend that radiation doses from CT scans be kept as low as possible and CT scanning should not be the preferred option if alternative procedures are available (10).

If we wanted to do a *prospective* cohort study of rare cancers associated with CT scans in young people, a procedure that only a relatively small proportion of young people undergo, we would have to enrol a very large number of participants over a period of several years. Then we would need to follow them up over the next several decades, as cancer takes quite a bit of time to develop. Not only would this require lots of funds and research personnel, but we wouldn't get any answers for quite some time. Assuming our scientific question was based on a theory (derived through critical thinking) about the potential dangers associated with childhood CT scans, it probably wouldn't be appropriately (or ethically) answered by a very drawn-out period of observation. Example 8.3 also touches on the tensions between relative and absolute differences, which we will hear more about in a later chapter. But when assessing the meaningfulness of findings and what preventive actions they might lead to, it is important to understand both the relative and absolute effects of exposures, then carefully consider the severity of potential health outcomes balanced against the implications (societal, financial, ethical) of acting (or not acting) to prevent these outcomes. We would have to decide whether preventing one additional case of cancer was worth avoiding CT scanning young people, even if the alternative procedures were more complex and expensive and despite any competing health priorities.

Researchers undertaking retrospective cohort studies don't always have to go on archaeological digs to collect their data, depending on how frequently the outcomes of interest occur and how quickly they develop. Cohort studies that are looking at infectious diseases, for instance, can be relatively quick and easy, especially if the infection of interest is a notifiable one and there is access to recent hospital records and surveillance data. One such cohort study, looking at post-COVID-19 health outcomes (11), is presented in Example 8.4.

EXAMPLE 8.4

A retrospective cohort study was conducted in the United Kingdom to measure organ-specific dysfunction in COVID-19 patients after discharge from hospital relative to people in the community who were matched on a range of demographic, socioeconomic and health-related variables (11). Nearly 50 000 people who had been discharged from NHS hospitals in England were individually matched (for sex, age, ethnicity, socioeconomic status and clinical characteristics) to 50 000 people who were initially randomly selected from the general population and who had not recently been hospitalised for COVID-19. The main outcomes of interest were rates of hospitalisation (readmission in the case of the COVID-19 group), all-cause mortality and diagnoses with respiratory, cardiovascular, diabetes, kidney or liver disease. All medical records for the follow-up period of nine months were reviewed.

After a mean (average) follow-up of 140 days, or just over 4.5 months, 14 060 of 47 780 discharged COVID-19 patients were re-hospitalised (29 per cent), which was four times the rate of hospitalisation in the not-exposed group. There were 5875 deaths in discharged COVID-19 patients (12 per cent), which was eight times the number of deaths in the not-exposed group. Rates of diagnosed respiratory and cardiovascular disease and diabetes were all significantly increased in discharged COVID-19 patients relative to the non-COVID-19 group ($p < 0.001$).

The researchers concluded that people who were discharged after hospitalisation with COVID-19 were at increased risk of multi-organ dysfunction relative to the general population and recommended greater integration of care around post-COVID-19 syndromes rather than relying on organ-specific approaches (11).

Hugo: So, if it is cheaper to do a retrospective cohort study, why don't people do them all the time?

Rachael: Does it all boil down to what the scientific question is?

Author (Emma): Retrospective cohort studies are generally faster and cheaper than prospective cohort studies but, as mentioned, they are restrained by what data are recorded and available. And, yes, it has a lot to do with the scientific question. If you were researching well-defined and well-documented exposures and outcomes, as was the study described in Example 8.4, data restrictions might not be much of a problem. But if your scientific question could only be answered by obtaining information that is not usually formally documented, (say, daily pizza and chip consumption), only a prospective approach would do.

Measuring outcomes in cohort studies

Cohort studies are perfectly designed for identifying and comparing the incidence of disease in exposed and not-exposed population groups. From reading earlier chapters in this book, we are now familiar with the idea of measuring rates of disease in populations. Cohort studies allow for increased accuracy in measuring incidence by accounting for the exact amount of time that people in the cohort spend at risk for the disease (or other outcomes). They do this by employing the concept of 'person-time at risk'. To compare what happens to exposed and not-exposed groups, the 'relative risk' is also calculated in cohort studies. The relative risk (also known as a 'rate ratio') is a ratio of the risk of an event in those exposed to the risk of the same event in those who are not exposed. We will be discussing more about the notion of risk in Chapter 10, but for now let's accept that risk and incidence are pretty much synonymous.

Incidence and person-time

In Chapter 2, we found out all about incidence and how incidence rates are calculated. So we know the incidence of an event is the rate at which new cases arise in an at-risk population over a specified period of time. In technical reports, such as those produced regularly by government-related agencies, incidence is usually estimated from the size of a specified population over a specified period of time. Cancer incidence, for example, is routinely reported in many countries. Most often, these are *cumulative* incidence rates, which express the proportion of a given population at risk in which new cancers arise over a specified of time – usually yearly. For instance, it is reported that the crude (observed or unadjusted) incidence of cancer in 2018 in Australia was 585.7 per 100 000 persons (12). This rate was calculated by dividing the number of new cancer cases notified in 2018 by the number of people in the Australian population in that year (146 335/24 982 688), which was then multiplied by 10^5 (100 000) to form a rate per 100 000 persons.

On a population level, and especially for the purposes of surveillance, annual cumulative incidence is totally appropriate as whole populations don't usually change much on a year-to-year basis and this allows us to easily compare disease occurrence from one year to the next. Crude incidence can be refined by looking at the incidence by sex or by age group – this is known as 'specific' incidence (no longer described as 'crude', but still cumulative!). For instance, the sex-specific incidence of cancer for females in Australia in 2018 was reported to be 523.3 per 100 000 (calculated by dividing the number of new cases in females by the number of females in the population that year) and the age-specific incidence of cancer in persons aged 20 to 24 years in 2018 was 2.6 per 100 000 (the number of new cases in people aged 20 to 24 years by the number in that age group in the 2018 population).

Another refinement to crude incidence can be made to account for the changes in the age structure of populations over time. The world's population is ageing – that is, people are living longer and making up a bigger proportion of the total population. According to the WHO, the proportion of the world's population that consists of people over 60 years of age will almost double between 2015 and 2050, from 12 per cent to 22 per cent (13). This all started in the wealthier countries of the world but has become a trend that is increasing even in poorer countries, which are now experiencing the fastest rate of change. The problem is that older people contribute most to the burden of illness, disability and mortality, but are also the least likely to be in full employment. So population ageing is associated with escalating costs to health and welfare systems and also with decreasing workforce capacity (the taxes that workers generate and the economic activity they drive) to support these costs.

Population ageing is a trend that represents one of the largest public health issues in the world today, but age also impacts the way health scientists collect, analyse and report data. In your reading of the scientific literature, you will often see incidence rates reported as being 'age-standardised'. This means the crude incidence rate has been weighted to account for changes in the age structure of the population over time, or even between countries. While we don't need to get into all the details of the process here, the usual method involves applying our observed age-specific rates to the age-specific proportions (weights) of a 'standard population' (in Australia, the 2001 population is generally used as the standard) to arrive at a summary, age-adjusted rate. The important thing is that if there looks to be a difference between reported age-standardised incidence rates (over time or between populations), whatever else is going on, we know that age plays no part in those differences. It turns out that age is actually associated with nearly all measurable health outcomes, especially mortality. So, although different statistical techniques are used, weighting or adjusting of outcome measures also happens in research studies. This is done for exactly the same reason: to reveal the true relationships between exposures and outcomes that are 'independent' of the effects of age and other potentially influencing variables or **confounders** – such as sex, socioeconomic status, comorbidities and so on – which we will hear a little more about later in this book.

Confounder: A variable that is associated with both a potential cause (*e*) and an outcome (*o*) that distorts the true relationship between *o* and *e*.

Regular reporting of cumulative incidence is great for the purposes of identifying and monitoring changes in the occurrence of disease and between populations that might be at risk for that disease. What cohort studies offer is a far more specific measure of incidence that takes into account the actual amount of time each person spends at risk for the outcome – known as 'person-time at risk'. As mentioned, cohort studies are essentially interested in the movement of people from the at-risk group to the group that develops the conditions to which they were at risk (the identified outcomes) – that is, movement from the denominator to the numerator. It makes sense that once people develop the condition of interest, they are no longer at risk for it. Further movement out of the at-risk group might occur if people drop out of the study, die or become lost to follow-up for any other reason. But all these people did spend at least some time at risk of the condition. Calculating person-time allows us to include the time spent at risk by everyone in the study to present as accurate an estimate as possible of the actual risk associated with the condition of interest in a specified population.

Let's say we went ahead with our cohort study of daily pizza and chip consumption. We set a study period of two weeks over which we weigh the participants daily, with the main outcome of interest being a weight gain of 5 per cent from baseline. Given the cohort we have to hand, we enrolled five people in our study: Rachael, Hugo, Emma (me), Steve and Patricia. In this hypothetical prospective cohort study, we noted one case of weight gain ≥5 per cent from baseline and only one participant was observed for the whole 14 days. Rachael lasted a week before weakening and switching to vegetables and fruit; Hugo became an incident case at day 12; Emma became violently ill early in the second week and could not sustain the diet; Steve decided to become a vegan by the second day; and Patricia maintained the diet for the full two weeks of the study period but did not meet the criteria for being a case (Figure 8.2).

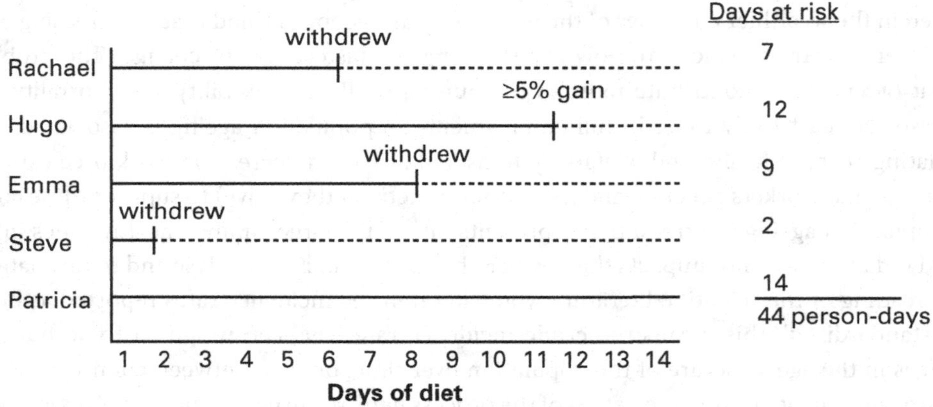

Figure 8.2 Person-time at risk – two-week pizza and chip diet and ≥ 5 per cent baseline weight gain

As you can see from Figure 8.2, each participant contributes the number of days they were observed to be at risk for the outcome to the total person-time. The amount of time they contribute is censored as soon as they stop being at risk, either by becoming a case or leaving the study or by completing the study without either event occurring. So, from this hypothetical example, we have identified one case of a 5 per cent weight gain in 44 person-days of follow-up. The person-time incidence rate is calculated by:

$$\frac{\text{Number of new specified events occurring in a specified period}}{\text{Sum of the length of time each person was at risk for the specified event}} \times 10^n$$

So, the incidence of a 5 per cent weight gain after a daily pizza and chip diet was: 1/44 = 0.0227 or 23 per 1000 person-days.

Rachael: Can that be interpreted to mean that 23 people will gain weight for every 1000 days of follow up?

Hugo: Or that 23 out of 1000 people following the diet for one day will gain weight? [Oh and, *mean*, by the way ...]

Author (Emma): Well, actually, you are both right. Using person-days, we could go back to our raw data and say one person gained weight in 44 person-days of follow-up or predict that we would see 46 cases of 5 per cent weight gain in 2000 person-days. But let's remember that this was a *hypothetical* exercise (and sorry about making you a case,

Hugo, but you have been very enthusiastic about pizza and chips), and we would probably need to recruit a lot more people who were into pizza and chips to really evaluate the risk of outcomes, including precise measures of weight gain per person-day. We would also need to recruit a suitable group of people who are on an alternative (probably more orthodox) diet as well to see how much weight they gained.

Relative risk

A cohort study generally includes two groups of interest that are classified according to their exposure to potential risk factors and are then followed up over time to compare their health outcomes. The most common way to accomplish this comparison is to calculate the incidence of the condition in each group and create a ratio of exposed to not exposed incidence – the relative risk (RR). The RR quantifies the excess risk associated with the exposure as is directly compared to the risk in the absence of exposure. RRs are calculated by dividing the incidence of a specified disease (or other event) in the exposed by the incidence of that disease in the not exposed. If there was no difference in incidence, this would return an RR of 1 since you are dividing one value by the same value. Just as is the case of odds ratios (which we met in Chapter 7), we interpret RRs by how much they differ from the value of 1 (the null value). The null value means there is no difference in incidence (or risk) between the two groups. An RR that is greater than the null (RR >1) indicates that the risk is higher in the exposed group, and an RR less than the null (RR <1) indicates that the risk is lower in the exposed group.

In Example 8.5, we return to the retrospective cohort study of post-COVID-19 health outcomes conducted by Ayoubkhani et al. in the United Kingdom (11).

EXAMPLE 8.5

In this retrospective cohort study (also described in Example 8.4), nearly 50 000 patients who had been discharged from hospital after having COVID-19 were individually matched with 50 000 people in the community and medical records for the period of nine months were reviewed for hospital admissions/readmissions, deaths and diagnosis with a range of organ-specific conditions (11).

Among other findings, the authors report that the relative risks they calculated for multiple outcomes comparing patients with COVID-19 and matched controls were higher in people aged under 70 years relative to older individuals, as well as for people belonging to 'ethnic minority' groups relative to the 'white' population. The largest relative risks were seen for respiratory disease in younger people (RR = 10.5, 95% CI: 9.7, 11.4) versus people aged 70 years and older (RR = 4.6, 95% CI: 4.3, 4.8); and respiratory disease in non-white people (RR = 11.4, 95% CI: 9.8, 13.3) versus white people (RR = 5.2, 95% CI: 5.0, 5.5)

As well as concluding that people who were discharged after hospitalisation with COVID-19 were generally more likely to develop multi-organ dysfunction (including respiratory disease) relative to the rest of the population, the authors point out that it was not just the elderly who were at risk and that risk also varied across ethnicities (11).

In Example 8.5, the relative risk for diagnosis of respiratory infections in discharged COVID-19 patients compared with the general community was reported for different age and ethnic groups. The RR of 10.5 can be interpreted to mean that the incidence of respiratory disease in discharged COVID-19 patients younger than 70 years of age was more than 10 times higher than in general community members of the same age, but only five times the incidence seen in those aged 70 years and older (RR = 4.5). In non-white discharged COVID-19 patients, the incidence of respiratory disease was more than 11 times that of the non-white general population. In white discharged COVID-19 patients, however, the incidence of respiratory disease was just over five times that of white community members. You might notice that all of the RRs reported in Example 8.5 are accompanied by confidence intervals that indicate the results are statistically significant as none of them overlap the null value (null = 1).

The way relative risk is calculated is described in Explanation 8.1.

EXPLANATION 8.1: Calculating relative risk

Construct a 2 x 2 table that cross-references the people with and without the health outcome by their exposure status – disease status in the columns and exposure status in the rows (see Figure 8.3).

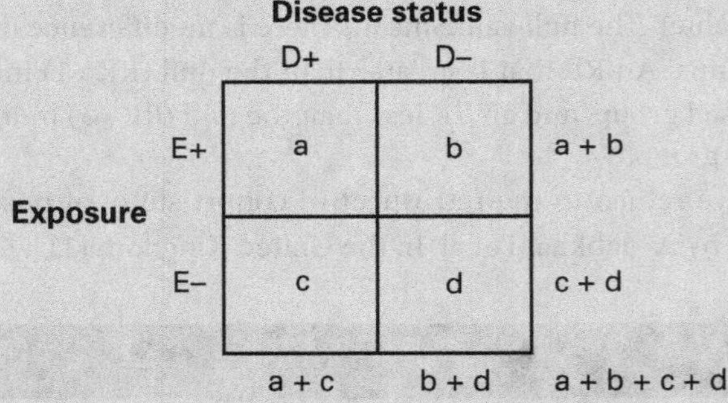

Figure 8.3 Cross-tabulation of disease and exposure status – set up to calculate relative risk (RR)

Cells:
a = number of people with the disease exposed to a particular risk factor
b = number of people without the disease exposed to a particular risk factor
c = number of people with the disease not exposed to a particular risk factor
d = number of people without the disease not exposed to a particular factor
a + c = number of people with the disease
b + d = number of people without the disease
a + b = number of people exposed to a particular risk factor
c + d = number of people not exposed to a particular risk factor
a + b + c + d = total number of people in the cohort
Risk of disease in the exposed = a divided by a plus b (a/a + b)
Risk of disease in the not exposed = c divided by c plus d (c/c + d)
RR = a/a + b divided by c/c + d

i.e. $RR = \frac{a/(a+b)}{c/(c+d)}$

Hugo: What is it with you and 2 x 2 tables!!

Rachael: A-huh ...

Author (Emma): There are just so many outcome measures in epidemiology that can be calculated using 2 x 2 tables. What's not to love?

Okay, let's have a go at working this out together ...

WORKED EXAMPLE 8.1

In their study of patients discharged after hospitalisation with COVID-19 (11), the researchers identified 2330 cases of diabetes diagnoses from the medical records of 47 780 patients who had previously been discharged after having COVID-19, and 1725 diabetes diagnoses from the medical records of 47 780 members of the general population over a period of nine months. We now have all the information we need to plug into our 2 x 2 table and calculate the relative risk as shown in Figure 8.4.

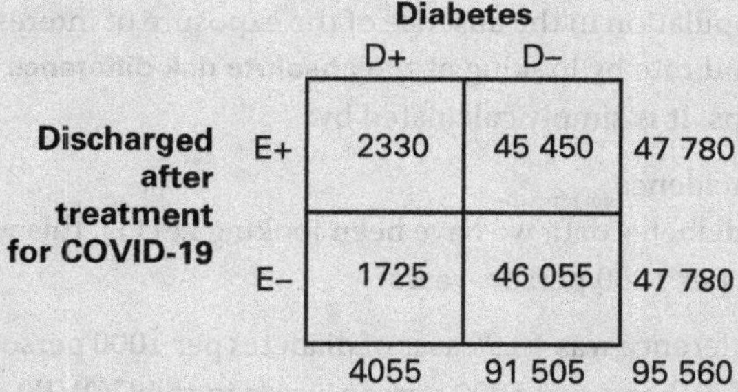

		Diabetes D+	Diabetes D–	
Discharged after treatment for COVID-19	E+	2330	45 450	47 780
	E–	1725	46 055	47 780
		4055	91 505	95 560

Figure 8.4 Diabetes diagnoses status cross-tabulated by exposure to COVID-19 hospitalisation status – set up to calculate relative risk (RR)

The RR is calculated by dividing the incidence of disease in the exposed by the incidence of disease in the not-exposed:

$$RR = \frac{a/(a+b)}{c/(c+d)}$$

$$= \frac{(2330/47\ 780)}{(1725/47\ 780)}$$

$$= \frac{0.049}{0.036}$$

$$= 1.36$$

The RR of 1.36 is larger than the null value (1.36 >1), so we know that recently discharged COVID-19 patients were at increased risk for diabetes compared with the general population. The RR indicates that discharged COVID-19 patients were 36 per cent more likely to develop diabetes than the general population. From the data in the table, we can say the cumulative incidence of diabetes in the exposed was 49 per 1000 persons over nine months, while the incidence of diabetes in the not-exposed was 36 per 1000 persons over nine months.

Rachael: Okay – not too bad!

Hugo: I think I got the idea, but I might need to practise this one a bit more ...

Author (Emma): It does take some thinking through, but the main thing is to understand the way incidence is involved in calculating relative risks and how to interpret relative risks when they are reported.

The authors (11) also calculated diabetes incidence per person-years of follow-up, which (as we now know) provides a more precise measure of exposure time than cumulative incidence. They reported that the incidence of diabetes in discharged COVID-19 patients was 126.9 per 1000 person-years versus 86.0 per 1000 person-years in the general population. These rates can be used to calculate an RR of 1.48 (126.9/86.0), suggesting a 48 per cent increased risk of diabetes in recently discharged COVID-19 patients relative to the general population.

You may have noticed that, while the COVID-19 patients had higher risk for diabetes, both groups had *some* risk for diabetes even when they might not have been exposed to COVID-19. Epidemiologists call the this the 'background rate' of the disease, which occurs anyway in a defined population in the absence of the exposure of interest. We can remove the effect of the background rate by looking at the **absolute risk difference** between the exposed and not-exposed groups. It is simply calculated by:

Absolute risk difference: (synonyms 'attributable risk', 'rate difference', 'excess rate', 'risk reduction') The absolute difference in effect – may be incidence, prevalence, mortality – quantifying the direct impact of an exposure.

$\text{Incidence}_{\text{exposed}} - \text{Incidence}_{\text{not exposed}}$

From the COVID-diabetes data we have been looking at (11), this would be:

126.9 – 86.0 = 40.9 per 1000 person-years

So, the absolute risk difference was 40.9 cases of diabetes per 1000 person-years. This suggests that nearly 41 cases of diabetes per 1000 person-years in the COVID-19 group was directly attributable to their exposure to COVID-19 (86 per 1000 person-years would have happened anyway). We are going to hear a bit more about interpreting risk and the ways risk can be attributed and presented in Chapter 10, but for now it is sufficient to be aware of yet another useful outcome measure associated with cohort studies.

Potential for bias in cohort studies

Among observational study designs, cohort studies are pretty much top of the range because they approach the strongest evidence for causal relationships between exposure and outcome. But it probably won't surprise you to learn that they might not be 'all that' when it comes to pesky things like potential bias, which can really mess with their strongest evidence 'rep'. Like all other research approaches, there are multiple ways in which bias can be introduced in even the best designed cohort study. Both major categories of bias – selection and measurement bias – can be introduced at any point and ultimately lead to erroneous conclusions.

Selection bias

In Chapter 7, we were introduced to the phenomenon of selection bias, which is any type of systematic error that causes any sample for your study to have characteristics that differ from those who were not selected. This can be a particular problem for case-control studies because the participants (cases and controls) are specifically recruited based on their status with respect to a particular condition of interest. Although participants in cohort studies are selected prior to the development of any health outcomes of interest, there are still multiple points at which selection bias may be introduced, as represented in Figure 8.5.

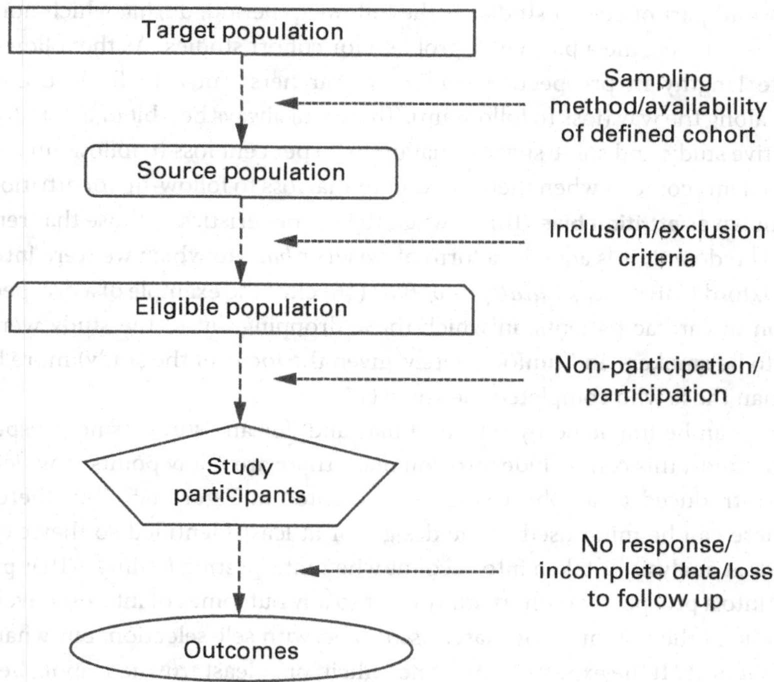

Figure 8.5 Levels or participant selection and potential sources of bias. Adapted from (14)

If we were planning to undertake a cohort study, we must first pose a scientific question, which would (we can presume) be based on great deal of critical thinking about a particular issue of interest. The population affected by that issue is what is defined in Figure 8.5 as the 'target population' – those to whom we would hope that our study would have particular relevance. The target population may well be the whole population of a city or country, all those involved in a specified industry or everyone in a specified population of a certain sex or age. It wouldn't ordinarily be possible to enrol all of the target population in our study, so we would need to identify a smaller defined population that could represent the target population – the 'source population'. This could be a suburb of a city, a single industry-specific workforce (e.g. a company) or sex- or age-related community groups. We might have chosen the source population on the basis of availability – for example, we might work with or for this population – but already they might look a little different from the target population, with characteristics that might influence outcomes in some way.

Once we have defined the source population, we would need to set about applying our inclusion or exclusion criteria to identify the eligible population. We might want to include only people of a certain age group, sex or employment status, and we may wish to exclude people who have poor health status or other issues that could impact their participation – for example, language proficiency or competing time priorities. People may even be classified as ineligible because of a lack of information about them – there may be inadequate documentation of particular blood test results for instance. For a number of reasons, there could be even more differences between our eligible population and the initial target population. Further differences could emerge should eligible people decline to be in the study, or if they are enrolled but then change their minds, or they do not fully complete the study requirements.

An important part of cohort studies is the follow-up period, during which non-response of participants can become a particular problem for cohort studies. As the follow-up period can be quite lengthy in prospective studies, researchers can actually lose contact with participants along the way (loss to follow-up). There will always be a bit of loss to follow-up in any prospective study, and some suggest that up to 20 per cent loss to follow-up is acceptable (15). The problems come in when there is a differential loss to follow-up (or attrition), leading to what is known as **attrition bias**. This is when the characteristics of those that remain differ from those who do not; it is actually a form of *survivor bias*, to which we were introduced in Chapter 7. Oxford University's *Catalogue of Bias* (16) cites the example of a prospective study of depression in cardiac patients, in which those dropping out of the study were younger, more likely to be smokers and (unfortunately, given the focus of the study) more likely to be depressed than those who completed the study (17).

Attrition bias: Occurs when the study participants who are lost to follow up have different characteristics than those who remain in the study (a form of selection bias).

All studies can be impacted by selection bias and, for any study using prospective data collection methods, this can include attrition bias. There are many points at which selection bias can be introduced to a cohort study (represented in Figure 8.5), but there are some ways that these can be minimised in the design, or at least identified so they can be either controlled for at analysis or taken into account when interpreting findings. That participants are enrolled into a prospective cohort study prior to any outcomes of interest developing may minimise some of the potential for biases associated with self-selection, but what about the exposure of interest? If the exposure concerned illicit, or at least frowned-upon, behaviours – such as drug use or smoking – people who engaged in these behaviours might be less likely to agree to participate. Clear information on the protection of confidentiality and the employment of strong interpersonal skills can be crucial for recruitment.

Choosing an appropriate comparison group is also an important strategy for minimising bias for both prospective and retrospective cohort studies. Comparison groups can be internal, in that they are members of the same source population prior to classification of exposure – for example, the Framingham Heart Study. An external group may also be selected for comparison, such as a different occupation or company. Or, as in the discharged COVID-19 patient example we looked at, people in the general population of the same age and sex (among other characteristics) might form the comparison group. The main thing is that the not-exposed comparison group should be as similar as possible to the exposed group with the exception of the exposure of interest. In retrospective studies, it is also important that the selection of exposed and not-exposed groups be accomplished without the investigators having any knowledge about participant outcomes.

Related to the above, here we reintroduce the phenomenon known as the 'healthy worker effect', which can particularly beset cohort studies that are comparing outcomes in occupational groups with those in the general population. The issue is that groups still in employment generally exclude those who are unwell, as sick people tend to leave the workforce. The general population, however, will include both sick and well people. Clearly, this form of selection bias will make it difficult to compare the outcomes between the two groups by diluting the health impact of any workplace exposure. Selecting general population comparison groups of working age and excluding those with comorbid conditions might help minimise the health worker effect in this situation.

Attrition bias can really only be addressed by taking steps to improve ongoing participation. This might include sending frequent reminders to participants, minimising as much as possible the information participants are required to provide (in surveys and physical testing) and promoting ongoing engagement through the use of higher-tech ways to interact with participants (such as apps, online blogs and surveys). Comparing what information has been collected about those lost to follow up with those who remain can also provide important insights on the nature and extent of potential selection bias.

Measurement bias

In the previous chapter, we learnt that measurement bias is a systematic error introduced by inconsistent measurement of study variables across comparison groups. In prospective cohort studies, and assuming the use of standardised data-collection instruments at baseline and follow-up, the measurement of exposure is generally unbiased. In retrospective studies, however, historical records are usually relied upon for information about exposure. As we have discussed, in this case we are stuck with any inaccurate, incomplete or missing data that may have been recorded, and probably will not have the capacity to chase down clarifying information from the original source. Depending on how long ago the data were recorded, it may well be that what is now considered an important risk factor was unrecognised at the time and so was only partially documented, if at all. In very large retrospective cohort studies, the main way to address this issue would be to exclude participants with missing exposure data. If a sizeable proportion of the members of an initially defined cohort are excluded due to missing data, this may again introduce the possibility of selection bias as the remaining participants may not end up being representative of the target population.

In some cohort studies, exposure information is collected from participants themselves, who may have inaccurate or incomplete recollections. Participants are usually informed about the focus of the study and its purpose, and this knowledge may influence memories about exposure in the past. Where the exposure of interest is ongoing, as some lifestyle risk behaviours are, participants may be reluctant to disclose or feel more comfortable responding in the way they perceive as socially acceptable (the potential for **social desirability bias**). Further, they may even change their risk behaviours because they are being observed, in a situation known as the **Hawthorne effect** (18). The Hawthorne effect takes its name from the first description of the phenomenon in a 1920s study of workers at the Hawthorne Works, an electric company in the United States, where worker productivity (the outcome of interest) was said to have increased during the investigation with changes in exposure to lighting (19). It was ultimately concluded that productivity increased due to the workers being observed rather than due to any lighting changes. Look at Example 8.6, in which the Hawthorne effect is examined in relation to handwashing by health practitioners.

Social desirability bias: Occurs when participants provide information in a manner they perceive will be favourable to the researcher; this is more likely to occur differentially between comparison groups (a form of measurement bias).

Hawthorne effect: Where participants change their risk behaviour due to being observed in a study (a form of measurement bias).

EXAMPLE 8.6

In a hospital in Taiwan, a prospective cohort study was undertaken over 15 months to investigate the Hawthorne effect in different types of healthcare provider groups (20). The researchers observed handwashing using two methods – overt and covert – across 31 522 handwashing events, which were matched 1:1 for overt and covert observations across occupation, department, time and location. There were 38 overt observers and 93 covert observers who observed 3047 matched pairs of events.

Overall handwashing compliance was higher in overt relative to covert observations (78 per cent versus 55 per cent, $p < 0.001$) and, using **risk differences**, the Hawthorne effect was measured at three times higher in nurses relative to doctors (30 per cent versus 11 per cent). The Hawthorne effect was larger in outpatient clinics relative to intensive care units (41 per cent versus 11 per cent). The magnitude of the Hawthorne effect differed among healthcare worker occupations and across locations, but not among departments.

The investigators concluded that the overt observation of handwashing compliance might not be that useful for accurate evaluation of infection-control practices.

Risk difference: (synonyms 'rate difference', 'excess rate', 'risk reduction', 'attributable risk') The absolute difference in effect – may be incidence, prevalence, mortality – quantifying the direct impact of an exposure.

Hugo: Only 78 per cent washed their hands even when they knew they were being observed!

Rachael: I think I'll go and wash my hands right now …

Author (Emma): It is important to note that a lot of handwashing events were observed in this study, yet most of the healthcare professionals were compliant. It is also worth remembering that healthcare workers in busy tertiary centres might wash their hands up to 100 times a day, so it is easy to see how it might get overlooked from time to time. Studies such as this help to remind us of the need for continuous attention to improving infection control in healthcare settings.

The real 'biggy' in terms of measurement bias in all cohort studies is in the measurement of outcomes. Inaccurate or inconsistent measurement of outcomes can occur due to incomplete reporting of outcome data in registries and clinical bases, which is particularly an issue for retrospective cohort studies that rely on historical data. Although not intentional, in prospective cohort studies it is possible that there might be more attentive examination of individuals known to be exposed to presumed risk factors relative to those who were not. Participants who are aware of the exposure–outcome relationship being investigated might also present more readily for diagnosis following exposure. When this problem affects both exposed and not-exposed groups more or less equally, no bias has been introduced – although it does tend to dilute the true relationship between the exposure and the outcome. When the misclassification of outcome occurs more frequently in one comparison group, however, bias is introduced.

Let's have a look at how measurement bias in relation to outcomes can distort the findings in cohort studies. Say we go ahead with a cohort study of a daily pizza and chips diet. We recruit 500 healthy health science students from one tertiary institution who eat pizza and/or chips that are available from their canteen almost every day. Our comparison group is 500 health science students (also healthy) at another tertiary institution where the canteen does not offer pizza or chips. At the beginning of a six-month follow-up period, we measure the participants' blood pressure and compare this with their blood pressure during follow-up and at the end of the study, with hypertension being our main outcome of interest. In Table 8.1, I have listed the possible outcomes that might occur if our classification of outcome is accurate in all cases (reflecting the 'true world'), is randomly misclassified (non-differential misclassification) or is affected by measurement bias (differential classification).

Table 8.1 Pizza and chips diet and the development of hypertension over six months in health science students (n = 1000)

	Hypertension (n)	No hypertension (n)	Relative Risk
True world*			
Exposed (n = 500)	83	417	1.6
Not exposed (n = 500)	52	448	
Non-differential misclassification			
Exposed (n = 500)	60	440	1.5
Not exposed (n = 500)	40	460	
Differential misclassification (bias)			
Exposed (n = 500)	83	417	2.1
Not exposed (n = 500)	40	460	

* Not really the true world

In Table 8.1, we can see that there is a 60 per cent increased risk of developing hypertension in the hypothetical 'true world' (RR = 1.6). If we have inaccurately measured the outcome but have done so in a random fashion in both exposed and not-exposed groups (i.e. non-differentially), we can see that the relative risk associated with pizza and chips each day decreases to 1.5. But if the misclassification only impacts one of the groups (here we have misclassified outcomes in the not-exposed group), the excess risk of hypertension associated with pizza and chips each day for six months has hypothetically almost doubled, now suggesting a 110 per cent increase in risk relative to the comparison group (RR = 2.1).

Hugo: I guess this means we probably shouldn't eat pizza and chips every day?

Rachael: So, does measurement bias always increase the RR?

Author (Emma): In this *hypothetical* example, daily pizza and chips doesn't look good in all three scenarios, but a bit of critical thinking would probably lead you to conclude it isn't a good idea in real life. In the case of non-differential misclassification, the effect measure (e.g. RR) is always reduced, but where a real bias exists (differential misclassification), the effect measure could increase or decrease, depending on which of the comparison groups is most affected.

There are some strategies that can minimise measurement bias in cohort studies, with the main one being to use the same methods to ascertain data on exposure and outcomes among all participants. These methods should involve the use of standardised definitions and data-collection forms by all data collectors. In retrospective cohort studies, the use of multiple sources of data can help to validate exposure status in both comparison groups. In prospective cohort studies, providing standardised training to interviewers who could also be kept unaware of the study aims can be helpful. This technique is known as blinding, which we will hear more about in Chapter 9. Those assessing study outcomes can also be kept unaware of the exposure status of participants. Keeping participants unaware of the study goals and exposure classification might also help but would be a bit ethically tricky. The use of memory cues and other interview techniques to enhance recall in participants, using additional sources of information to validate exposure as well as using objective measurements to validate outcomes would be a preferable approach.

A related problem touched on in previous chapters (and discussed in more detail later in this book) is the issue of confounding. This is when other variables (characteristics or risk factors) associated with both the exposure of interest and the outcome can distort the true relationship between that exposure and the outcome. The best way to deal with this in all study types is to identify and measure all potential confounders at the beginning of a study so they can be controlled for at the time of analysis, or even design the study in a way that limits the influence of confounders in the first place (e.g. restrict eligibility to people of a certain age or sex). Prospective cohort studies can be quite inflexible to evolving understandings about the influence of particular risk factors and characteristics over the life of the study. Any information on potential confounders that would have been collected may only be measurable at one point in time – that is, at the beginning of the study. In the situation of unmeasured confounders, statistical methods may be the only way to work out their effect on your findings. For instance, the Mantel-Haenszel technique provides a summary RR (or OR) of the relationship of interest that is weighted (there's that word 'weight' again) according to strata of the confounding variable (21). Or an '*E*-value' calculates the potential magnitude of the effect of unmeasured confounders required to return the RR estimated in your study to the null (22). Anyway, the take-home message here is that confounding is bad – very, very bad – which is why consideration of confounding lies at the forefront in the design and analysis of most high-quality studies.

I have listed the link to the *Catalogue of Bias* (16) in the 'Further reading' section for those that want to learn more about sources of, and remedies for, bias and confounding in health science research.

Strengths and limitations of cohort studies

Aren't cohort studies great? They really deserve their reputation as top-shelf observational research designs. If we have a scientific question like 'What happens to people when they are exposed or not exposed to a particular risk factor?', cohort studies are really the 'go to' design. If we have a good understanding of an exposure, we can follow people along and find out what happens to them. Because the exposure is measured first, we can be pretty sure the exposure happened before the outcome did. This represents a huge advantage on cross-sectional studies and moves us much closer to determining causality. It doesn't go all the way to claiming causation, however, as it is unlikely that we have accounted for all possible risk factors involved in the outcome and we wouldn't usually have a lot of control over the actual levels of exposure involved (23). Nonetheless, we can study some rare exposures with cohort studies. In prospective cohort studies, we can use standardised measures of exposure and get information about types of exposures that only active participants can provide. There are many exposures that are not generally documented in clinical records or collected routinely elsewhere, such as individual alcohol consumption or levels of activity. One downfall with evaluating risk behaviours as exposures is that these behaviours usually change over time. The risk behaviours may be modified or even ceased by individuals in the exposed group or the practices may be taken up by people in the comparison group. This can all take some high-level surveillance by investigators to sort out during follow-up. Thankfully, methods such as deriving 'person-time at risk' can help out in this situation.

Due in part to the person-time at risk thing, really top-notch estimates of incidence and mortality can be derived from cohort studies, and these can be used to calculate relative and absolute risks for multiple outcomes. Unless the follow-up of participants is particularly active over the study period, most cohort studies rely on good data linkages between various state registries (birth, deaths, cancers, etc.) and clinical databases, which mainly only have consistent quality and completeness in higher-income countries. It has been estimated that population-based cancer registries, for instance, cover pretty close to 70 per cent of the population in highincome countries, but only around 17 per cent nationally in lower-income countries (24). This means that many cancers and other outcomes might not be identified even in high-income countries, and cohort studies requiring data linkage might not even be possible in lower-income countries.

Of course, if we were seriously into studying outcomes such as cancer, which takes a really long time to develop and remains quite rare across populations as diseases go, we would need to enrol a very large number of people and follow them up for a very long period of time. If we were to conduct a prospective cohort study such as this, we would be talking about a lot of research funding. We would need a fortune just to pay for the research personnel, not to mention office facilities and consumables, costs associated with medical assessments and so on (and on). We could always opt for a retrospective cohort study, which is much cheaper to conduct and has results available sooner, and reserve the prospective cohort approach for the study of much more common phenomena of shorter duration – for example, COVID-19. Retrospective cohort studies do have the disadvantage of being restricted to the information documented in the past, so must rely on data recorded by multiple persons, possibly inconsistently, with few available avenues for chasing up missing, incomplete or equivocal data. Many of these problems are not as pressing in the case of shorter cohort studies investigating events occurring in recent history.

In the previous section, we discussed the potential for different kinds of bias and, as is the case for all study designs, the potential introduction of bias is an ever-present threat for cohort studies. As we now know, the not-exposed group in cohort studies may be internal (selected from the same population as the exposed group), external (a similar population selected from elsewhere, such as a different occupation group) or a similar group selected from the general population. Although the aim is to recruit a comparison group that differs from the exposed group only with respect to their exposure status, the potential for selection bias remains due to potentially unmeasured risk factors. In fact, some say it is actually not possible to be fully confident that any difference between comparison groups can be controlled for in cohort studies (25).

Attrition bias is another form of selection bias to which prospective cohort studies are prone, particularly when the study involves long follow-up periods. Longer prospective studies are also restricted to the exposure information collected at the beginning of the study, which may also open the door to the problem of unmeasured confounders. Retrospective studies also have issues in relation to selection bias. Because they look at historically documented data, they are unaffected by attrition bias, but missing or incomplete data can really rain on their parade. Further, it is likely that standardised reporting was not utilised by the potentially multiple clinicians recording data back then. Inconsistent documentation of exposure and outcome can also introduce the potential for misclassification which, if it occurred differentially across comparison groups, could result in measurement bias.

The main advantages and disadvantages of cohort studies are summarised in Table 8.2.

Table 8.2 Advantages and disadvantages of cohort studies

Type of cohort study	Advantages	Disadvantages
Both prospective and retrospective	Approaches causality by establishing temporality. Can study rare exposures. Allows investigation of multiple outcomes. Provides precise estimates of disease occurrence and mortality over time. Can estimate absolute and relative risks.	Not possible to fully assess causality. Misclassification of risk behaviours (exposures) that may change over time (e.g. alcohol or other drug use). May be subject to availability of good data linkage between clinical and population registries. Usually requires large numbers of participants. Identifying suitable comparison groups can be problematic (potential for selection bias).
Prospective	Provides the strongest evidence for temporality. Allows for consistent measurements of specific exposure. Provides information about exposures that are not usually documented in clinical records or registries. Allows investigation of outcomes that were identified subsequent to the start of the study.	Subject to 'attrition bias'. Not suitable for the investigation of rare outcomes or diseases with long progression. Can be very expensive and may take a long time to conduct. May include unmeasured confounders. Restricted to exposure information collected at the start of the study.
Retrospective	Relatively inexpensive and quick to conduct. Can study rarer outcomes.	Prone to selection bias (via missing data). Prone to measurement bias. Restricted to previously recorded data.

Rachael: There always seem to be long lists of advantages and disadvantages about every study design.

Hugo: And it seems that we always come back to what design works best for the scientific question.

Author (Emma): Well, exactly! This is all part of learning to think critically and how to apply this process to problem-solving. When we identify an issue, we can look at the problem from multiple angles, frame an appropriate scientific question, then select the best way to answer it. So we need to know the strengths and weaknesses of each study design to be able to make this decision.

Conclusion

In this chapter, we have learnt all about cohort studies and how they can be used to find out what happens to groups of people who are exposed or not exposed to a particular risk factor. We learnt that cohort studies are considered pretty much top of the range for observational studies because of their ability to confirm temporality (exposure precedes outcome), which moves closer to establishing causality in a way that other observational study designs cannot.

Learning objective 1: Describe the main features, types and uses of cohort studies

We learnt that the two main types of cohort studies are prospective and retrospective designs and what types of information these studies can provide. We heard about the well-known, and ongoing, prospective cohort study, the Framingham Heart Study, as well as other prospective and retrospective studies of various lengths in relation to their appropriateness for the scientific questions posed.

Learning objective 2: Interpret the common outcome measures of cohort studies

Here we revisited the concept of incidence rates and how they are calculated, when different types of rates are used, and also explored the notion of person-time at risk. In this section, we introduced the relative risk (RR) and had a go at interpreting and calculating RR through a worked example. We also introduced the concept of risk difference and looked at how it is important to consider both absolute and relative risk.

Learning objective 3: Identify the main types of potential sources of bias in cohort studies and understand some of the methods used to address these

In addressing this objective, we discussed the two major categories of bias – selection and measurement bias – as they apply to cohort studies and strategies for addressing bias. We discussed the main points at which selection bias can be introduced from the identification of the target population through to information being analysed at the end of the study, and the types of selection bias to which each type of cohort study (prospective and retrospective) is most prone. We also learnt about different sources of measurement bias and specifically looked at the impact of misclassification of outcomes.

Learning objective 4: Discuss the strengths and limitations of cohort studies

Finally, we summarised the ability of cohort studies to confirm the temporal pathway between exposures and outcomes, determining precise measures of incidence and comparing risk between exposed and not-exposed groups. We pointed out the limitations of cohort studies, particularly prospective designs, for the study of rare diseases (or those of long duration) and the problems associated with using historical data in retrospective cohort studies. As with all study types, cohort studies are prone to different types of bias; these are also summarised in meeting this objective.

Further reading

Bankhead C, Aronson JK, Nunan D. *Catalogue of Bias*. 2017. https://catalogofbias.org

Framingham Heart Study. Three generations of health research. 2023. www.framinghamheartstudy.org

Questions

Answers are available at the end of the book.

Multiple-choice questions

1. A study of the relationship between mobile phone use and brain tumours was undertaken in Japan. A very large cohort of young people (aged 15 to 21 years) were recruited to the study and underwent a number of clinical tests, including a CT scan of the head. An app recorded their time spent actively making phone calls. These data were uploaded to the research team every week and two-yearly health assessments (including CT scans) were conducted over a follow-up period of 30 years. What sort of study design does this sound like to you?
   A – Retrospective cohort study
   B – Not possible to identify the direction of study from the information given
   C – Prospective cohort study
   D – Randomised controlled trial
2. Which of the following is *not* a feature of cohort studies?
   A – Cohorts are sorted into groups based on their exposure.
   B – There must be equal numbers in each comparison groups.
   C – At enrolment, all participants are free of the condition/s of interest.
   D – Comparison groups should have similar characteristics apart from their exposure status.
3. In a cohort study of childhood asthma and home heating appliances in Germany, investigators reported that the relative risk (RR) of asthma was 0.51 ($p < 0.05$) for reverse-cycle air-conditioning relative to unflued gas heating. Which statement most accurately interprets this RR?
   A – Unflued gas heating was associated with a 51 per cent reduction in childhood asthma relative to reverse-cycle air-conditioning.
   B – The increased risk of asthma associated with reverse-cycle air-conditioning was statistically significant.
   C – More than half of the risk of asthma (51 per cent) was directly attributable to unflued gas heating.
   D – The risk of childhood asthma associated with reverse-cycle air-conditioning was half that of unflued gas heating.

4. To what types of selection bias are prospective cohort studies particularly prone?
   A – Allocation bias
   B – The 'health worker' effect
   C – Attrition bias
   D – Recall bias.
5. Which of the following is *not* a strength of prospective cohort studies?
   A – Study rare exposures
   B – Establish temporal relationships between exposure and outcomes
   C – Study rare outcomes
   D – Study multiple outcomes.

Short-answer questions

1. A team of researchers investigated excess all-cause and cardiac-specific mortality experienced by people who were born prematurely and cared for in neonatal intensive care units (NICUs). They accessed the hospital records of NICU patients admitted from 1930 to 1940 and those of infants born at full term during the same period in the same hospitals. They then reviewed deaths registry data from time of birth to present day, collecting data on cause of death and comparing these outcomes between the pre-term and full-term groups. What type of study design do you think was employed here and why do you think so?
2. Go to the Australian Institute of Health and Welfare page 'Cancer data in Australia' (www.aihw.gov.au/reports/cancer/cancer-data-in-australia/contents/cancer-mortality-by-age-visualisation) to look at cancer mortality data for Australia. Under 'Select a cancer site/group', pick a topic of interest. What were the crude and age-standardised mortality rates for all persons (not sex-specific) for the cancer you have chosen in 2020, and what do you think might account for the difference in the crude and age-specific rates you observe? *Hints: you can change between crude and age-standardised mortality at the 'Please select the age group' menu. Hovering your cursor over the data point on the chart brings up the precise rates information.*
3. In the United Kingdom, a cohort study has been going for 60 years and is called the National Child Development Study (NCDS). This study enrolled over 17 000 people in England, Scotland and Wales who were born in a single week of 1958. They continue to collect information on the cohort's physical health, psychosocial development, education and employment status, home and social lives, and attitudes (26). Look at the NCDS site (https://ncds.info). After you have got your bearings, select a topic from the 'What have we learned?' menu. Briefly (with the emphasis on *briefly*) summarise what knowledge the NCDS has contributed.
4. A very famous long-running cohort study was the British Doctors Study, which Richard Doll (a physician), Richard Peto and Austin Bradford Hill (both epidemiologists and statisticians) began in the 1950s. The study recruited a large cohort of doctors (>40 000) and followed them up for 50 years. The study looked at the exposure of tobacco smoking and its links with multiple health outcomes, including lung cancer. Table 8.3 shows preliminary results reporting lung cancer deaths after six years of follow-up in the proportion of the cohort who were male and aged 35 years and over (approximately 24 000). Describe how you interpret the information in Table 8.3.

Table 8.3 Mortality in British doctors in relation to level of smoking in men aged 35 years or older (27)

Cause of death	Deaths (n)	Age-standardised mortality rates (per 1000)			
		Non-smokers	Daily average smoking (grams)		
			1-14	15–24	≥25
Lung cancer	84	0.07	0.47	0.86	1.66
Other cancer	220	2.04	2.01	1.56	2.63
Respiratory disease	126	0.81	1.00	1.11	1.41
Coronary thrombosis	508	4.22	4.64	4.60	5.99
Other causes	779	6.11	6.82	6.38	7.19
All deaths	1714	13.25	14.92	14.49	18.84

5. Looking at Table 8.3, calculate and interpret the absolute difference in all-cause mortality for non-smokers and men smoking 25 grams of tobacco per day.
6. Using the information in Table 8.3, what was the relative risk of death from all causes for those in the highest category of smoking relative to non-smokers, and how do you interpret the RR?
7. Again using information in Table 8.3, calculate the RRs associated with the different levels of smoking to complete Table 8.4.

Table 8.4 Relative risk of mortality in British doctors in relation to level of smoking in men aged 35 years or older. Adapted from (27).

Cause of death	Non-smokers	Daily average smoking (grams)		
		1-14	15-24	≥25
Lung cancer	1 [reference]	6.7	?	?
Other causes	1 [reference]	?	?	?
All-cause death	1 [reference]	?	?	?

In Table 8.4, the non-smokers are the reference category, so the mortality in each category of smoking is divided by the mortality observed in non-smokers. For example, I have calculated the RR for the lung cancer in the lowest category of smoking as:

Mortality in non-smokers = 0.07 [reference category]
Mortality in those smoking 1–14 grams daily = 0.47
RR= 0.47/0.07 = 6.7

Now you can calculate the RRs for lung cancer mortality in those smoking 15–24 grams daily (relative to non-smokers) and in those smoking ≥25 gram daily (relative to non-smokers). Then repeat the exercise for mortality from other causes, and all causes.

8. Ten people were recruited to a cohort study and were followed up for 20 months to see whether they became a new case of interest. During that time, there were three cases and four participants withdrew. The length of time they all spent in the study is presented in Figure 8.6. Calculate the total person-time at risk represented in Figure 8.6 and also the incidence per 1000 person months.

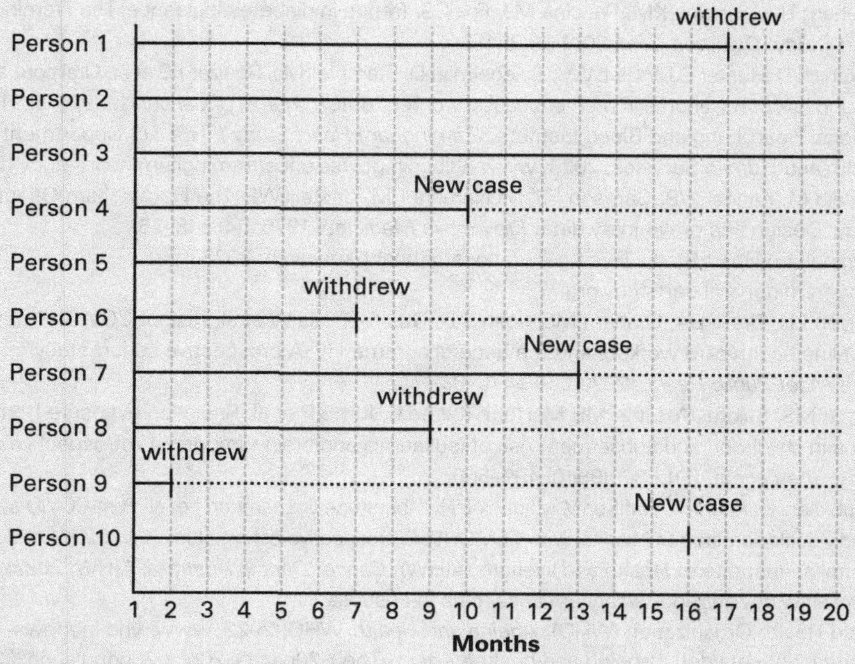

Figure 8.6 Time of observation and outcomes in a hypothetical cohort study

9. Say you want to investigate the relationship between stress at university and later health status in middle age (45 to 64 years). You recruit all new undergraduate entrants to your study and administer surveys that are designed to measure stress levels at two-monthly interviews throughout their journey through university and then sort them into 'high-stress' (exposed) and 'low-stress' (not exposed) groups on the basis of their results by the time of graduation. You subject your participants to a range of psychosocial and physiological testing at baseline, at the end of their studies, and then at two-yearly intervals for 40 years. What major and specific types of bias might your study be prone to here?
10. Researchers want to investigate the relationship between exposure to a specific type of solvent used in a particular industry and the later development of chronic disease. Only one particular industry uses the solvent in its manufacturing processes but there is currently some evidence that prolonged exposure might lead to the development of a range of chronic illnesses. There is some evidence that exposure to the solvent is associated with autoimmune arthritis, chronic kidney disease and degenerative eye diseases that occur in early life relative to the general population. Do you think a prospective cohort study design would be appropriate for this investigation and what is your reasoning?

References

1. Tsao CW, Vasan RS. Cohort profile – the Framingham Heart Study (FHS): Overview of milestones in cardiovascular epidemiology. *International Journal of Epidemiology*. 2015;44(6):1800–13.
2. Freund KM, Belanger AJ, D'Agostino RB, Kannel WB. The health risks of smoking. The Framingham Study: 34 years of follow-up. *Annals of Epidemiology*. 1993;3(4):417–24.
3. Vasan RS, Pencina MJ, Cobain M, Freiberg MS, D'Agostino RB. Estimated risks for developing obesity in the Framingham Heart Study. *Annals of Internal Medicine*. 2005;143(7):473–80.

4. Abraham TM, Pencina KM, Pencina MJ, Fox CS. Trends in diabetes incidence: The Framingham Heart Study. *Diabetes Care*. 2014;38(3):482–7.

5. Feskanich D, Hunter DJ, Willett WC, Spiegelman D, Stampfer MJ, Speizer FE et al. Oral contraceptive use and risk of melanoma in premenopausal women. *British Journal of Cancer*. 1999;81(5):918–23.

6. National Heart Lung and Blood Institute. *Framingham Heart Study (FHS)*. US Department of Health and Human Services; 2023. www.nhlbi.nih.gov/science/framingham-heart-study-fhs

7. Feinleib M, Kannel WB, Garrison RJ, McNamara PM, Castelli WP. The Framingham Offspring Study: Design and preliminary data. *Preventive Medicine*. 1975;4(4):518–25.

8. Framingham Heart Study. Three generations of health research. 2023. www.framinghamheartstudy.org

9. Nguyen LH, Drew DA, Graham MS, Joshi AD, Guo C-G, Ma W et al. Risk of COVID-19 among front-line health-care workers and the general community: A prospective cohort study. *The Lancet Public Health*. 2020;5(9):e475–83.

10. Pearce MS, Salotti JA, Little MP, McHugh K, Lee C, Kim KP et al. Radiation exposure from CT scans in childhood and subsequent risk of leukaemia and brain tumours: A retrospective cohort study. *The Lancet*. 2012;380(9840):499–505.

11. Ayoubkhani D, Khunti K, Nafilyan V, Maddox T, Humberstone B, Diamond I et al. Post-COVID syndrome in individuals admitted to hospital with COVID-19: Retrospective cohort study. *BMJ*. 2021;372:693.

12. Australian Institute of Health and Welfare (AIHW). *Cancer Data in Australia*. AIHW; 2022. www.aihw.gov.au/reports/cancer/cancer-data-in-australia

13. World Health Organization (WHO). *Ageing and Health*. WHO; 2022. www.who.int/news-room/fact-sheets/detail/ageing-and-health#:~:text=The%20pace%20of%20population%20ageing,from%2012%25%20to%2022%25

14. Elwood MJ. *Causal Relationships in Medicine: A Practical System of Critical Appraisal*. Oxford University Press; 1992.

15. Song JW, Chung KC. Observational studies: Cohort and case-control studies. *Plastic and Reconstructive Surgery*. 2010;126(6):2234–42.

16. Bankhead C, Aronson JK, Nunan D. *Catalogue of Bias*. University of Oxford, Center for Evidence-Based Medicine; 2017. https://catalogofbias.org/biases/attrition-bias

17. Damen NL, Versteeg H, Serruys PW, van Geuns RJ, van Domburg RT, Pedersen SS et al. Cardiac patients who completed a longitudinal psychosocial study had a different clinical and psychosocial baseline profile than patients who dropped out prematurely. *European Journal of Preventive Cardiology*. 2015;22(2):196–9.

18. Ramirez-Santana M. Limitations and biases in cohort studies. In: Barría RM, ed. *Cohort Studies in Health Sciences*. IntechOpen; 2018. pp. 29–45.

19. Landsberger HA. *Hawthorne Revisited: A plea for an Open City*. Cornell University Press; 1957.

20. Wu K-S, Lee SS-J, Chen J-K, Chen Y-S, Tsai H-C, Chen Y-J et al. Identifying heterogeneity in the Hawthorne effect on hand hygiene observation: A cohort study of overtly and covertly observed results. *BMC Infectious Diseases*. 2018;18(1):369.

21. Last J. *A Dictionary of Epidemiology*. 2nd ed. Oxford University Press; 1988.

22. Ananth CV, Schisterman EF. Hidden biases in observational epidemiology: The case of unmeasured confounding. *British Journal of Obstetrics and Gynaecology*. 2018;125(6):644–6.

23. Euser AM, Zoccali C, Jager KJ, Dekker FW. Cohort studies: Prospective versus retrospective. *Nephron Clinical Practice*. 2009;113(3):c214–17.

24. Pramesh CS, Badwe RA, Bhoo-Pathy N, Booth CM, Chinnaswamy G, Dare AJ et al. Priorities for cancer research in low- and middle-income countries: A global perspective. *Nature Medicine*. 2022;28(4):649–57.

25. Healy P, Devane D. Methodological considerations in cohort study designs. *Nurse Researcher*. 2011;18(3):32–6.

26. National Child Development Study. *The National Child Development Study (NCDS)*. Centre for Longitudinal Studies, UCL Social Research Institute; 2023. https://ncds.info/home/about

27. Doll R. Lung cancer and smoking. *Journal of the Royal Society of Health*. 1957;77(6):247–54.

Controlling exposure

9

Is it worth taking that medicine?

Learning objectives

After studying this chapter, you will be able to:

1. Describe the main features of randomised controlled trials
2. Understand the importance of randomisation and allocation concealment
3. Discuss the ethical issues related to randomised controlled trials
4. Describe the strengths and limitations of randomised controlled trials

Introduction

So far in this book, we have found out all about observational study designs, including cross-sectional studies, case-control studies and cohort studies. Observational (non-experimental) studies describe and investigate what is happening to people, and the things that might be related to what is happening to people, in the 'natural world' – that is, they don't involve actually *doing* things to people. In this chapter, we are moving across to the experimental branch of the epidemiological research tree (you might want to review Figure 1.2) and focusing specifically on randomised controlled trials (RCTs).

RCTs are often referred to as the 'gold standard' of health research designs (1), and are ranked pretty much at the top of the hierarchy of scientific evidence (2). Representations of the hierarchy of evidence in the form of pyramid are more or less ubiquitous on the internet and in textbooks, and one more is presented here. Figure 9.1 shows the ranking of the strength of evidence provided by different methods of inquiry from weak to strong from the base of the pyramid to its peak.

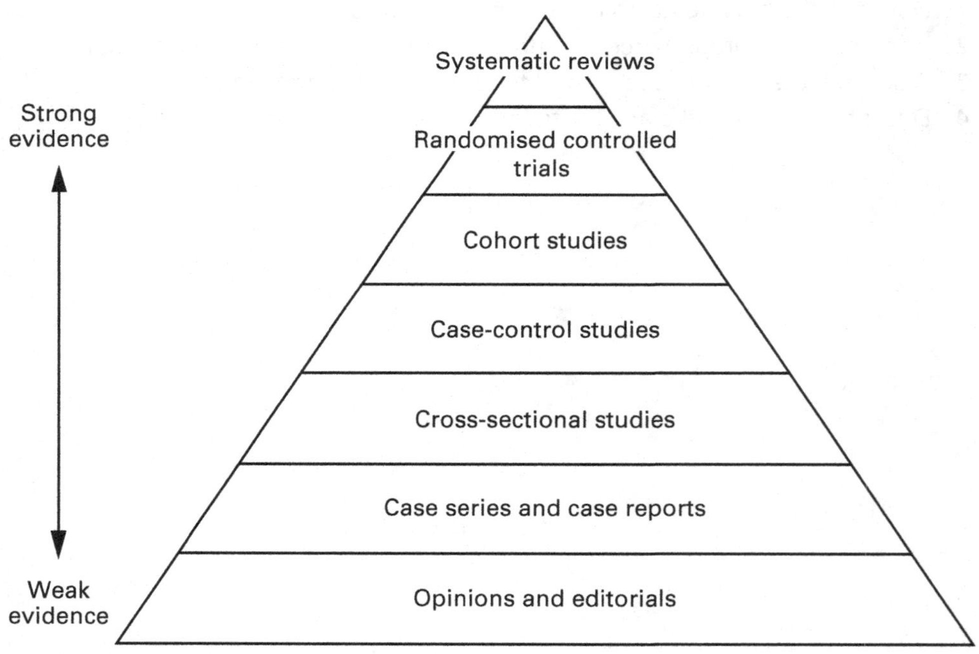

Figure 9.1 Hierarchy of evidence. Adapted from (2).

According to the hierarchy of evidence pyramid, the only study design deemed to provide more convincing evidence than an RCT is the systematic review. We will hear a little bit more about this type of study below, but it is worth noting for now that systematic reviews traditionally (though not always) rely on pooling data from multiple RCTs.

Hugo: So are you saying that none of the designs we have heard about so far provides decent evidence?

Rachael: Are experimental studies considered more important than observational studies?

Author (Emma): These are valid questions about of the 'hierarchy of evidence' concept – which, it could be argued, stems from a very 'positivist' view of scientific research. There is, in fact, a growing recognition that the perfect study design is the one that provides the sort of evidence that specifically addresses the scientific question posed (3), which doesn't really fit the whole unidirectional ranking thing. So all the study designs we have discussed can provide 'decent' and 'important' evidence, as long as they are the right design for the question.

So far, this book has focused on evaluating and interrogating high-quality evidence to reach an understanding or solve a problem through the process of critical thinking. This process is always embarked on as a response to an identified problem or issue that we need to address in order to arrive at a solution. In the health sciences, the problem or issue is expressed as a scientific question, which can only be answered with the use of an appropriate research design. As we saw in Chapter 1, questions related to the rich breadth of human experience and the meaning these experiences have for individuals can only be addressed adequately by qualitative methods. When it comes to quantitative methods, observational studies are immensely useful for identifying and describing health or social issues. They can provide information about exposures and risk factors associated with the occurrence of health and social conditions, and this information is crucial for informing the development of evidence-based interventions that can address those issues or prevent them occurring in the first place. Experimental studies, such as RCTs, use rigorous methods (the thing for which they are most famous) to evaluate the performance of the interventions themselves. So RCTs are likely to be the best way to address the question of this chapter: 'Is it worth taking that medicine?'

Randomised controlled trials

RCTs start with recruiting a sample of participants from a well-defined population, often (though not always) a clinical population, who are randomised to either receive some sort of intervention or not. The intervention may be a medication or other therapy, a surgical procedure or even an education or exercise program. The 'not' group (otherwise known as 'controls') may receive an inactive medication that looks similar (a 'placebo') or pretend intervention that appears to follow the same process (e.g. sham surgery) or be given the standard treatment or therapy. The participants are then 'followed up' during and after the study to see what impact the intervention had, which is determined by comparing outcomes in the intervention and non-intervention groups. These outcomes might include an improvement in, or cure of, the clinical or social issues the intervention was intended to address; the safety of the intervention; side-effects or complications associated with the intervention; determination of the optimal dosage and duration of treatment; and any long-term outcomes.

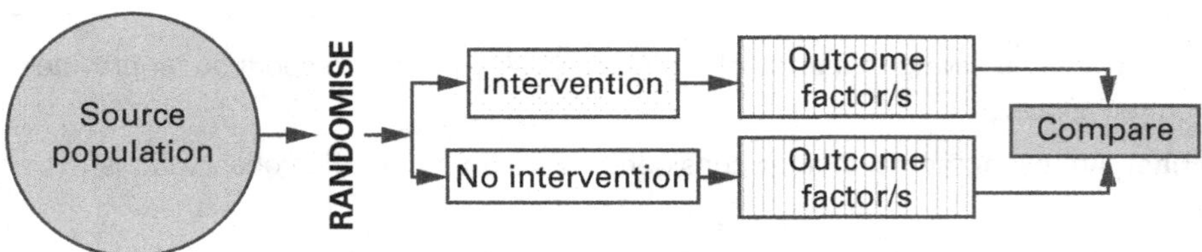

Figure 9.2 Direction of investigation for randomised controlled trials

The direction of study for your basic RCT is outlined in Figure 9.2, although RCT designs can be more complex depending on how many intervention groups are being compared and whether there are any 'crossover' elements (e.g. when intervention and control groups swap over after a period of follow-up during the study). For now, we will focus on the most important things about RCTs, which actually appear in the name of the study design itself – people are randomly assigned (the 'randomised' bit) to receive an intervention in order to test the performance of that new intervention (the 'trial' bit) against what happens to the comparison group (the 'controlled' bit).

EXAMPLE 9.1

In what is thought to be one of the very first clinical trials way back in the eighteenth century, Scottish physician James Lind investigated treatments for the condition of scurvy on naval ships (4). Scurvy was once a devasting affliction of sailors around the world, caused (as we now know) by a deficiency of vitamin C. Scurvy causes a breakdown of capillaries leading to abnormal bruising, bleeding gums, internal bleeding and (if untreated) death. During their sometimes many months at sea in the early days of sea voyaging, sailors did not have access to fresh fruits and vegetables – particularly citrus fruits, which contain high quantities of vitamin C. Scurvy became a scourge that sometimes resulted in the deaths of the majority of the sailors on board. It was after reading about the deaths of 380 of 510 sailors on one ship that Lind became interested in studying scurvy at sea (5).

Aboard the *Salisbury* in 1747, Lind identified 12 sailors with scurvy. After making sure the stage of their condition and their normal diets were similar, Lind administered six different treatments to the sailors over a six-day period. Two patients were given cider; two received the now obsolete, but then common, scurvy treatment of 'elixir vitriol' (sulfuric acid and alcohol); two received vinegar; two received salt water; and two received oranges and lemons to eat each day.

After six days of treatment, Lind reported that only the two sailors receiving citrus fruit had recovered, one of whom had recovered sufficiently to be deemed fit for duty by the sixth day (4).

Unfortunately, it would be decades until the findings of Lind actually improved nutritional practice at sea (5), but ultimately the performance of citrus against scourge of scurvy was confirmed and the condition became a bad memory, at least among sailors.

Scientific rigour: The application of the highest standards of the scientific method, particularly with reference to minimising bias.

As possibly the world's first clinical trial (or at least the first published one), the Lind example presented in Example 9.1 is certainly worthy of attention. The study design exhibited some of the features of today's clinical trials but did lack a certain amount of **scientific rigour** –

the application of the highest standards of the scientific method, particularly with reference to minimising bias. Absent from Lind's investigation, and one of the more important ways that RCTs minimise bias, is the **randomisation** bit – which we will hear a bit more about later. Lind's work did, however, provide a template for clinical trials, a design that really took off during the twentieth century. One early effort published in the 1930s compared sanocrysin (a salt compound containing gold and thiosulphate that was a recognised treatment at the time) with injections of distilled water for treating tuberculosis in the United States (6). Twenty-four tuberculosis (TB) patients were pair-matched to two groups and a single flip of a coin was used to assign the groups to receive the sanocrysin or be the control group. The investigators did try to keep the treatment allocation secret, but it is unlikely they were successful as sanocrysin had terrible side-effects, to the extent that one patient died of liver necrosis during the study. In any event, the sanocrysin was ultimately found to have little benefit over the three-year period of follow-up.

Randomisation: A process of allocating participants to intervention and control groups by chance to ensure the similarity of study groups at the start of the study, in order to minimise the potential for selection bias and validly measure the impact of the intervention being investigated.

One of the very first truly randomised controlled studies was published in 1950, again investigating TB treatments, this time the antibiotic Streptomycin (7). This was a multicentre study in the United States, which involved the determination of participant eligibility and prognosis rankings by an independent expert panel whose members did not know the patients' names or the hospital they were in. Strict study protocols assured consistent methods across institutions, so that the participants were as similar as possible when allocated to the study groups (270 in the intervention group and 271 controls). All participants received the same treatment regimen in each hospital, and clinical outcomes were measured in the same way. The intervention group ('subjects') and control group both received standard tuberculosis therapies, but subjects also received streptomycin for 91 days. For the record, it turned out the streptomycin was very beneficial for TB patients, with improvements noted across all measures and throughout the study in the intervention group relative to the controls (8). The meticulous design and attention to detail of this study was a standout compared with earlier and then contemporary efforts at clinical trials, and really set the scene for RCTs into the future.

Hugo: What happened to the sailors who didn't get the citrus fruit during the study?

Rachael: Yes, and what about the TB patients who didn't get the antibiotics?

Author (Emma): Lind reports little about the other patients, mostly stating that they didn't recover – although the cider-treated sailors did improve slightly over the period of observation (4). The authors of the streptomycin study report greater deterioration and higher mortality in controls over the first six months of the study. An update at 12 months showed that the deaths in controls were by then double those of the streptomycin group (7), indicating that the study continued unchanged despite the clear benefits of the treatment. But yours are pretty important questions, which really speak to the ethics of these clinical trials. We are going to hear a little bit more about this later in this chapter but, I'm sorry to say, if ethical issues were considered at all by the investigators of these studies, they were not highlighted at the time and no formal ethical oversight was involved the conduct of the studies.

Incidentally, tuberculosis is often thought of as an old threat to human health, a distant memory due to the introduction of antibiotic treatments and vaccines in the early twentieth century (9). However, TB never really went away in developing countries, has re-emerged in lower socioeconomic populations in wealthier countries and continues to be a worldwide threat due to the emergence of multi-drug resistant TB (10). Second only to COVID-19, TB is a leading cause of death to infectious diseases globally (11) and its management and treatment continue to be the focus of many RCTs to this day.

Types of randomised controlled trials

While all RCTs contain the essential elements of randomisation and the trialling of interventions in comparison groups, the ways different types of studies are described in the scientific literature may cause confusion. RCTs can be classified by how they deliver the intervention to their participants – whether they have a 'parallel' or 'crossover' design. In parallel designs, each participant group only receives one of the interventions or treatment regimens throughout the study. As mentioned above, in crossover designs participant groups may swap over during the study – in effect, intervention group participants become their own control in the study. Crossover designs are a bit more complex as there could be carryover effects of the first treatment (or subsequent treatments, if there are more than one) that must be taken into account. This can be accomplished by allowing time for a 'wash-out' period between treatments (a period without the initial treatment to allow for all of its effects to dissipate), and randomising the treatment sequence is also used if multiple interventions are being investigated (12).

Blinding: (synonym 'masking') A process whereby participants and/or investigators are kept unaware of the allocation of interventions in an experimental study to prevent the introduction of bias in measuring the effect of the intervention.

As well as being classified by design type, RCTs can be classified according to who knows what during the investigation. When people are kept unaware of aspects of a study, it is called **blinding**, which is done to prevent the potential for bias in measuring the effect of the intervention. An 'open' trial is one in which everybody is aware of which group is randomised to the treatment and its outcome. This happens most often when the intervention involves some sort of surgery. Most of the time, however, at least someone is blinded and just how many are blinded defines the classification of the RCT. A 'single-blind' trial is where one group in the study does not know who received the experimental treatment. This is usually the participants themselves, but the single-blinded group may also be the investigators measuring outcomes of the intervention. For instance, it might be difficult to blind participants receiving surgical or program-based interventions, but it is possible to blind the investigators or clinicians evaluating the treatment outcome. As the name suggests, in double-blind RCTs, at least two groups involved in the study are unaware of who received the treatment, and usually these are the participants and the investigators or those responsible for assessing the outcome of the trial. There are also triple-blind and quadruple-blind RCTs, which can involve blinding patients, the investigators, the outcome assessors and even the data analysts. More about blinding later!

Rachael: So, now we know what it means when we hear about a study called something like a 'randomised, placebo-controlled, double-blind, parallel-study'!

Hugo: Those quadruple-blind RCTs sound like nobody knows what is going on!

Author (Emma): Most blinded trials have very clear and rigorous protocols governing every aspect of the recruitment, allocation to study groups, intervention administration, assessment of outcome and so on. At the end, once there is no possibility of introducing bias, there is usually a prescribed method of unblinding. So it's not like they are all just stumbling around with blindfolds on!

In the earlier days of the COVID-19 pandemic, there was some evidence that a parasite treatment (specifically, a treatment for intestinal worms) called 'ivermectin' could stop the SARS-CoV-2 virus replicating in cell cultures. Everyone got really excited at first, but it turned out that the concentration of the drug required to have the same effect in humans would be toxic, at 100 times the usual recommended dose for treating parasites (13). Perhaps representing a strange human attraction to parasite treatments, the drug hydroxychloroquine (prescribed mostly for malaria, but also for rheumatoid arthritis) was feted as a potential saviour, but also turned out to cause more harm than good in COVID-19 patients (14). Possibly due to increasing societal mistrust in authority and scientists in the United States at that time, and despite the growing evidence pointing to the lack of any benefit to the treatment, many people championed the use of both ivermectin and hydroxychloroquine for COVID-19 and pitted themselves against the authorities in promoting their 'miracle cures' (15, 16). One of the many RCTs involving treatment for COVID-19 with these medications is described in Example 9.2. See if you can recognise some of the terminology used.

EXAMPLE 9.2

Beltran Gonzales and colleagues undertook a randomised, double-blind, placebo-controlled clinical trial to evaluate the performance of ivermectin and hydroxychloroquine in patients hospitalised with severe COVID-19 in Mexico (17).

The participants had an average age of 53 years, and 62 per cent were males. Eligible patients, 106 in total, were randomised to one of three treatment groups: hydroxychloroquine (33 participants), ivermectin (36 participants) or placebo (37 participants). The main outcomes of interest were length of stay due to improvement, worsening respiratory illness and death during the follow-up period.

There was no statistically significant difference in duration of stay due to improvement between the three study groups ($p = 0.43$). There were also no differences in worsening respiratory illness or death ($p = 0.83$). The authors concluded that there was no benefit in treating non-critical hospitalised patients with severe COVID-19 with either hydroxychloroquine or ivermectin (17).

Randomised control trials in the community

So far, we have talked about RCTs conducted in clinical settings and/or focused on disease and treatments. However, RCTs can be conducted in all sorts of settings and for all types of social or health issues, as long as the method suits both the intervention and the population in which it will be trialled. For instance, in Saudi Arabia, a single-blind community-based RCT investigated the quality of life and physical effects of low- and high-intensity aerobic and resistance training in community-dwelling older men who had exacerbated loss of muscle-mass and strength post-COVID-19 (18). Another single-blind, community-based RCT looked at the effects of immediate versus delayed access to a nutrition education program in low-income parents in the United States (19). In fact, whole communities can take part in randomised controlled community trials. For instance, a randomised controlled, single-blind community trial was conducted in Uganda, investigating whether home-based treatments for sexually transmitted infections would reduce the incidence of HIV (20). In this study, four to seven adjoining villages were clustered into one of 10 groups (56 villages in all), which were then randomly allocated to the intervention or control groups (i.e. five clusters in each).

Systematic reviews

Mentioned a few times in this book, systematic reviews are a type of study that is strongly associated with RCTs. Systematic reviews essentially pool together the evidence presented in well-conducted RCTs, themselves often seen as the pinnacle of scientific rigour. The aim is to identify, evaluate and synthesise all the available evidence from high-quality studies using predetermined explicit and systematic methods to address specific research questions. Systematic reviews are considered to be objective and less prone to bias, as the literature searches they undertake are comprehensive, exhaustive and repeatable; they use explicit criteria for choosing and excluding studies; and they include an assessment and discussion of the quality of the 'primary studies' included in the review. Primary studies, incidentally, are those conducted and described by the authors of the published report, so most systematic reviews include the information from the original study and not studies that are described in papers published at another time.

Systematic reviews synthesise the information in all the included studies and *may* include a 'meta-analysis'. This is a statistical way to pool the data from two or more quantitative studies to produce a single estimate of effect (e.g. a relative risk, an odds ratio, a difference in mean scores). The results of each study are weighted (a statistical manoeuvre that assigns greater value) so that larger studies contribute more to the pooled estimate relative to smaller studies. If the studies are very different from each other (e.g. differences in methods used, population groups or measurement taken), it is not appropriate to conduct a meta-analysis, which is why many systematic reviews don't include one. If a meta-analysis is possible, the larger numbers in a pooled sample allow for smaller effects to be detected, which is due to increased statistical power (a little more on power later). No meta? No matter! It is the 'systematic' part of systematic reviews that is of most importance, so a well-conducted review without a meta-analysis (meta-analysis-less?) will still produce a meaningful synthesis of the evidence.

One of the best-known collections of systematic reviews is the Cochrane Library, which is accessible on the internet (21). The Cochrane Library contains everything you want to know about systematic reviews and how they are conducted. Importantly, it provides a searchable database of high-quality systematic reviews on an enormous range of topics. Rather than spending a lot of time sifting through the published literature and evaluating the quality of the information yourself, systematic reviews essentially provide a 'one stop shop' of information about most health issues of interest, assuming that there have been some high-quality primary studies published on the topic to review (one of the big down-sides of relying on systematic reviews). Nonetheless, for a busy health professional (or student), systematic reviews can be a valuable and time-saving resource. I have included the link to the Cochrane Library in the 'Further reading' section. In many countries, the Cochrane Library is publicly available or can be accessed via your university or college.

Methodological aspects of randomised controlled trials

One reason why RCTs are held in such high regard is the effort taken to ensure they are validly measuring the effects of the intervention they are trialling. It is no good going through all the effort and expense of conducting a study to evaluate a new therapy or program if it is not possible to isolate the impact of the intervention from the effects that participant characteristics might have on outcomes. Here we come to the most famous part of RCTs: the process of randomisation.

Randomisation

At the end of an RCT, we want to compare outcomes and we want to be sure it is the intervention alone that is causing any differences between the groups. Randomisation provides a way to accomplish this through evenly distributing participant characteristics that might influence outcomes. For the whole thing to work, each eligible participant has to have an equal chance of being assigned to any of the comparison groups. Although there will always be an element of variation due to chance, the whole purpose is to ensure that the control and intervention groups look as similar as possible at the start of the study without the potential for selection bias that may arise should investigators or clinicians (who are frequently actively involved in the investigation) find themselves in a position to influence the allocation process.

Rachael: Why would people want to influence the allocation process if that could mess up the trial?

Hugo: Yeah, is there something dodgy about researchers and clinicians that we should know about?

Author (Emma): Everybody comes with inbuilt preconceptions and prejudices that influence our personal judgements, whether we are aware of them or not. As well as this, the main motivation of health providers is to provide care for their patients. If a new treatment has come along that might help them (otherwise, why would the investigators be going to the trouble and expense to trial it?), it can be difficult for clinicians to objectively enrol their patients in the RCT knowing they had an even chance of not getting the experimental treatment.

Earlier, we heard about the 1930s study of sanocrysin in 24 TB patients, who were pair-matched and then randomised to intervention and control groups by a single flip of a coin (6). Assuming the coin toss was a fair one, this was a reasonable attempt to randomise the two groups. However, you would want to ensure that every possible characteristic that might influence treatment was matched before that single toss. Another way to ensure random assignment to study groups would be to flip a coin for each eligible participant. The idea would be that the groups would end up looking similar as the long-run probability is that

50 per cent of the coin tosses would turn up heads and 50 per cent would turn up tails. However, this would not work very well for small studies. If you were to repeatedly flip a coin and note the outcome (and it is worth trying this for yourself), you would likely find that heads and tails outcomes don't start being evenly distributed right away, and sometimes not until very many tosses have occurred. Tossing a coin might work better for large studies but there are more suitable, and less tiring, ways to randomise both smaller and larger numbers of participant into study groups.

There are essentially three main types of randomisation: simple randomisation, block randomisation and stratified randomisation (22). Okay, there are other and (predictably) more complex types of randomisation, but here we will mainly consider the three major categories.

Simple randomisation is chance allocation based on a single sequence – coin flipping is an example of this. These days, most researchers use a computer program to accomplish simple randomisation, but people can use tables of random numbers that are often published in statistics books or on the internet, select sealed envelopes or even choose cards from a shuffled deck. The main thing is that the allocation must not be predictable. Order of presentation at a clinic or date of birth would not be suitable, for instance, because the sequence of allocation is difficult to conceal and could be predicted by those recruiting or even the participants themselves (23). Simple randomisation is not that great for studies involving small numbers of participants because, as mentioned in relation to coin tossing, probability is a long-run game and small study groups can get quite unbalanced using these techniques.

In *block randomisation*, all the participants are assorted into small groups ('blocks') that each contain a number divisible by the number of comparison groups. In a study of one intervention, there are two study groups (the intervention and the control group) so the number of participants per block could be two, four or six, and so on. If there are three study groups (e.g. two intervention and one control group), the number per block could be three, six, nine and so on. Once the block sizes are determined, all possible combinations of study group allocations are then worked out for each block. Say you had 40 participants and two study groups, and you had decided on blocks of four people. The six possible combinations would be: (1) treatment–control–treatment–control; (2) control–treatment–control–treatment; (3) treatment–treatment–control–control; (4) control–control–treatment–treatment; (5) control–treatment–treatment–control; and (6) treatment–control–control–treatment. The block numbers (1–6) would then be randomised to generate a sequence to assign your recruited participants. Block randomisation is great for achieving balanced numbers in each treatment group, which is particularly desirable if you only have small numbers, but there can be unequal distribution of characteristics in each block that might introduce bias at analysis (24).

If we are pretty sure that certain participant characteristics might influence the outcome of the investigation, we might consider *stratified randomisation*. In this process, we would sort our participants into groups (or 'strata') based on the characteristics we have identified and then randomise participants to intervention and control groups within each stratum. So, if we were worried about sex and age, we would first sort the participants into male and female groups and then further sort these sex strata into age groups (say 'below 65 years' and '65 years or older'). This would give us four groups (young males; older males; young females; older females) that can each be randomised to the intervention or control group. Stratified randomisation provides a way to ensure that study groups are balanced for numbers and composition. Depending on the number of people involved, you could stratify for several potentially influential characteristics and confounders, but it is not a suitable method for small participant numbers (25).

Stratified randomisation is clearly worth considering if you have a good number of participants all recruited and ready to go, but it doesn't suit the very many (probably the majority) of ongoing RCTs that recruit, allocate to treatment and control groups, and implement interventions as soon as eligible participants are identified. For our purposes, it is sufficient to be aware that there are methods to deal with this scenario (e.g. covariate adaptive randomisation) and they follow the main principles of ensuring that our comparison groups are as similar as possible and that each eligible participant has to have an equal chance of being assigned to any of the comparison groups. A flowchart of when to use the various types of randomisation is presented in Figure 9.3.

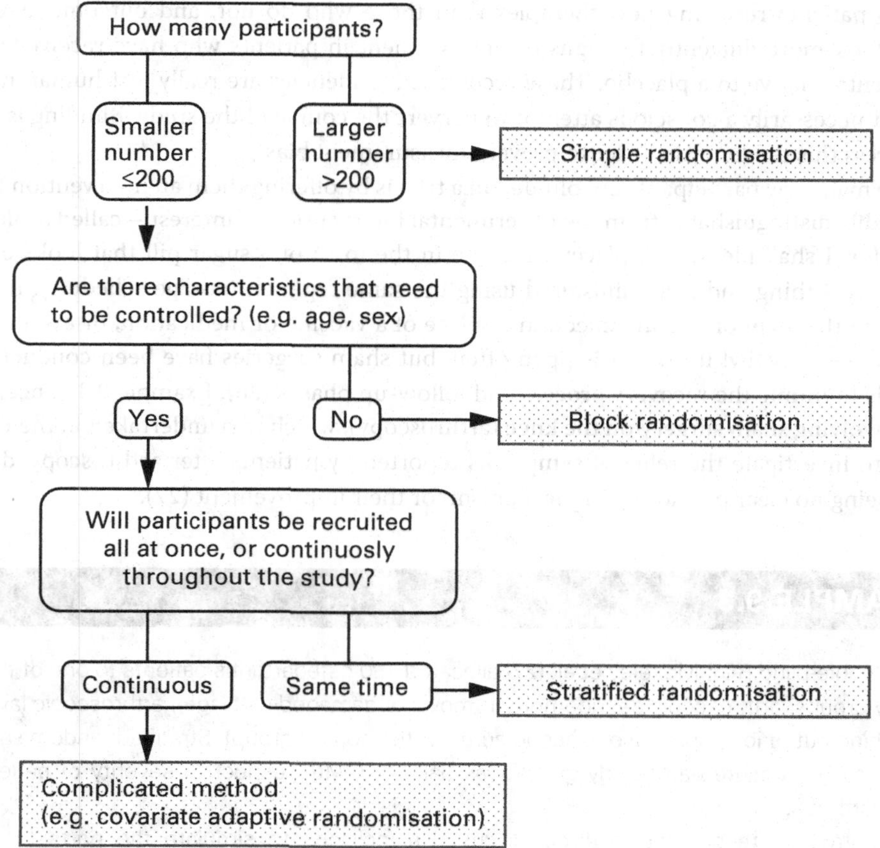

Figure 9.3 Flowchart for randomisation method selection. Adapted from (24).

Blinding and allocation concealment

We have talked about how RCTs can be classified by the number of people who are kept unaware of aspects of the study – for example, single- or double-blind studies – and we now know that blinding is done to prevent the potential for bias in measuring the effect of the intervention. A form of blinding also occurs right at the beginning of the study, before anyone has been randomised to the intervention and control groups, and this is

Concealment of allocations: A process by which the random allocation sequence of RCTs is kept secret to prevent knowledge of which participant is assigned to which study group (intervention or control).

the important process of **concealment of allocations**, which is critical for minimising the potential for selection bias. Here we will take a closer look at blinding and allocation concealment.

Blinding

As we now know, blinding in RCTs is done to prevent people's (participants, investigators, outcomes assessors) expectations influencing their assessments of outcomes. This can be a particular issue when the outcome is measured subjectively. For instance, a participant who knew they were taking a new medication for chronic headaches may respond positively, be more relaxed and be more hopeful in general, which (for a whole host of psychological and social reasons) may cause them to perceive greater benefit to the treatment than might actually exist. Health professionals may be more enthusiastic or optimistic while providing care to patients receiving new therapies than those who do not, and outcome assessors might look more diligently for signs of improvement in patients who have received active treatments relative to a placebo. These recognised tendencies are really just human nature, and not necessarily a conscious attempt to pervert the course of the study. Blinding is a way to address this tendency in order to prevent measurement bias.

The main way participants are blinded in a trial is by offering them an intervention that is not readily distinguishable from the experimental intervention of interest – called a 'placebo' (Latin for 'I shall please'). A placebo may be in the form of a sugar pill that looks exactly like the real thing and is administered using the same regimen (dosage schedule). It could also be in the form of a saline injection in place of a vaccine or medication, or even a sham surgery – yes, really! It doesn't happen often, but sham surgeries have been conducted on controls to mimic the recovery process and follow-up phases (26). Example 9.3 concerns an RCT involving sham surgery on the knee (arthroscopy), which was undertaken in the United States to investigate the relief of symptoms reported by patients after arthroscopy, despite there being no clear physiological mechanism for their improvement (27).

EXAMPLE 9.3

In a double-blind RCT, Moseley et al. (27) allocated 180 osteoarthritis patients to one of three study groups: arthroscopic debridement (removal of damaged cartilage), arthroscopic lavage (washing out of joint spaces) or placebo surgery (the control group). Stratified randomisation was used to ensure each study group was balanced with respect to severity of patients' osteoarthritis.

Controls were subject to three, 1 cm skin incisions to simulate the ports for the arthroscope, although arthroscopes were not actually inserted into the knee. Sham surgery participants were sent to recovery areas and cared for by nursing staff who were blinded, as were patients and outcome assessors. Two control patients suffered minor complications, such as wound infection and painful swelling of the leg. Follow-up involved assessing outcomes (e.g. pain level and functional ability) several times over 24 months.

No significant differences in pain or function between the two intervention and control groups was reported at any follow-up assessment. The authors concluded that outcomes of arthroscopic lavage or arthroscopic debridement were no better than those of the placebo procedure (27).

Hugo: I don't know how I would feel about having fake surgery!

Rachael: And you wouldn't even know what study group you were going to be in!

Author (Emma): Thinking of the pain and risk that those in the control group might experience explains a lot about how infrequently sham surgery is used in placebo-controlled RCTs.

In the Moseley et al. study (Example 9.3), 13 per cent of the controls correctly guessed that they had sham surgery, but 13 per cent of the lavage and debridement groups (combined) incorrectly guessed that they had the sham surgery. So it seems that the sham surgery was pretty convincing as a placebo, at least among the patients themselves. In this particular study, none of the groups experienced improvement, but many RCTs have observed improvement in control groups, in what is known as the **placebo effect**. The placebo effect was initially thought to be purely a psychological response to participant expectations of positive treatment effects triggered by the deception represented by administration of the placebo (28). It now seems, however, that the effects are not just psychological but likely involve a range of complex neurobiological mechanisms and the release of neurotransmitters (such as endorphins, which reduce pain and stress) that directly impact physiological function (29). The placebo effect can be a very powerful influence on human health, and its now quantifiable neurological impact (demonstrated via neurological imaging) is increasingly being investigated to uncover its potential for improving health outcomes (30).

Placebo effect: When people receiving a placebo experience an improvement in physical or mental health despite receiving an inactive treatment.

Another aspect of the placebo effect, often referred to as the 'nocebo' affect, is when participants report side-effects to treatment despite having received only the placebo (31). A review of 120 systematic reviews (yes, reviews of reviews are a thing) that synthesised the findings of 1271 RCTs that used placebos found that almost half the trials described adverse effects reported by placebo-control groups (32). In this review, 5 per cent of the adverse effects attributed to the placebo were so serious that the control participants dropped out of the study. Nocebo effects clearly can impact the ability of a trial to evaluate safety and acceptability of new treatments by making it difficult to see true differences between study groups. Through the same complex psychosocial and neurobiological processes, even those receiving active treatments have been known to exhibit nocebo effects (i.e. more severe side-effects than would be expected), which could ultimately impact on the use of clinically beneficial treatments due to perceptions of unacceptable side-effects (33).

Concealment of allocations

Allocation concealment is a process that occurs prior to, and is distinct from, blinding, but which has the similar objective of preventing bias that may be introduced by the knowledge of who receives what treatment in the trial. It has the special purpose of concealing the actual sequence of randomisation so that the investigators or clinicians who are enrolling patients have no idea what group the next participant is to be assigned to. Detorri (34) gives the example of a spine surgeon working on a new treatment that they believe is more beneficial than standard care and is undertaking an RCT to demonstrate this. From the random sequence, they know that the next patient on the list should receive the treatment. When that patient arrives, they seem to have lots of other illnesses (comorbidities), which the surgeon thinks would negatively impact any treatment they were to receive and thus not show the true benefit of the new treatment. Although the patient might meet the RCT eligibility criteria, the surgeon might subconsciously look for justifications not to enrol them. As Detorri suggests, perhaps the surgeon notices slight hesitation and offers more time to think about it, decides to order more tests, or uses any number of other subtle ways to subvert the randomisation sequence (34).

Concealment of allocations is critical to the unbiased conduct of the research as even beautifully designed randomisation sequences can be undermined should these sequences be deciphered, even by those with non-malign intent. Schulz and Grimes (35) write about real cases where investigators held up allocation envelopes to bright lights, and even opened sealed allocation envelopes, until the desired treatment group was revealed. Opaque envelopes or coded containers, centralised trial coordinators or pharmacies, and computer-assisted systems are accepted methods of allocation concealment. The critical thing is that those directly implementing the randomisation sequence should not be able to decipher it.

Just as important, the secret code determining who gets what treatments should be safely retained so that un-blinding can occur at the end of the study. A mechanism for unbreaking the code before the end of the trial is also required should something go seriously wrong, such as serious adverse events in participants.

Outcome measures of RCTs

You may have noticed that the basic design of an RCT is pretty similar to that of a prospective cohort study (see Chapter 8), with the exception of the randomisation bit and the fact that the 'exposure of interest' is deliberately administered to the participants. So it probably won't surprise you to know that some of the outcome measures are also pretty similar and include estimating relative risks. Just to remind you: the relative risk is a ratio of the incidence of an event in the exposed group relative to the incidence of the same event in the not-exposed group. It is actually not uncommon for odds ratios to be calculated in some trials (we met odds ratios in Chapter 7, in relation to case-control studies), but relative risks (RR) are pretty common in RCTs. Other common RCT outcome measures include **mortality rate ratios (MRR)** and **number needed to treat (NNT)** (among many more). Let's have a closer look at some of these measures using data from a published RCT on tuberculosis prevention in people living with HIV infection (36), described in Example 9.4.

Mortality rate ratio (MRR): A ratio of the incidence of death in the exposed group relative to the not-exposed group.

Number needed to treat (NNT): The number of patients who need to be treated to prevent one specified outcome (e.g. death, stroke, improvement, cure).

EXAMPLE 9.4

Tuberculosis (TB) occurs more often in people with HIV infection relative to those without HIV infection. A randomised double-blind, placebo-controlled trial was conducted in South Africa to evaluate isoniazid (a common treatment for established TB) for preventing TB in people currently taking antiretroviral therapy for HIV infection (36).

Of 1329 HIV patients, 662 were randomised to receive isoniazid treatment and 667 to receive a placebo for 12 months. The main outcome of interest was the incidence of TB and the secondary outcomes were death and side-effects.

Across the approximately three and half years of the study, the 1329 participants contributed to 3227 person-years of follow-up. There were 95 incident cases of TB, of whom 37 were in the intervention group (2.3 per 100 person-years) and 58 in the control group (3.6 per 100 person-years).

The therapy was discontinued due to raised alanine transaminase serum levels (an enzyme released by damaged liver cells) in 19 intervention group participants and 10 of the controls (RR = 1.9; 95% CI: 0.90, 4.09). There were 37 deaths during follow-up, 16 in the intervention group and 21 in the placebo group, but these deaths were due to 'all causes' and not necessarily due to TB. The all-cause mortality for both groups was one per 100 person-years, slightly (but not statistically significantly) lower in the intervention group (0.9 per 100 person-years) relative to controls (1.2 per 100 person-years).

The authors concluded that 12 months of isoniazid treatment reduced the incidence of TB, and that it was well tolerated and safe. They recommended that all HIV patients on antiretroviral therapy in moderate to high TB incidence areas should be offered isoniazid preventive treatment.

There is enough information in Example 9.4 to have a go at calculating all we want to cover in this section: the relative risk of TB; the mortality rate ratio; and the number needed to treat. We already had a look at calculating relative risks in Chapter 8, so hopefully it will be quite fresh in your mind that the relative risk is calculated by dividing the incidence of disease (or other condition) in the exposed by the incidence in the not-exposed. And the mortality rate ratio? MMR provides a way to directly compare the specific occurrence of death in the intervention and control groups and is simply the relative risk of death. Have a go with the help of Worked example 9.1 to see whether you get the same answers.

WORKED EXAMPLE 9.1

$RR = I_{exposed}/I_{not\text{-}exposed}$

From the information from Example 9.4:

RR = 2.3 per 100 person years/3.6 per 100 person-years
= 0.64

The RR is less than 1, indicating a protective effect for isoniazid and suggesting that a 36 per cent relative reduction in TB in HIV patients relative to placebo.

$MRR = M_{exposed}/M_{not\text{-}exposed}$

From the information from Example 9.4:

MRR = 0.9 deaths per 100 person years/1.2 deaths per 100 person-years
= 0.75

The MRR is lower than 1, which indicates a protective effect from the isoniazid treatment. Relative to the controls, the risk of death was 25 per cent lower in the treatment group; however, these were deaths due to all causes and not TB specifically. From the information provided in Example 9.4, it is possible that the difference in the number of deaths could have occurred by chance alone.

Hugo: Okay – that seems to all make sense.

Rachael: Well, we did do a lot of that in the last chapter.

Author (Emma): There is no harm reviewing what we know before moving on!

The other outcome measure to be considered here is the number needed to treat (NNT), which is often calculated in RCTs. At the end of our RCT, we want to know how many people will benefit (or be at risk) from our new treatment. NNT calculates the number of patients that need to be treated to prevent or allow one additional specified outcome (e.g. death, stroke, improvement, cure). Having this information is really important for answering questions such as the one at the start of this chapter: *Is it worth taking that medicine*? Implicit in this question are other questions, such as: Will the treatment actually help to address the health issue? How likely is it that treatment benefits will be achieved? And are benefits worth any risks or side-effects of the treatment? Such information is useful for individuals, clinicians and health policy-makers. If governments are considering funding the provision of interventions or health programs, they will want to know how many people will ultimately benefit from providing expensive health resources, which is exactly what NNT allows us to quantify.

EXAMPLE 9.5

An open-label, randomised controlled, single-blind trial was undertaken in Mexico, looking at the use of vitamin D in children hospitalised with COVID-19 (37). Among 45 such patients, 20 were randomised to receive vitamin D and 25 to the control group, who received no vitamin D. They were followed up during their hospitalisation to assess their progress by assessors who were unaware of who had received the vitamin D.

Ten per cent of the intervention group (2/20) progressed to requiring ventilation, as did 36 per cent (9/25) of the controls ($p = 0.10$); one of the intervention patients died (5 per cent) relative to six (24 per cent) controls ($p = 0.23$). For progression, the absolute risk reduction (RD) was 26 per cent (95% CI: 8.8%, 60.2%) and NNT was 3 (95% CI: 2, 11). The RD for death was 19 per cent (95% CI: −3.9%, 42.8%) and the NNT was 6 (95% CI: 2, 26) for death. No adverse effects were noted in patients receiving the vitamin D supplements.

The researchers concluded that vitamin D seemed to be associated with decreased risk of COVID-19 progression and death in these paediatric patients, although more studies were required to confirm their findings (37).

You might recognise some of the terminology used in Example 9.5. This is an open-label randomised controlled, single-blind study. So, everyone knew who got the vitamin D apart from the outcome assessors and perhaps some of the youngest children (if not intentionally), all of whom were randomised to intervention and control groups. They did see a difference in disease progression and deaths that favoured the intervention, but the numbers were quite small and this might explain the reported p values of 0.10 and 0.23 (p >0.05). The risk reduction (the difference between the outcome occurring in either group) was calculated as 26 per cent for COVID-19 progression (i.e. ventilation required), meaning that 26 per cent fewer children required ventilation in the vitamin D group relative to controls. The risk reduction for death was 19 per cent, but the reported confidence interval suggests that this was not significant since it included the null value of 0 per cent (−3.9 per cent to 42.8 per cent). The number needed to treat (NNT) was reported to be 3 for progression and 6 for death (and please check out the 95% confidence intervals – did they include the null value?). This means that you would need to treat three children with vitamin D to prevent one additional occurrence of requiring ventilation and six children would need to be treated with vitamin D to prevent one additional death due to COVID-19.

The way the NNT is calculated is described in Explanation 9.1.

EXPLANATION 9.1: Calculating number needed to treat

Construct a 2 x 2 table that cross-references the occurrence of the event of interest (e.g. death, stroke, improvement, cure) in intervention participants and controls – participant status in the columns and event status in the rows (see Figure 9.4).

		Participant status		
		Intervention	Controls	
Event	E+	a	b	a + b
	E–	c	d	c + d
		a + c	b + d	

Figure 9.4 Cross-tabulation of participant in an event of interest status – set up to calculate NNT

Cells:

a = number of intervention group participants who experienced the event
b = number of controls who experienced the event
c = number of intervention group participants who did not experience the event
d = number of controls who did not experience the event
a + b = all of those experiencing the event
c + d = all of those not experiencing the event
a + c = number of intervention group participants
b + d = number of controls
Risk of the event in the intervention group = a divided by a + c (a/(a + c))
Risk of the event in the control group = b divided by b + d (b/(b + d))
Risk difference (RD) = the difference between the larger risk and the smaller risk
So:

$$\frac{a}{(a+c)} - \frac{b}{(b+d)}$$

or

$$\frac{b}{(b+d)} - \frac{a}{(a+c)}$$

NNT = 1/RD

If everyone who was treated experienced the event (death, cure, etc.) and nobody in the control group did (an RD of 100 per cent or 1.0), the NNT would equal the maximum of 1 – equivalent to the maximum likelihood of 100 per cent, meaning you would only need to treat one person to observe the event. So the NNT is essentially a ratio of the maximum probability divided by the observed difference between the groups.

Rachael: That's a lot to think about!

Hugo: I think we are going to need some help on this one …

Author (Emma): Happy to oblige – you know 2 x 2 tables are my thing!

Let's have a go at calculating NNT using more data from the RCT of isoniazid treatment in HIV patients for tuberculosis prevention that was first described in Example 9.4 (36).

WORKED EXAMPLE 9.2

There were 1329 HIV patients in total, 662 of whom were randomised to receive isoniazid treatment and 667 to receive a placebo for 12 months. The main outcome of interest was the incidence of TB, so let's calculate the NNT for that.

There were 95 incident cases of TB in total, 37 were in the intervention group and 58 in the control group. So, using the magic of marginal totals (they must all add up), our 2 x 2 table will look something like Figure 9.5.

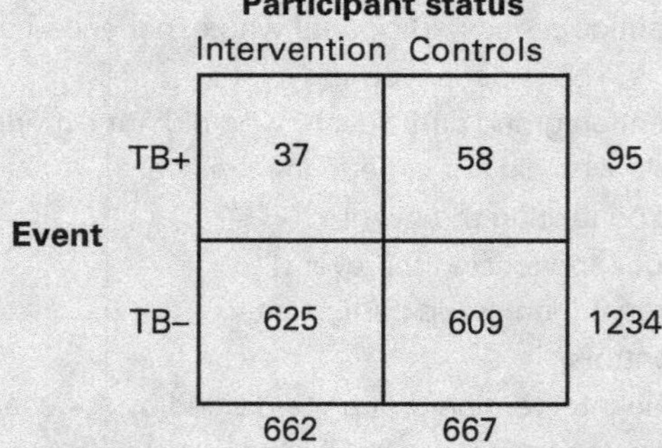

		Participant status		
		Intervention	Controls	
Event	TB+	37	58	95
	TB–	625	609	1234
		662	667	

Figure 9.5 Intervention group of HIV patients (izoniazid treatment or not) cross-tabulated by new TB diagnosis – set up to calculate NNT

NNT is calculated by dividing 1 by the risk difference

Risk of developing TB in the intervention group = 37/662 = 0.056 (5.6%)

Risk of developing TB in the control group = 58/667 = 0.087 (8.7%)

RD = 0.087 – 0.056 = 0.031

NNT = 1/RD

= 1/0.031

= 32.3

You would need to treat 32 HIV patients with isoniazid for 12 months to prevent one additional case of tuberculosis.

Rachael: I did it!

Hugo: Me too! But that seems a lot of people to treat to prevent one extra case of TB!

Author (Emma): It is here that you would need to carefully weigh up the cost of the treatment or procedure, any associated side-effects or complications, and the seriousness of the event you are trying to prevent or condition you are trying to improve. If isoniazid is fairly inexpensive and any side-effects are generally tolerated, it may be deemed worth prescribing it to all HIV patients to prevent one extra tuberculosis case, a serious infectious disease, arising in 32 treated with isoniazid.

Other statistical fun

As we have been at pains to emphasise, this is not a book on biostatistics, as interesting as that might be. Nonetheless, there a few biostatistical-like concepts that it is worth being aware of in relation to research in general, and RCTs in particular. These concepts build on our earlier discussions and include things such as developing hypotheses, statistical power and sample size.

The hypothesis

If you haven't come across this term in all the health science literature you have now read, I am sure someone at some stage (possibly with a smug expression on their face) has used the term 'hypothesis' while explaining their world-view to you at length. And the term sure gets a workout on a lot of those legal drama series on television. The truth is that the actual use of the hypothesis in research doesn't stray so far from its popular usage. In essence, a hypothesis is a statement proposing an explanation that is usually arrived at following observation and reflection. This sounds a lot like all that critical thinking stuff we have been hearing about, doesn't it? In research, the hypothesis reflects the scientific question and will be stated in a form that is a testable – that is, the form of the hypothesis should allow it to be supported or rejected through the analysis of data.

In RCTs, the primary hypotheses are generally developed ahead of the actual study, which will inform the study design and development of the study protocol (the document that outlines the study plan that form the rules for all those involved in conducting the study). Generally, those hypotheses will be something like, 'This new treatment will be better at preventing poor outcomes than the old treatment in patients suffering from early stages of that disease.' Obviously, this hypothesis would be solidly informed by comprehensive researching of the literature and other clinical evidence, as it would be very difficult to get the funds and formal approvals to go ahead with the study otherwise.

Another type of hypothesis generation occurs at the point of analysing the data collected in the trial. These hypotheses are specifically stated to inform the interpretation of statistical tests. Frequently, these are in the form of the 'null hypothesis' – the hypothesis that declares that there is nothing interesting going on (denoted as H_0). If you were looking at a new treatment for tuberculosis compared with the performance of an established treatment, for instance, your hypothesis might use the improvement rate of the older treatment as the null value – for example, H_0: There is no difference in rate of hospitalisations for tuberculosis when comparing the new and old treatments. The hypothesis can be tested by comparing the observed number of hospitalisations in our study and generating a statistic, such as a *p* value, that will estimate how likely it would be to see the number of hospitalisations observed in the intervention group if the null hypothesis was true. Depending on the likelihood of this, we can then accept or reject the null hypothesis.

Opposite to the null hypothesis that states that the intervention has no effect, sometimes the hypothesis proposes that there *is* an effect. This is known as the 'alternative hypothesis' (denoted as H_A, or sometimes H_1). In our hypothetical RCT of a new tuberculosis treatment, we might formulate an alternative hypothesis such as:

H_A: Hospitalisation rates for tuberculosis differ between new and old treatments.

Whether we construct null or alternative hypotheses, the main thing is that we are setting up a situation to statistically evaluate differences. This may be a difference in incidence, prevalence, disease status or improvement, mortality or whatever our outcomes of interest are. Whether we are aiming for really big differences, or small but clinically meaningful differences, mostly we want to know whether those differences are likely to be real. In the health sciences, we want to know whether those differences are statistically significant – our best evidence for a real effect of the intervention versus an outcome that might have arisen by chance.

Power and sample size

We have already been introduced to ways that quantify the probability of findings arising from studies (specifically, *p* values and confidence intervals) and we will not concern ourselves here with how they are actually calculated. However, it is important to remember that the size of the sample is critically linked to the ability of the study to statistically demonstrate a difference if it really exists. This ability is known as the 'power' of a study, which has several components including how frequent the outcome of interest is, how large the effect of the intervention is and how many participants there are (sample size). In Example 9.5, the researchers saw a difference in COVID-19 progression and deaths in children who were randomised to receive vitamin D supplements or not, but the *p* values (0.10 and 0.23 respectively) were not significant (37). What we don't know is whether the observed difference was just due to chance, or could actually be a real difference only requiring a larger number of participants to demonstrate this statistically. It was a pretty small study as RCTs go, and serious outcomes such as deaths due to COVID-19 are actually fairly rare in younger children – they only saw one in the intervention group and six in the controls, and these children were sick enough to be hospitalised. It is possible that vitamin D is ineffective in preventing serious COVID-19 outcome in children hospitalised with COVID-19; however, it is also possible that the study was 'under-powered' to show the difference in progression and mortality between treated and untreated groups.

Before the study even starts, right at the planning stage, there is a way to work out how many people you need to recruit for each group in a study to have the required statistical power. The formula for this is based on the size of the difference you want to show between groups (magnitude of effect) and your willingness to accept the chances of being wrong. There are two ways you might be wrong when interpreting findings, and these are known as type 1 and type 2 errors. Type 1 errors are made when the null hypothesis is rejected when it is actually true (very embarrassing). A type 2 error is the error of missing something exciting and accepting the null hypothesis when it is actually false. Power is actually the probability that the study can avoid making a type 2 error. The type 1 error is basically what the *p* value is set at (e.g. $p < 0.05$). For example, when reading the methods section of many published RCTs, you will almost definitely come across terminology such as that in the RCT described in Example 9.4:

> A final sample size of 1368 had 80% power to detect a 35% reduction in the incidence of tuberculosis in the intervention versus control group assuming a rate of 8·5 per 100 person-years in the control group, a type I error of 0·05 and a 30% loss to follow-up in each group ... (36, p. 685).

In human language, the authors are saying that they used a fancy formula to work out they needed to recruit 1368 participants to be able to show a difference of 35 per cent in TB incidence between the patients receiving isoniazid and the patients who didn't (based on assumptions of the usual, untreated incidence of TB in this group, and accounting for how many participants experience tells them will drop out of the study for various reasons). These numbers would mean their study would have an 80 per cent probability of avoiding making the type 2 error of accepting the null hypothesis when it is false (i.e. they would be prepared to be wrong 20 per cent of the time, or one in five). They have set a 5 per cent probability of making the type 1 error of rejecting the null hypothesis when it true (i.e. they would be prepared to be wrong 5 per cent of the time, or one in 20).

Hugo: Mmm, I may need to think about this a bit more ...

Rachael: Why are they prepared to make a type 2 error more often than a type 1 error?

Author (Emma): Remember, Hugo, it is just the broad concepts to be aware of here – so that you recognise them when you do all that reading of the scientific literature. The reason for increased tolerance of type 2 errors is due to the general conservatism of scientists, who are reluctant to challenge existing beliefs and theories without strong evidence. A bit like the assumption of innocence in a legal trial, it is less harmful to acquit than send someone to prison in error. In science, it is far less embarrassing to accept the status quo than to mistakenly make a claim to have found something new.

Ethical issues and randomised controlled trials

In our earlier examples, some of us became a bit concerned about the sailors who didn't get the citrus fruit and the TB patients who didn't get the antibiotics (4, 8), were worried by the TB patients who were treated with the almost toxic sanocrysin (6), and were positively alarmed by the idea of sham surgery (27). If we feel this way, it is because practices such as those described seem somehow at odds with how we think people should be treated – depending on our own personal frameworks for deciding what is fair and unfair, right or wrong. This framework essentially acts as a moral code for guiding our own behaviour, and responses to the behaviours of others, as we live our lives – our own personal ethics. This ethical framework may be based on particular religious beliefs, the example of our families and friends, educational or work institutions and/or our own observations and experiences in life. Personal ethics exert a powerful influence on the way we conduct ourselves and interact with the world, whether or not we have noticed their existence.

Some people have definitely taken notice of ethics, which actually has its roots in Greece, way back in the fifth century BCE. In fact, the word 'ethics' is taken from the Greek word *ethos*, which initially meant 'habitual meeting place' but subsequently evolved to mean 'character' (38, 39). Growing from ancient times, the study of ethics has become a whole field of philosophical study with various specialisations including the application of ethical standards and principles to real-world activities, such as research.

As discussed, the whole RCT thing is relatively new and has its origins at a point in history where there wasn't a whole lot of connection between the expanding fields of ethical philosophy and the emerging one of clinical experimentation. Because RCTs are about trialling new (perhaps even previously untested) treatments, or withholding potentially beneficial treatment, the whole thing can seem as if investigators are into treating people like guinea pigs (40). There is a lot of gruesome history of human experimentation (worse than the studies described in this chapter) occurring before, but especially during, World War II that kind of shocked the world into mandating ethical practice in research from the latter half of the twentieth century onwards. The main impetus for this change arose from the publication of two main documents: the Nuremberg Code, which was a legally framed ethical code on human experimentation arising during the trials of Nazi physicians in Nuremberg after World War II; and the Declaration of Helsinki, which was an ethical guideline for medical research widely adopted in 1964 and subsequently revised numerous times, most recently in 2013. The Nuremberg Code set out 10 principles to ensure that human experimentation should only be conducted if it actually benefited society, and it had a really strong emphasis on informed consent. The Declaration of Helsinki stresses the fundamental right to self-determination and to make informed decisions about participation, and the supremacy of participant welfare over the needs of science or society (41).

We have now reached a point where all research, not just clinical research, must have formal approval and oversight from established Human Research Ethics Committees (HRECs). These committees are usually affiliated with universities, institutes and anywhere else where research involving humans is conducted. In Australia, for instance, there are around 200 individual HRECs that rigorously review applications for all studies proposed around the country. Australia has developed a national guideline that builds on the Nuremberg Code and Declaration of Helsinki by governing all aspects of research, not just its implementation (42). This National Statement outlines mandatory ethical obligations for researchers, institutions where research is conducted, funding organisations, governments and even HRECs themselves. It sets out the requirements and rights of research participants, researchers and authors of research papers – basically every aspect of the research process and all people involved. I have included the National Statement in the 'Further reading' section at the end of this chapter so you can see for yourself how comprehensive it is. For most research conducted around the world these days, formal applications covering all ethical aspects of the conduct of the proposed study are considered by relevant HRECs, and without such approval the study may not proceed. Without appropriate HREC approvals for a given research project, hard-won research funds are not released to the investigators in many countries and most quality scientific journals will not publish study findings.

Randomisation and equipoise

RCTs necessarily involve doing things to people – 'experimenting on people' who are required to risk themselves, possibly with no direct benefit to themselves. Patients who are randomised to receive new treatments risk the potential for as yet unknown side-effects or complications. Alternatively, patients who require treatment just as much as everyone else in the study may be randomised to receive a possibly less beneficial treatment. The fact that the participants taking these risks are not necessarily the same people who will ultimately benefit from the study is an inherent ethical issue of RCTs in general, which has caused some to question whether RCTs can ever really be ethically acceptable (43). Others propose that RCTs can be ethically justified as long as participants understand, and experts honestly agree, that there is no evidence for the benefit of one treatment over another, a situation that is known as **equipoise** (44). It is further argued that, assuming equipoise, participation in a trial may have a physical and psychological benefit regardless of which study group patients are assigned, due to increased care and monitoring that usually occurs during the study (40). If evidence emerges during the study that one treatment is clearly superior to the other (or less safe), this disrupts equipoise and the trial would have to be stopped. In this case, one strategy might be to later offer the superior treatment to the study group that didn't receive it during trial.

Equipoise: In clinical trials, a situation where participants understand, and experts honestly agree, that there is no evidence for the benefit of one treatment over another.

Deception involving placebos

RCTs work best when people involved in the study are kept in the dark about who has what treatment. Blinding helps to reduce bias in the study by reducing subjective assessments of treatment effect and can be applied to the participants, those administering the treatment and those measuring the outcomes. When it is the patients being blinded, it is often with the use of a placebo – a deception that essentially means withholding treatment. The deception itself might be considered psychologically harmful and therefore unethical, although potentially justified given that the participants are told this might happen at the outset (a bit more on this later). Yet a placebo in place of an active treatment could mean a threat to health for those in the control group, such as progression of illness or even death (and how about any potential complications that might arise from sham surgery!). For this reason, it has been suggested that placebos not be used at all in RCTs unless no standard treatment for the condition exists (40). In Australia, the use of placebos cannot be ethically approved unless there is no standard treatment, or there is evidence that the standard treatment is more harmful than the experimental treatment (42). Elsewhere, HRECs (also informed by the Helsinki Declaration) additionally approve the use of placebos when, 'for compelling and scientifically sound methodological reasons', the placebo is 'necessary to determine the efficacy or safety of an intervention' (45).

One way to deal with any harms that might be associated with placebos is to use cross-over RCT designs (described earlier in this chapter), which would enable all participants to ultimately receive treatment. Another is to use an 'add-on' design, in which all participants receive standard care and the experimental treatment and placebo are randomly assigned as additional treatments (41). Otherwise, ethical research practice would demand only limited use of placebos after consideration of the possibility of harm to participants, the availability of standard care and whether standard care presents a more serious threat to health than the experimental intervention.

Informed consent

It could be argued that the issues involved with randomisation and placebos could be negated by the process of obtaining informed consent from all participants. Informed consent is now required from all participants in any type of study following the provision of a language-appropriate description of the study purpose, what will be required of participants and any risks to the participant and how these might be addressed. In RCTs, participants are also informed about the whole randomisation and blinding thing. In most types of studies, the participant will have the opportunity to think about their potential participation for a while and may even have the chance to discuss the whole thing with friends and family before signing up. In RCTs, however, recruitment and entry to the study tend to be far more immediate, and occurring during some sort of clinical contact. The participant may be still reeling in shock from a diagnosis (or that of their child), may be unwell with complications from ongoing illness or may have squeezed in an outpatient appointment before dashing off to work or some other commitment. Valid questions might be asked about how much information could realistically be absorbed under any of these scenarios.

Further legitimate questions might be raised about the extent to which RCT participants fully understand that the purpose of the study is not really all about them. RCTs essentially aim to benefit future patients and are not specifically focused on treating the participants in the study. Because recruitment is generally undertaken by a medical-type person in a clinical context, it is easy to see why patients might misunderstand the purpose of the RCT in what is known as 'therapeutic misconception' (41). The problem with therapeutic misconception is that participants may sign up because they have over-estimated the benefits of their involvement in the study, which naturally goes against the grain in terms of the whole informed consent thing, and can also lead to later distress should participants not derive the anticipated therapeutic benefits (46). The same phenomenon can also act as a recruitment magnet (and may even have been exploited for this purpose) for people anxious to join clinical trials related to their condition, despite the treatments being unproven and the randomisation procedures involved (47). Many have concluded that truly informed consent is probably unattainable, but that rigorous efforts should be made to strive for all ideals of informed consent whilst relying on the guidance and oversight of HRECs (40).

When thinking some of the earliest RCT efforts, as we have done in this chapter, it is important to note that any ethics applied would have reflected the perceptions about research and science prevailing at the time. We have come a long way towards improving the ethical conduct of research through HRECs describing and enforcing the application of ethical principles. It is really important that these principles continue to be reviewed over time to ensure practice keeps up with contemporary ethical standards.

Strengths and limitations of randomised controlled trials

At the beginning of this chapter, we asked whether it was worth taking a particular medicine or not, a question for which RCTs are literally made. So many advances in treatment and care, but also in community-based education and health programs, have occurred due to the information provided by RCTs. As we have heard, the rigorous methods for which

RCTs are famous have enthroned this study design near the peak of the 'hierarchy of evidence' pyramid, hailed as the 'gold standard' level of evidence. The only study design thought to surpass the level evidence from RCTs is a systematic review, and even this design chiefly relies on the information provided by RCTs. What more could we possibly need than an RCT?

As we know, a properly conducted RCT can provide evidence to assess the effectiveness of an intervention, its safety and its value for money. The main feature of an RCT that allows it to do this is randomisation, which minimises the impact of any participant characteristics that might influence or bias findings. Blinding of participants and/or others involved in the study further minimises the potential for measurement bias. Because these things are so tightly controlled, however, RCT participants start to look a little different from real-world populations and, as a result, RCTs are not usually able to provide evidence for many other important impacts of healthcare that can directly influence the clinical usefulness of many interventions. A treatment may be effective and safe, but how will patients of the future access it? There are many health and wealth disparities among different groups in all societies, yet many RCTs do not report on the performance of interventions against key socioeconomic indicators (48). As discussed by Furler et al. (49), it is often unclear whether socioeconomically disadvantaged groups are even represented as RCT participants. Since these groups are known to have lower health status to begin with, this might impact evaluations of intervention effectiveness. Given known economic disparities and health inequities within and between countries, the overall impact of new treatments can only be diminished further if those most at risk are not able to access them at all due to economic factors.

So, while the methods of RCTs are specifically about minimising bias, selection bias cannot be ruled out. Further, there is still a possibility that people will agree to participate, or even request to be in a study that is perceived to provide a therapeutic benefit, which we talked about earlier. This type of bias is known as **volunteer bias,** and can really mess with all phases of a study from recruitment, retention and follow-up (50). Enthusiastic volunteers might comply more readily with treatment protocols and can be unrepresentative of the population in relation to a number of important characteristics that could impact treatment outcome (e.g. education level, socioeconomic level, smoking status, alcohol consumption).

Volunteer bias: Occurs when persons volunteering to participate in a trial have clinical and other characteristics that may differ from those of non-volunteers (a form of selection bias).

Through the careful control of the timing and exposure to interventions, RCTs are pretty much unparalleled among study designs for demonstrating causal relationships. Strict study protocols ensure the precise administration of treatments or therapies even across large multicentre studies. However, it is not possible to replicate these tight controls in all settings, which raises the issue of generalisability. Future administration of the intervention will occur in multiple situations and sometimes by patients themselves, and it is unlikely that treatment impacts would not vary with the circumstances. There are also many situations where an RCT would be unsuitable, or even unethical, for investigating potential relationships – causal or otherwise. If you wanted to understand the effect of COVID-19 lockdowns on the mental health of children, for instance, a cohort study would be a far more suitable design. If you wanted to know what factors might lead people to be incarcerated (sentenced to a term in prison), a case-control study would probably work better. Even where the scientific question is essentially clinical, an RCT might not necessarily be the right way to go. For instance, a placebo-controlled trial of post-surgical pain management treatments would not be a study in which I would be keen to be involved!

In our discussion of some of the ethical issues associated with RCTs, we mentioned the proposal that all participants might benefit from the study due to the increased care and monitoring that occur during the study, although there were many other potential harms, particularly for those assigned as controls. Another potential issue is the cost to society represented by the cost of RCTs in the context of finite health and research resources. RCTs can be very large, involving multiple centres, which is a strategy to increase statistical power, and we rely on this ability to identify new health interventions and treatments that improve health outcomes. But RCTs are *very* expensive, consume a lot of human resources to organise and implement, and are generally funded at the expense of non-clinical (less expensive) research that may also improve population health. It is worth spending a bit of time thinking about what research and programs do not get funded in this reality. Nonetheless, an Australian government report estimated that every dollar invested in RCTs returned $5.80 of benefit across the economy (51).

Some of the advantages and disadvantages of RCTs are presented in Table 9.1.

Table 9.1 Advantages and disadvantages of randomised controlled studies

Advantages	Disadvantages
• Provides strong evidence of effectiveness, safety and cost-effectiveness via minimising bias and confounding through randomisation and blinding	• Rarely provides evidence on accessibility and equity • Subject to volunteer bias
• Strongest evidence for causality (i.e. carefully controlled to show directional relationship between exposure and outcome) • Carefully controlled exposure through precise administration of treatment/therapy	• Not suitable for many public health issues • Problems with generalisability
• Potential benefit to all participants due to increased care and monitoring occurring during the study	• Ethically problematic at times
• Can involve multiple centres and very large numbers of participants to achieve statistical power	• Expensive: time and money

Rachael: So, deciding on an RCT is really about what scientific question you have, but also whether you can get funding?

Hugo: I vote we don't decide to ask questions about surgical procedures!

Author (Emma): There certainly are a number of ethical and other issues to think about, but at least we now know why RCTs are the best study design for finding out if it is worth taking a particular treatment or medicine (you ask, we answer ...).

Conclusion

This chapter has introduced the main features and uses of RCTs, including how they developed and rose to be considered the 'gold standard' in research designs due to their rigorous methods. The learning objectives of this chapter are listed below together with summaries of how they were addressed.

Learning objective 1: Describe the main features of randomised controlled trials

We learnt about the basic direction of study in RCTs, starting with a population that is randomised to receive an experimental treatment or to be in the control group, who are followed up in order to compare health and treatment outcomes. We heard about the way RCTs are classified by the way the intervention is delivered (parallel or cross-over designs) and by which people were kept unaware of who got the active treatment (e.g. single- or double-blind). We also had a brief discussion about community-based trials and systematic reviews.

Learning objective 2: Understand the importance of randomisation and allocation concealment

Here we covered some of the important methodological aspects of RCTs. The purpose and methods of randomisation were described, including different randomisation approaches (simple, block and stratified randomisation). The importance of allocation concealment and blinding was discussed, as well as the phenomenon of placebo effects. We revisited the calculation and interpretation of relative risk (RR), applying this method to calculating mortality rate ratios (MRR), and learnt about number needed to treat (NNT) and the significance of this measure for policy-makers. Hypotheses generation and testing were briefly introduced, and the concepts of statistical power and sample size determination were also a feature of this section.

Learning objective 3: Discuss the ethical issues related to randomised controlled trials

In meeting this objective, we learnt about the origin of ethical thinking, the development of human research ethics committees (HRECs) and their role in the guidance and oversight of research today. We also highlighted some of the important ethical issues associated with RCTs, including issues associated with randomisation, the use of placebos and informed consent.

Learning objective 4: Describe the strengths and limitations of randomised controlled trials

Finally, we identified that RCTs are fantastic for providing strong evidence for the effectiveness and safety of interventions but, despite being famous for their efforts to reduce bias, are still subject to the potential for volunteer bias. They provide perhaps the strongest evidence of causation of any study design, but can be really expensive and are not suitable for researching many health issues that might occur in the population. We also acknowledged the strong potential for RCTs to provide clinical benefit, counterbalanced with some associated ethical issues.

Further reading

Cochrane Library of Systematic Reviews. Cochrane Library; 2023. www.cochranelibrary.com

National Health and Medical Research Council (NHMRC). *National Statement on Ethical Conduct in Human Research 2007*. NHMRC; 2018. www.nhmrc.gov.au/about-us/publications/national-statement-ethical-conduct-human-research-2007-updated-2018

Questions

Answers are available at the end of the book.

Multiple-choice questions

1. Which of the following best describes the direction of investigation for an RCT?
A – Randomisation, allocation concealment, intervention, compare outcomes
B – Allocation concealment, intervention, randomisation, compare outcomes
C – Recruitment, randomisation, intervention, compare outcomes
D – Recruitment, randomisation, blinding, meta-analysis.

2. An RCT is undertaken to look at ivermectin as a treatment for mild to moderate COVID-19. Clinic COVID-19 patients are randomised to either receive the treatment or standard care. Outcomes for both patient groups are compared at the end of the study period. What broad type of RCT is this?
A – A cross-over RCT design
B – Insufficient information to identify the RCT type
C – A parallel RCT design
D – A single-blind RCT design

3. What is the main purpose of randomisation in an RCT?
A – To make sure each study group is representative of the population
B – To make sure the study groups are of equal size from the start of the study
C – To help balance the groups with respect to characteristics that might influence the outcome of the intervention
D – To enable accurate assessment of treatment outcomes

4. Among the following strategies, which would you say would be most likely to achieve randomisation in an RCT?
A – Odd and even hospital record numbers
B – Use alternate presentations to an outpatient clinic
C – Toss a coin
D – Allocate to study groups based on severity of illness.

5. Which of the following is *not true* about systematic reviews?
A – Systematic reviews require a comprehensive search of the scientific literature.
B – The quality of studies is assessed and reported in systematic reviews.
C – Predetermined and explicit methods are used to address specified research questions in systematic reviews.
D – Systematic reviews always include a statistical pooling of data in a meta-analysis.

Short-answer questions

1. An RCT was conducted in Qatar, looking at the impact of hydroxychloroquine (parasite treatment) administered with or without azithromycin (an antibiotic), relative to placebo in patients with mild COVID-19 (52). After enrolment, 456 patients were blinded and randomised into one of three study groups: placebo, hydroxychloroquine (HC) alone, or HC and azithromycin together (152 patients in each group). SARS-CoV-2 PCR testing occurred after six and 12 days of treatment to see whether patients had either been 'cured' or had reduced viral load at either time point. There was no difference in proportions virologically cured between groups ($p = 0.821$) by day 6, or by day 14 ($p = 0.072$) and there were no serious adverse events. What are some of the main features of RCTs that you can discern from this description?

2. Go to the Cochrane Library (www.cochranelibrary.com, or access the Cochrane Library via your institution). Use the search function to find a systematic review on any COVID-19 topic of interest to you. How many systematic reviews did you find? You might also want to look at the number of trials registered with Cochrane on the same topic (you can access trials information from the tab at the top of the search result window). *Note: accessibility to the Cochrane Library is described at* www.cochranelibrary.com/help/access#:~:text=One%2Dclick%20free%20access%20in,requirement%20for%20individual%20login%20information.
3. You want to undertake an RCT looking at the impact of a new TB treatment. You plan to recruit a large clinic population with TB at the same time and randomise them to either a treatment or a control group. However, you are concerned that there a quite a few older people, people with comorbidities, and current and former smokers in the clinic population, and all these factors might influence treatment outcomes. What sort of randomisation procedure might you consider using here, and why?
4. In your own words, explain the purposes of allocation concealment and blinding in randomised controlled trials.
5. After seeing good results in rodents, a new drug called 'exenatide' was trialled in people with alcohol use disorder to see whether it would reduce their drinking (53). The study design was a randomised, double-blind, placebo-controlled trial with 62 participants in the intervention group and 65 controls. In the end, exenatide did not influence alcohol consumption overall but did significantly reduce the number of heavy drinking days and the total alcohol consumed in a sub-group of the participants who were classified as obese. Some of the outcomes they reported are presented in Table 9.2. There were more reports of side-effects of the gastrointestinal type in the intervention group relative to the placebo group, but all participants reported experiencing adverse events even though the control group received only an inactive treatment. Comment on what you think might be happening here.

Table 9.2 Adverse events in patients taking exenatide versus controls. Adapted from (53).

Adverse event	Placebo – n = 65 count (%)	Exenatide – n = 62 count (%)
Any serious adverse event (hospitalisation due to alcohol withdrawal; death; suicidal behaviour)	8 (18.5)	11 (24.2)
Weight loss from baseline	26 (40.0)	42 (67.7)
Nausea	10 (15.4)	23 (37.1)
Loss of appetite	6 (9.2)	15 (24.2)
Fatigue	3 (4.6)	8 (12.9)
Generalised itching	7 (10.8)	2. (3.2)
Headache	4 (6.2)	1 (1.6)

6. A multicentre, open-label RCT of high- versus low-dose vitamin D in the treatment of older patients with COVID-19 was conducted in France (54). Of 254 participants, 127 were randomised to receive supplementation with high-dose vitamin D and 127 were randomised to receive standard vitamin D supplements. The primary outcome was 14-day overall mortality and the secondary outcome was 28-day overall mortality, and these outcomes are

presented in Table 9.3. Using the information, calculate and interpret the mortality rate ratio for each outcome. [*Hint:* MRR = $M_{exposed}/M_{not\text{-}exposed}$.]

Table 9.3 Mortality in patients taking high-dose vitamin D supplements versus controls. Based on (54).

Adverse event	Low dose – n (%)	High dose – n (%)
14-day mortality	14 (11.0)	8 (6.2)
28-day mortality	21 (16.5)	19 (15.0)

7. After some fancy statistical testing that controlled for potential confounders, Annweiler and team (54) report the single dose of extra vitamin D early in the course of infection significantly reduced mortality at 14 days (p = 0.049), but this benefit was not sustained as similar mortality between groups was observed at 28 days (p = 0.29). Using the data provided in the previous question, calculate the number needed to treat with high-dose vitamin D to prevent one additional death by 14 days. [*Hint*: NNT = 1/RD.]
8. A research group published the protocol for a planned randomised, double-blind, placebo-controlled trial in Vietnam (55). This study would have two parallel arms, comparing standard treatment for tuberculous meningitis (for the control group) with standard treatment *plus* increased doses of rifampicin and levofloxacin (lower doses being part of standard treatment). The authors stated: 'The study will include 750 patients (375 per treatment group) including a minimum of 350 HIV-positive patients. The calculation assumes an overall mortality of 40% vs. 30% in the two arms, respectively (corresponding to a target hazard ratio of 0.7), a power of 80% and a two-sided significance level of 5%. Randomization ratio is 1:1.' (55, p. 1). How do you interpret the author's statement?
9. Using your own words, comment on some of the ethical issues associated with the use of placebos in RCTs.
10. An investigator wants to conduct an RCT to look at the effects of a new treatment for patients hospitalised with COVID-19 and asks you to help design the study. The possible choices of study groups include the following:
    a. new treatment alone in one group, placebo for the controls
    b. new treatment alone in one group, standard treatment for the controls
    c. new treatment plus standard treatment in one group, standard treatment for the controls.

    Thinking these through, what would you consider the pros and cons of each option?

References

1. Jones DS, Podolsky SH. The history and fate of the gold standard. *The Lancet*. 2015;385(9977):1502–3.
2. Bondemark L, Ruf S. Randomized controlled trial: The gold standard or an unobtainable fallacy? *European Journal of Orthodontics*. 2015;37(5):457–61.
3. Tugwell P, Knottnerus JA. Is the 'evidence-pyramid' now dead? *Journal of Clinical Epidemiology*. 2015;68(11):1247–50.
4. Lind J. *A Treatise of the Scurvy in Three Parts. Containing an inquiry into the Nature, Causes and Cure of that Disease, together with a Critical and Chronological View of What has Been Published on the Subject*. A. Millar; 1753.
5. Tröhler U. Lind and scurvy: 1747 to 1795. Journal of the Royal Society of Medicine. 2005;98(11):519–22.

6. Amberson JBJ, McMahon BT, Pinner M. A clinical trial of Sanocrysin in pulmonary tuberculosis. *American Review of Tuberculosis*. 1931;24(4):401–35.

7. Streptomycyin in Tuberculosis Trials Committee. Streptomycin Treatment of pulmonary tuberculosis. *British Medical Journal*. 1948;2(4582):769–82.

8. Long ER, Shirley HF. A controlled investigation of streptomycin treatment in pulmonary tuberculosis. *Public Health Reports (1896–1970)*. 1950;65(44):1421–51.

9. Ducati RG, Ruffino-Netto A, Basso LA, Santos DS. The resumption of consumption: A review on tuberculosis. *Memórias do Instituto Oswaldo Cruz* 2006;101(7).

10. Satapathy P, Itumalla R, Neyazi A, Mobin Nabizai A, Nazli Khatib M, Gaidhane S et al. Emerging Bedaquiline resistance: A threat to the global fight against drug-resistant tuberculosis. *Journal of Biosafety and Biosecurity*. 2024;6(1):13–15.

11. World Health Organization (WHO). *Global Tuberculosis Report 2023*. WHO; 2023.

12. Spieth PM, Kubasch AS, Penzlin AI, Illigens BM, Barlinn K, Siepmann T. Randomized controlled trials – a matter of design. *Neuropsychiatric Disease Treatment*. 2016;12:1341–9.

13. National Institutes of Health. COVID treatment guidelines: Ivermectin. 2023. www.covid19treatmentguidelines.nih.gov/therapies/miscellaneous-drugs/ivermectin

14. Therapeutic Goods Administration. Amendments to the new restrictions on prescribing hydroxychloroquine for COVID-19. 2020. www.tga.gov.au/news/safety-alerts/amendments-new-restrictions-prescribing-hydroxychloroquine-covid-19

15. Saag MS. Misguided use of hydroxychloroquine for COVID-19: The infusion of politics into science. *JAMA*. 2020;324(21):2161–2.

16. Schraer R, Goodman J. Ivermectin: How false science created a COVID 'miracle' drug. *BBC News*. 2021. www.bbc.com/news/health-58170809

17. Beltran Gonzalez JL, González Gámez M, Mendoza Enciso EA, Esparza Maldonado RJ, Hernández Palacios D, Dueñas Campos S et al. Efficacy and safety of ivermectin and hydroxychloroquine in patients with severe COVID-19: A randomized controlled trial. *Infectious Disease Reports*. 2022;14(2):160–8.

18. Nambi G, Abdelbasset WK, Alrawaili SM, Elsayed SH, Verma A, Vellaiyan A et al. Comparative effectiveness study of low versus high-intensity aerobic training with resistance training in community-dwelling older men with post-COVID 19 sarcopenia: A randomized controlled trial. *Clinical Rehabilitation*. 2022;36(1):59–68.

19. Dollahite JS, Pijai EI, Scott-Pierce M, Parker C, Trochim W. A randomized controlled trial of a community-based nutrition education program for low-income parents. *Journal of Nutrition Education and Behavior*. 2014;46(2):102–9.

20. Wawer MJ, Sewankambo NK, Serwadda D, Quinn TC, Kiwanuka N, Li C et al. Control of sexually transmitted diseases for AIDS prevention in Uganda: A randomised community trial. *The Lancet*. 1999;353(9152):525–35.

21. Cochrane Library of Systematic Reviews. Cochrane Library. 2023. www.cochranelibrary.com

22. Kim J, Shin W. How to do random allocation (randomization). *Clinical Orthopedic Surgery*. 2014;6(1):103–9.

23. Beller EM, Gebski V, Keech AC. Randomisation in clinical trials. *Medical Journal of Australia*. 2002;177(10):565–7.

24. Kang M, Ragan BG, Park JH. Issues in outcomes research: An overview of randomization techniques for clinical trials. *Journal of Athletic Training*. 2008;43(2):215–21.

25. Broglio K. Randomization in clinical trials: Permuted blocks and stratification. *JAMA*. 2018;319(21):2223–4.

26. Wolf BR, Buckwalter JA. Randomized surgical trials and 'sham' surgery: Relevance to modern orthopedics and minimally invasive surgery. *Iowa Orthopedic Journal*. 2006;26:107–11.

27. Moseley JB, O'Malley K, Petersen NJ, Menke TJ, Brody BA, Kuykendall DH et al. A controlled trial of arthroscopic surgery for osteoarthritis of the knee. *New England Journal of Medicine*. 2002;347(2):81–8.

28. Last J. *A Dictionary of Epidemiology*. 2nd ed. Oxford University Press; 1988.

29. Kaptchuk TJ, Miller FG. Placebo effects in medicine. *New England Journal of Medicine*. 2015;373(1):8–9.

30. Colagiuri B, Schenk LA, Kessler MD, Dorsey SG, Colloca L. The placebo effect: From concepts to genes. *Neuroscience*. 2015;307:171–90.

31. Colloca L, Barsky AJ. Placebo and nocebo effects. *New England Journal of Medicine*. 2020;382(6):554–61.

32. Howick J, Webster R, Kirby N, Hood K. Rapid overview of systematic reviews of nocebo effects reported by patients taking placebos in clinical trials. *Trials*. 2018;19(1):674.

33. Colloca L, Panaccione R, Murphy TK. The clinical implications of nocebo effects for biosimilar therapy. *Frontiers in Pharmacology*. 2019;10:1372.

34. Dettori J. The random allocation process: Two things you need to know. *Evidence Based Spine Care Journal*. 2010;1(3):7–9.

35. Schulz KF, Grimes DA. Allocation concealment in randomised trials: Defending against deciphering. *The Lancet*. 2002;359(9306):614–18.

36. Rangaka MX, Wilkinson RJ, Boulle A, Glynn JR, Fielding K, van Cutsem G et al. Isoniazid plus antiretroviral therapy to prevent tuberculosis: A randomised double-blind, placebo-controlled trial. *The Lancet*. 2014;384(9944):682–90.

37. Zurita-Cruz J, Fonseca-Tenorio J, Villasís-Keever M, López-Alarcón M, Parra-Ortega I, López-Martínez B et al. Efficacy and safety of vitamin D supplementation in hospitalized COVID-19 pediatric patients: A randomized controlled trial. *Frontiers in Pediatrics*. 2022;10.

38. Halloran SM. Aristotle's concept of ethos, or if not his somebody else's. *Rhetoric Review*. 1982;1(1):58–63.

39. Malik K. *The Quest for a Moral Compass: A Global History of Ethics*. Atlantic Books; 2014.

40. Edwards S, Lilford R, Braunholtz D, Hewison J, Jackson J, Thornton T. Ethical issues in the design and conduct of randomised controlled trials. *Health Technology Assessment*. 1999;2(15):1–132.

41. Nardini C. The ethics of clinical trials. *Ecancermedicalscience*. 2014;8:387.

42. National Health and Medical Research Council (NHMRC). *National Statement on Ethical Conduct in Human Research 2007*. NHMRC; 2018. www.nhmrc.gov.au/about-us/publications/national-statement-ethical-conduct-human-research-2007-updated-2018

43. Royall RM. Ethics and statistics in randomized clinical trials. *Statistical Science*. 1991;6(1):52–62, 11.

44. Nix HP, Weijer C. Uses of equipoise in discussions of the ethics of randomized controlled trials of COVID-19 therapies. *BMC Medical Ethics*. 2021;22(1):143.

45. World Medical Association (WMA). *WMA Declaration of Helsinki: Ethical Principles for Medical Research Involving Human Subjects*. WMA; 2023 www.wma.net/policies-post/wma-declaration-of-helsinki-ethical-principles-for-medical-research-involving-human-subjects

46. Henderson GE, Churchill LR, Davis AM, Easter MM, Grady C, Joffe S et al. Clinical trials and medical care: Defining the therapeutic misconception. *PLOS Med*. 2007;4(11):e324.

47. Dresser R. The ubiquity and utility of the therapeutic misconception. *Social Philosophy and Policy*. 2002;19(2):271–94.

48. Jull J, Whitehead M, Petticrew M, Kristjansson E, Gough D, Petkovic J et al. When is a randomised controlled trial health equity relevant? Development and validation of a conceptual framework. *BMJ Open*. 2017;7(9):e015815.

49. Furler J, Magin P, Pirotta M, van Driel M. Participant demographics reported in 'Table 1' of randomised controlled trials: A case of 'inverse evidence'? *International Journal for Equity in Health*. 2012;11:14.

50. Jordan S, Watkins A, Storey M, Allen SJ, Brooks CJ, Garaiova I, et al. Volunteer bias in recruitment, retention, and blood sample donation in a randomised controlled trial involving mothers and their children at six months and two years: A longitudinal analysis. *PLOS One*. 2013;8(7):e67912.

51. Australian Clinical Trials Alliance. *Economic Evaluation of Investigator-initiated Clinical Trials Conducted by Networks*. Australian Commission on Safety and Quality in Health Care; 2017.

52. Omrani AS, Pathan SA, Thomas SA, Harris TRE, Coyle PV, Thomas CE et al. Randomized double-blinded placebo-controlled trial of hydroxychloroquine with or without azithromycin for virologic cure of non-severe COVID-19. *eClinical Medicine*. 2020;29–30:100645.

53. Klausen MK, Jensen ME, Møller M, Le Dous N, Jensen A, Zeeman VA et al. Exenatide once weekly for alcohol use disorder investigated in a randomized, placebo-controlled clinical trial. *JCI Insight*. 2022;7(19).

54. Annweiler C, Beaudenon M, Gautier J, Gonsard J, Boucher S, Chapelet G et al. High-dose versus standard-dose vitamin D supplementation in older adults with COVID-19 (COVIT-TRIAL): A multicenter, open-label, randomized controlled superiority trial. *PLOS Medicine*. 2022;19(5):e1003999.

55. Heemskerk D, Day J, Chau TTH, Dung NH, Yen NTB, Bang ND et al. Intensified treatment with high-dose Rifampicin and Levofloxacin compared to standard treatment for adult patients with Tuberculous Meningitis (TBM-IT): Protocol for a randomized controlled trial. *Trials*. 2011;12(1):25.

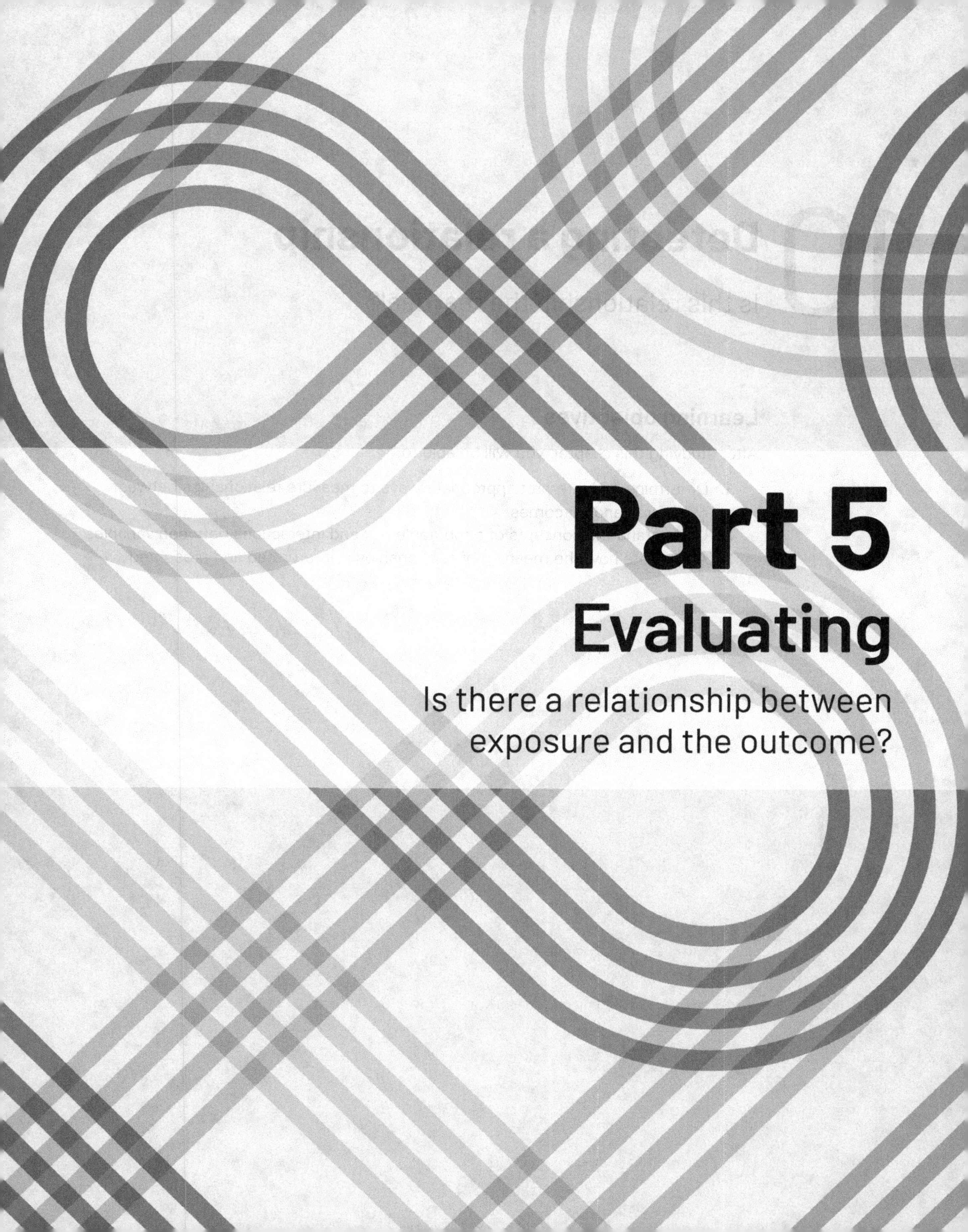

Part 5

Evaluating

Is there a relationship between exposure and the outcome?

10 Detecting a relationship

Is this relationship the real deal?

Learning objectives

After studying this chapter, you will be able to:

1. Determine and interpret appropriate ways to measure relationships between exposures and outcomes
2. Understand the concepts of attributable risk and interactions between variables
3. Appreciate how the meaning of relationships is interpreted and presented

Introduction

We have come a long way so far in this book, by now having developed a good understanding of the various ways in which epidemiology can be used to answer scientific questions. We have had a close look at the some of the more common epidemiological designs and the sorts of findings they can generate. In the study approaches we have looked at, the main purpose of investigation has been to understand and quantify relationships – those between exposures and outcomes, or between interventions and effects. And, just like the common plot-line of a romantic tale, in this chapter we consider how we can work out whether those relationships are the 'real deal'. How do we know we have measured what we think we have (is this really love?) and how much of the effect we have measured is entirely due to the exposure or intervention (or just a holiday thing?)?

Hugo: Ha-ha – is your relationship all that!

Rachael: But don't the statistical testing and *p* values tell us that?

Author (Emma): Statistical significance tells us that, on the given parameters, the result is unlikely to have arisen by chance. But it can't tell us whether we have made valid measurements or adequately taken into account all the relevant circumstances when we have set those parameters. As we will hear later, statistical significance also does not necessarily mean the same as clinical or public health significance.

There are quite a few things that we need to consider when deciding whether a relationship really exists and, if so, whether it is meaningful. This is important to establish if our findings are ultimately to inform an appropriate health or other response. In this chapter, we will revisit some of the ways we have now learnt to identify and quantify epidemiological relationships before considering how we might account for factors that may contribute to or influence those relationships. Finally, we are also going to take a closer look at statistical versus public health or clinical significance and this thing called 'risk', and the various ways it can be represented.

Measuring relationships and their effect

In Part 4 of this book, we spent a lot of time looking at different epidemiological approaches for identifying and quantifying associations depending on which side of the relationship we were interested in. In Chapter 6 we were interested in investigating exposures and outcomes together (analytical cross-sectional and ecological studies); in Chapter 7 we focused on exposures that were associated with defined outcomes (case-control studies); and in Chapter 8 we were all about exploring outcomes associated with defined exposures (cohort studies). Moving away from observational studies, we also looked at the outcomes associated with exposures that were deliberately introduced in Chapter 9 (randomised controlled trials). Each study type is specifically designed to accommodate the main focus of study and require a range of specific ways to measure the relationships investigated. Let's take a little time here to review some of those measures.

Correlation and prevalence ratios

If we wanted to know how much an outcome changes as the level of exposure changes, we might consider undertaking an analytical cross-sectional study and measure the correlation present in the relationship. Correlations are typically measured between two variables that take the form of continuous data (data that can take any value across a scale – for example, height or temperature). For instance, we might want to see how much weight increases along with increasing consumption of pizza and chips. The best way to graphically represent such a relationship is to plot it on a scatter plot. In scatter plots, each individual is represented by a single dot that demonstrates their position in relation to two variables shown on the x- and y-axes. Once all the individuals' dots are plotted, you can see whether there tends to be a pattern among the dots. Statistical methods (which we do not need to concern ourselves with here) can even plot a 'line of best fit', which minimises the differences between the data points to better show the trend, as has been included in the scatter plots showing potential correlations in Figure 10.1.

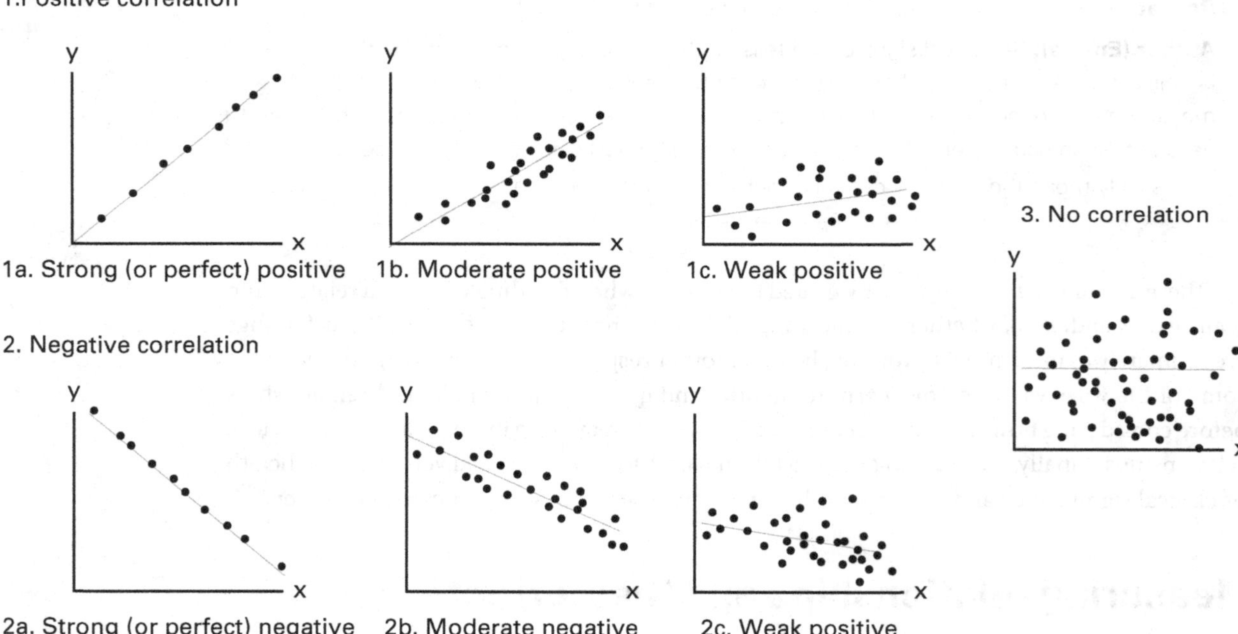

Figure 10.1 Scatter plots of potential correlation scenarios

To create a scatter plot for weight and daily pizza and chips, we might plot weight (in pounds or kilograms) on the y-axis, and average daily units of energy consumed in the form of pizza and chips (in calories or kilojoules) on the x-axis. Possible outcomes to this hypothetical investigation are represented in Figure 10.1 – ranging from strong positive correlations to strong negative correlations, and everything in between. For instance, we could hypothetically identify a positive correlation in which the more daily energy consumed in the form of pizza and chips, the heavier the individual. The positive correlation may be very strong, where the individual dots cluster closely to the line of best fit, or may be weak, with the dots showing a wider spread around the line of best fit. Although it is highly unlikely in this case, there remains a (*hypothetical*) chance that we might see that energy from pizza and chips was negatively correlated with weight – with individuals being lighter the more energy from this source that is consumed. Or there may be no correlation between pizza and chips and weight at all (again, unlikely!). Additional mysterious statistical processes can be used to calculate a **correlation coefficient** named 'r'. The main thing to know here is that this 'r' quantifies the correlation and ranges from −1 to +1, with 0 being the 'null' value. In Figure 10.1, for instance, the perfect positive relationship (1.a) could be r = 1 and the perfect negative relationship (2.a) could be r = −1, with the no-correlation scatter plot (3) potentially being r = 0. The rule of thumb for interpreting r is something like:

Correlation coefficient: A statistical measure of the linear correlation between variables that is represented by 'r', taking the value −1 to +1 to indicate the strength and direction of the relationship.

- 0.0 to 0.4/−0.4 = weak relationship
- 0.4/−0.4 to 0.7/−0.7 = moderate relationship
- 0.7/−7 to 1.0/−1.0 = strong relationship.

It is worth noting that almost no biological relationships will achieve a perfect correlation, and the reader should be deeply suspicious if an r of 1 (or −1) is reported. The other point to be aware of is that our examples have only talked about potential *linear* relationships – and involve drawing straight lines. Relationships between variables can be real without being consistent across changes in value. For example, crowd size at the local park could be strongly positively correlated with warmer weather, but if the temperature increases to extreme levels, fewer people will decide to venture out. Further, the extent to which a line of best fit can be plotted depends on the range of data collected in the first place, with lower correlation estimates associated with less-comprehensive data sets (1).

In cross-sectional studies, we often measure prevalence – which is the proportion of a specified population affected by a specified condition or event at one point in time. Proportions essentially describe types of variables known as 'categorical data' (data that are defined by exclusive categories – for example, male/female, disease/no disease). As we discovered in Chapter 6, analytical cross-sectional studies can compare the prevalence of a condition in exposed groups to the prevalence in not-exposed groups by developing a 'prevalence ratio' (PR), in which the prevalence in the exposed population is divided by the prevalence in the not-exposed population. As with all ratios, the null value is 1 (arising from dividing a number or one value by a number of the same value), so:

- PR is 1 = no difference in prevalence between exposed and not-exposed groups
- PR >1 = increased prevalence in the exposed group relative to the not-exposed group
- PR <1 = decreased prevalence in the exposed group relative to the not-exposed group.

A cross-sectional study using both correlations and prevalence ratios is summarised in Example 10.1. The study looked at whether a hormone (adiponectin) that is known to play a role in regulating glucose levels and is secreted by fat cells (adipose tissue) could be protective for the development of 'metabolic syndrome' (2). Metabolic syndrome is a bunch of conditions that occur together in individuals, including obesity, hypertension, high cholesterol and insulin resistance. Metabolic syndrome increases the risk of heart disease, stroke and type 2 diabetes (3). Look at Example 10.1 and see whether you agree with the conclusions.

EXAMPLE 10.1

In two groups of consecutive patients presenting for outpatient care in Brazil, von Frankenberg et al. (2). investigated the relationship between low serum adiponectin levels and the development of metabolic syndrome. First, in one hospital they conducted a cross-sectional study in 172 patients with and without metabolic syndrome who had all undertaken a glucose tolerance test. Then, to confirm their findings, they replicated the analysis in a larger group of patients (n = 422) who were undergoing cardiac care at another hospital. In both groups, they obtained a range of biochemical and immunological blood test results, including serum adiponectin.

Looking at the various indicators associated with metabolic syndrome, serum adiponectin levels were positively correlated with HDL-cholesterol serum levels (r = 0.452, p <0.001), and negatively correlated with waist circumference (r = –0.269, p <0.001), fasting glucose levels (r = –0.289; p = 0.001) and serum triglycerides (r = – 0.252, p <0.001). After adjusting for age and sex, the prevalence ratio (PR) of adiponectin and metabolic syndrome in the smaller patient group was 0.84 (95% CI: 0.75, 0.93; p = 0.001). The age- and sex-adjusted PR in the larger patient group was 0.94 (95% CI: 0.90, 0.97; p = 0.001).

The authors concluded that decreased adiponectin levels were associated with metabolic syndrome and that adiponectin levels decreased with increasing signs of metabolic syndrome (2).

In Example 10.1, we saw both positive and negative correlations. HDL-cholesterol was positively correlated with adiponectin levels. HDL-cholesterol ('high density lipoprotein' cholesterol) is known as a 'good' component of cholesterol (as opposed to low density lipoprotein, or LDL cholesterol), as it assists in cholesterol absorption, preventing it from building up and clogging arteries (4). So it is no surprise that increased HDL might also be associated with increased levels of other good stuff, like adiponectin. In this case, the correlation of r = 0.45 was calculated and indicates (according to the above 'rule of thumb') a moderate positive correlation. It was all downhill from there with weak negative (but statistically significant) correlations between different criteria for metabolic syndromes. These negative correlations are also called 'inverse relationships' because increases in one factor are associated with decreases in another factor. For instance, this study found that as waist circumference increased, adiponectin levels decreased (2), which would ultimately lead to impaired glucose regulation.

Prevalence ratios were also calculated in the study described in Example 10.1. For both populations studied by von Frankenberg's group (2), prevalence ratio for metabolic syndrome was less than the null (<1) for those with increased adiponectin relative to those with low adiponectin levels, indicating a protective affect for adiponectin.

Rachael: Okay, I think I got that!

Hugo: I'm going to go straight home and make my father go on a diet!

Author (Emma): In addition to this one cross-sectional study, there is now quite a bit of evidence about the cluster of conditions that make up the metabolic syndrome and the risk for diabetes and cardiovascular events. All of which is becoming much clearer given global population trends for increasing obesity, a major component of metabolic syndrome as well as being considered a serious chronic and progressive disease in its own right (5).

Odds ratios

In Chapter 7, we found out all about case-control studies and how they are great for looking at the relationships between a range of exposures and a defined outcome. If we wanted to find out what was causing a major outbreak of a communicable disease, or the long-ago exposures that might be associated with a current chronic condition, case-control studies are a cheap and rapid way to go (relative to prospective approaches). As we know, the design means selecting people with the condition of interest (the cases), then comparing their exposure histories with those of people with similar characteristics who don't have the condition (controls). Because we are selecting participants based on their case status, case and control groups are essentially two artificial population groups, which means they are not representative of a population where the cases would have arisen naturally. Moreover, the participants have already been determined to have experienced (or not experienced) the outcome or condition. This situation means we can't estimate disease incidence or calculate relative risks. What we can do is estimate the odds of exposure in cases and controls and compare these odds by calculating an odds ratio (OR).

Hopefully without confusing the issue here, OR is sometimes used to approximate relative risk (RR) in large studies, but it is always important to be aware that OR and RR are actually comparing completely different things (odds of exposure versus risk of an outcome). It has also been shown that ORs under-estimate RR when the ratio of odds is less then 1, but over-estimate RR when the ratio of odds is greater than 1 (6). Providing another potential source of confusion, it is worth noting that ORs are not the exclusive domain of case-control studies, as they are used in many other types of studies, including other cross-sectional and even randomised controlled trials. The important thing is to keep in mind what an OR actually represents – strictly, the odds of exposure in one group relative to the odds of exposure in another group (7).

The OR is calculated by dividing the odds of the exposure in the cases by the odds of exposure in the controls. You might revisit Chapter 7 to find out how to calculate an OR using a 2 x 2 table (love those things!), but here we can simply remind ourselves of how they are interpreted. Being a ratio, the interpretation of OR might look a bit familiar to you:

- OR is 1 = no difference in the odds of exposure between cases and controls
- OR >1 = increased odds of exposure in cases relative to controls
- OR <1 = decreased odds of exposure in cases relative to controls.

Case-control studies are used for all sorts of research and, given the focus on investigating exposures and the fast pace with which they can be conducted, they are used to great advantage wherever a rapid public health response is required, such as the investigation of outbreaks. Have a look at the case-control study summarised in Example 10.2 and see whether the study design and outcome measures are familiar to you. This study investigated a cholera outbreak in Ethiopia, with the disease still being a major public health concern in more than one-third of countries globally (8).

EXAMPLE 10.2

With cholera outbreaks becoming more common in Addis Ababa, Ethiopia, Dinede and colleagues (8) undertook a case-control study to uncover the source and risk factors of an active cholera outbreak in 2017.

Using data from multiple health centres, cases were defined as patients aged ≥5 years of age with acute watery diarrhoea, with or without vomiting. Controls were recruited from the same healthcare centre in which the cases were identified but did not have a history of acute watery diarrhoea. Participants were interviewed using a questionnaire that collected demographic and risk factor data.

The researchers recruited 25 cases with a median age of 38 years (ranging from 15 to >44 years) and 50 controls who had a median age of 35 years (also ranging from 15 to >44 years). All cases had acute watery diarrhoea and dehydration requiring intravenous fluids in cholera treatment centres, but all recovered. Cholera was confirmed by the detection of *Vibrio cholerae* (the bacteria that causes cholera) in stool samples, as well as in samples of holy water and raw vegetables. After adjusting for a range of other factors, the authors reported that drinking contaminated holy water had an OR of 20.5 (95% CI: 3.5, 119.6), consumption of raw vegetables had an OR of 15.3 (95% CI: 3.0, 81.5) and washing hands with soap after visiting the latrine had an OR of 0.04 (95% CI: 0.01, 0.3).

The authors concluded that cholera transmission in this outbreak was associated with the consumption of contaminated raw vegetables and holy water, but that washing hands with soap after going to the bathroom was a good idea.

Looking at Example 10.2, two of the reported ORs were greater than the null value (null = 1), which indicated higher odds of exposure in cases relative to controls. Drinking contaminated holy water had an OR of 20.5, which indicates that the odds of exposure in cases was more than 20 times that of controls. The odds of exposure to contaminated raw vegetables in cases was more than 15 times the odds of exposure in controls. One of the ORs was smaller than the null value, which may indicate a protective effect of the exposure. The OR associated with handwashing after using the toilet in cases was only 4 per cent of that of controls (OR = 0.04). Despite some wide confidence intervals associated with the ORs (did you note these?), it is not surprising that cooking vegetables and washing hands after going to the bathroom were recommended by the authors (8), and I would probably consider refraining from drinking the holy water in future, too!

Rachael: It is really bad that so many countries still have to worry about cholera.

Hugo: Yeah – so much for the 'epidemiological transition'!

Author (Emma): Very impressive, Hugo! Yes, Rachael, in wealthier countries there is a tendency to think that things like cholera are just stories from the pages of history. Studies such as the one described in Example 10.2 further demonstrate the patchiness of the so-called epidemiological transition (discussed in Chapter 1) and the great inequities in health that persist within and between countries.

Relative risk

Case-control and cross-sectional study designs make it possible to measure relationships between exposures and outcomes, but none of these provides a way to measure the incidence or risk of disease in a given population. The best study design to do this is a cohort study, as we heard in Chapter 8. Cohort studies also establish temporality and therefore move us much closer to considering causal relationships than other study designs. In cohort studies, a population without the outcome of interest is selected, then individuals are sorted into groups based on their exposure to one or more potential risk factors (or a separate, unexposed comparison group is used), then exposed and unexposed groups are followed up over time to compare what outcomes develop. The whole process can be done in real time (prospectively) or by reviewing historical records (retrospectively), but the direction or investigation always moves from exposure to outcome. The fact that the participants are not selected on the basis of their outcomes means that incidence can be measured precisely as it naturally occurs following their exposure. Incidence can be compared according to exposure classification by calculating a relative risk (RR) – the risk of a specified outcome in those exposed divided by the risk of the same outcome in those not-exposed. The way RR is calculated is explained in Chapter 8, and the way it is interpreted follows a similar pattern to all ratios:

- RR is 1 = no difference in the risk of the outcome between exposed and not-exposed groups
- RR >1 = increased risk of the outcome in the exposed group relative to the not-exposed group
- RR <1 = decreased risk of the outcome in the exposed group relative to the not-exposed group

Let's look at an example of a cohort study. HIV has been with us for a long time and, although no vaccines or cures have yet been developed, its medical management has now improved so much that this disease (thought to be responsible for more than 35 million deaths worldwide) has essentially been reclassified as a chronic disease (9) and people with HIV are now living long enough to start getting conditions usually associated with ageing. One such condition is osteoporosis, which causes bones to progressively lose density, becoming more brittle and fracturing more easily. As well as the effects of actual ageing, osteoporosis in people living with HIV can be exacerbated by the long-term use of an antiviral medication, highly active antiretroviral therapy (HAART) (10). Summarised in Example 10.3 is a Danish cohort study that investigated the incidence of bone fractures in people with and without HIV infection (11).

EXAMPLE 10.3

A cohort study in Denmark investigated the risk of fracture in people living with HIV on HAART relative to the general community (11). The researchers selected participants from an ongoing nationwide population cohort study, the Danish HIV Cohort Study, which is a collaboration involving all HIV treatment centres in Denmark. They age- and sex-matched people from the general population to each HIV patient using the Danish Civil Registration System, which stores information on all Danish residents. Information on fractures was obtained from the Danish National Hospital Register.

EXAMPLE 10.3 Continued

The main outcomes of interest were any first fracture, fracture of sites typically requiring low-energy events (e.g. wrists, humerus, hips, vertebral fatigue fracture) and fracture at sites typically requiring high-energy events or trauma (e.g. multiple fractures at once, multiple fractures of the femur, thoracic spine, pelvis). They compared time to first fractures in 5306 HIV-infected patients and 26 530 matched members of the general population. The period of follow-up was approximately 14 years and participants contributed a total of 38 456 person-years of follow-up (median follow up was 6.5 years).

Compared with the general population, HIV-infected patients had an increased risk of bone fractures (RR = 1.5; 95% CI: 1.2, 1.4). Where the patients were infected only with HIV (mono-infected), the risk relative to population controls was lower (RR = 1.3; 95% CI: 1.2, 1.4), but the risk was higher in patients co-infected with hepatitis C (HCV) (RR = 2.9; 95% CI: 2.5, 3.4).

The risk for low-energy fractures was greater in both HIV mono-infected (RR = 1.6; 95% CI: 1.4, 1.8) and HIV/HCV co-infected patients (RR = 3.8; 95% CI: 3.0, 4.9) compared with the general population. The risk of high-energy fractures was only increased in HIV/HCV-co-infected patients (RR = 2.4; 95% CI: 2.0, 2.9) and the risk of low-energy fractures among HIV mono-infected patients was only increased when the patient was taking HAART (RR = 1.8; 95% CI: 1.5, 2.1).

The authors concluded that the risk of fractures was higher in HIV-infected patients relative to the general population, particularly for low-energy fractures in HIV mono-infected patients taking HAART (11).

From Example 10.3, we can see that HIV-infected patients had a 50 per cent increased risk of any type of fracture relative to the general population (RR = 1.5). The increased risk was 30 per cent in patients with HIV mono-infection (RR = 1.3) but it was almost three times in patients co-infected with HCV (RR = 2.9). The fracture risk for HIV mono-infected patients on HAART rose to 80 per cent above the fracture risk of the general public (RR = 1.8). See whether you can interpret the other RRs reported in Example 10.3 for yourself!

Hugo: So, does that mean that being infected with both HIV and hepatitis C was nearly two and a half times the risk of high-energy fractures compared with being infected with HIV alone?

Rachael: But having HIV alone and being on antiviral medications increased the risk of low-energy fractures by 80 per cent?

Author (Emma): Well done, you two! That is exactly what was reported in the example, remembering that these are the risks of fractures *relative* to the risk observed in members of the general population of the same age and sex (more on *absolute* differences later).

RRs are also among various outcome measures that are calculated in randomised controlled trials (RCTs). Unlike observational studies, RCTs are part of the experimental study design family, as they involve doing things to people rather than just observing what happens to them without intervention. Despite this, the direction of study is the same for both RCTs and cohort studies. The exposure in the case of RCTs is in the form of an intervention, medication or procedure, the comparison groups are randomly selected using rigorous methods, but the RR is interpreted in exactly the same way as in cohort studies – comparing the outcome in the 'exposed' relative to the outcome in those 'not-exposed'.

A note on causal relationships

Because of the direction of study, RCTs and cohort studies allow us to calculate incidence and relative risk. For this reason, unlike the other types of studies described in this book, cohort studies and RCTS give us confidence about the temporality of the relationship between exposure and outcome – that is, we are assured that the exposure happened before the outcome developed. This takes us forward from identifying associations between exposures and outcomes and moves us closer to considering causality. It doesn't get us all the way there, but there are a number of approaches we might use to assess whether the relationships we have identified could potentially be causal ones.

While strong epidemiological evidence alone can sometimes be sufficient to intervene even in the absence of identification of the precise cause (e.g. John Snow and the Broad Street Pump), there are a number of public health and medical reasons, and even commercial and legal ones, to uncover the precise cause of a particular condition. So, people have been working on how to establish causation from epidemiological studies for years. Some of the more famous systems for doing so include the Bradford Hill criteria for causation (12) and Rothman's causal pies (13). We will hear a bit more about causal pathways in Chapter 11 but, in brief, Bradford Hill proposed nine criteria for assessing causality as follows:

1. *Strength* of the effect size: a small RR does not mean there is no causal relationship, but the probability of a causal relationship increases with the size of the RR.
2. *Consistency* of the relationship: repeated observation of the same phenomenon by different people on different occasions.
3. *Specificity*: the relationship is specific to a particular population (or site) and a particular outcome.
4 *Temporality*: the exposure occurs before the outcome does.
5. *Biological gradient*: the existence of a dose–response relationship – as the exposure increases so does the incidence of the outcome (the relationship can also be inverse, with increasing exposure reducing the incidence of the outcome).
6. *Plausibility*: that there is some sort of biologically logical mechanism linking the exposure and outcome (although Bradford Hill admits this criterion can be limited by existing scientific knowledge).
7. *Coherence*: consistency across different types of evidence – for example, epidemiological and laboratory findings.
8. *Experiment*: confirmation of associations by conducting experiments.
9. *Analogy*: good comparison of the relationship to known relationships existing between similar exposures and outcomes.

Bradford Hill did not suggest that all of the criteria must be met to establish causation, but suggested that weighing up how well any of the criteria are met can help to determine whether a causal relationship best explains what has been observed (12).

Rothman's model of causation (13) proposed that multiple individual factors are required to cause disease and these are called 'component causes', each of which acts as a slice of a complete 'causal pie', or mechanism of 'sufficient cause'. More than one sufficient cause may lead to a particular disease, with different components in each pie. If one component appears in every pie, it is considered a 'necessary' cause, because the disease will not develop without it regardless of how many other components are implicated in disease development. Rothman's conceptual scheme is presented in Figure 10.2, presenting three causal mechanisms for a single hypothetical disease, including all the components of a sufficient cause for the outcome. Component A is in all of the causal pies and so represents a necessary cause.

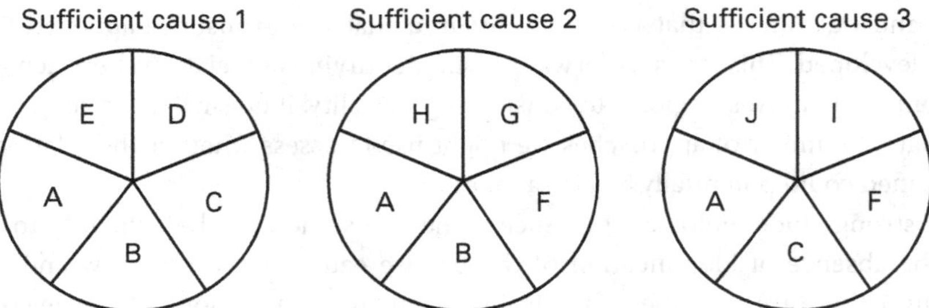

Figure 10.2 Conceptual scheme of three sufficient causes of hypothetical disease. Adapted from (13).

For an example of how this model can be used to explain a causal relationship, let's return to our Chapter 1 quandary about colds and open windows. If you recall, we applied critical thinking to the question of whether sitting next to open windows could cause you to catch a cold. We couldn't find direct evidence that sitting next to open windows caused colds, but we did learn that more colds happen in winter, cold air might damage the mucosal lining of the respiratory system and make a person more susceptible to viral infection, and the virus is more stable in cold weather so it might hang around in the environment for longer. Further, higher transmission of respiratory viruses such as colds occurs where there is reduced air circulation, and when people are more likely to huddle together indoors during the winter months. Socioeconomic or other predisposing factors are almost certainly involved and it is likely that there are other, unidentified factors at play that increase the risk of transmission (Why? Because there always are!). Figure 10.3 shows three potential sufficient causes for catching a cold, using Rothman's model.

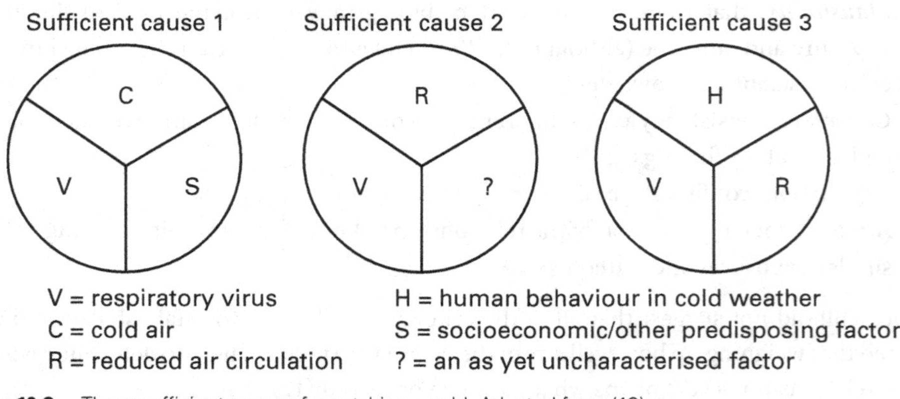

Figure 10.3 Three sufficient causes for catching a cold. Adapted from (13).

In sufficient cause 1, I propose that a respiratory virus, cold air and socioeconomic and other predisposing factors can cause respiratory infections. Sufficient cause 2 has the virus, reduced air circulation and an unknown factor as causal components. Finally, the virus, human behaviour (e.g. huddling together indoors) and reduced air circulation are proposed as sufficient cause 3. We could actually propose all the nominated components (and probably others) in a single sufficient cause mechanism, as long as we include the necessary cause – the respiratory virus itself. It is also worth noting that not all sufficient causes will have equal effect, with some causal mechanisms being responsible for a greater proportion of the total cases of disease than others.

Rachael: Do you have to address all of the components of a sufficient cause to prevent disease?

Hugo: Or do you just have to get rid of the necessary cause?

Author (Emma): Remember that all the components of a sufficient cause work together to cause disease. The necessary cause (e.g. the virus) must be present, but it needs all the other components as well to cause the condition. So, if you can't get rid of the necessary cause, removing one or more of the others in the mechanism should help. A bit like wearing masks in the COVID-19 pandemic – the SARS-CoV-2 virus is a necessary cause of COVID-19 but wearing masks, adequate ventilation and social distancing all reduce the ability of the virus to enter the respiratory system of a susceptible individual.

What else might be affecting this relationship?

In earlier chapters, we have touched on the idea of risk differences and introduced the notion of background rates of disease. In this section, we are going to find out how these concepts can be used to understand how much of an effect is actually due to the exposure itself. We will also look at how different exposures might work together to result in an outcome that differs from what would normally be expected from their individual effects.

Attributable risk

We were introduced to the idea of background rates of disease in Chapter 8. The background rate is the disease that is assumed to occur naturally in a given population, irrespective of our particular exposure of interest. To see how much disease a particular exposure is responsible for, we can remove the background rate by calculating an absolute risk difference (RD) or **attributable risk** – the difference between the incidence in the exposed and the incidence in the not-exposed:

Attributable risk: (synonyms 'absolute risk difference', 'rate difference', 'excess rate', 'risk reduction') The absolute difference in effect – may be incidence, prevalence, mortality – quantifying the direct impact of an exposure.

$$RD = I_{exposed} - I_{not\text{-}exposed}$$

In an example presented in Chapter 8, Ayoubkhani et al. (14) estimated diabetes incidence per person-years of follow-up in recently discharged COVID-19 patients relative to members of the general public who had not been diagnosed with COVID-19. The incidence of diabetes in discharged COVID-19 patients was 126.9 per 1000 person-years versus 86.0 per 1000 person-years in the general population. The absolute risk of diabetes in discharged COVID-19 patients is:

126.9 – 86.0 = 40.9 per 1000 person-years

So, almost 41 cases of diabetes per 1000 person-years in the COVID-19 group could be directly attributable to their exposure to COVID-19 (86 per 1000 person-years would have happened anyway). Absolute risk differences can be calculated using incidence, mortality or prevalence, and can provide a way to measure the actual impact of an exposure in a population group that is exposed to that risk factor.

Attributable proportion: (synonyms 'attributable risk percent', 'attributable fraction (exposed)', 'etiologic fraction') The percentage of disease occurrence (or risk) in an exposed group that can be directly attributed to the exposure.

It is often easier to think about the proportion of disease attributable to a particular exposure rather than absolute rate differences. We can do this by calculating the percentage of disease incidence (or risk) in the exposed group that is attributable to their exposure, which is known as the **attributable proportion** (also known by various other names, including 'etiologic fraction' and 'attributable risk percent'). Implicit in this measure is the notion that not all disease can be attributed to a single exposure, not even in exposed groups. For example, smoking is strongly associated with lung cancer but not all lung cancer is caused by smoking and there remains a chance that other risk factors (e.g. genetics) may contribute to some of the risk even in smokers. The attributable proportion (AP) is calculated by dividing the absolute risk difference by the risk in the exposed:

$AP = RD/I_{exposed}$

Using the data from Ayoubkhani et al. (14) on diabetes in discharged COVID-19 patients:

40.9/126.9 = 0.32

The attributable proportion was 0.32, or 32 per cent – so nearly one-third of the diabetes seen in discharged COVID-19 patients could be attributed to their exposure to COVID-19.

Population attributable proportion: (synonyms 'etiologic fraction/proportion', attributable risk percent (population)') The percentage of disease occurrence (or risk) in the population that can be directly attributed to a particular exposure.

And what if we wanted to know how much diabetes we could prevent across the whole population? This information could be really useful to health policy planners. There are many reasons to spend health resources on COVID-19 prevention, but what if we wanted to work out the impact of preventing COVID-19 on the total population incidence of diabetes? To do this, we can calculate the **population attributable proportion** – also known by many synonyms but let's stick with this one! Population attributable proportion (PAP) is calculated by dividing the difference between the risk in the population and the risk in the not-exposed subset of the population (also known as the 'population risk difference') by the risk in the population, as follows:

$PAP = (I_{population} - I_{not\text{-}exposed})/ I_{population}$

Of course, this means you need to have a good idea of what the risk/incidence is in the whole population (not just the participants of your study), but you can see how it would be useful to know what removing the risk factor would do for your overall diabetes health budget.

Hugo: Not really!

Rachael: I think we are going to need an example here!

Author (Emma): It can be confusing, especially with all the synonyms, but I'm happy to work this through using a 2 x 2 table …

Let's work through this together using the familiar, but *hypothetical,* topic of health science-related headaches that we considered in Chapter 7 ...

WORKED EXAMPLE 10.1

Let's say we had a university with a total enrolment of around 30 500 students. The university offers study programs in four faculties – two of which are the Faculty of Arts and Humanities and the Faculty of Health Sciences. These two faculties have 21 800 students, 3800 of whom are enrolled in health science programs. A lot of the university students have been complaining about headaches (estimated to be about 160 per 1000 students per month), with the loudest complaints coming from arts and humanities and health science students, so you decide to take a closer look these two faculties. A total of 3850 headaches were reported by students in these faculties over one month and, of these, 1150 were reported by health science students.

Using the magic of marginal totals, we now have all the information we need to plug into a 2 x 2 table of our cohort study, as shown in Figure 10.4.

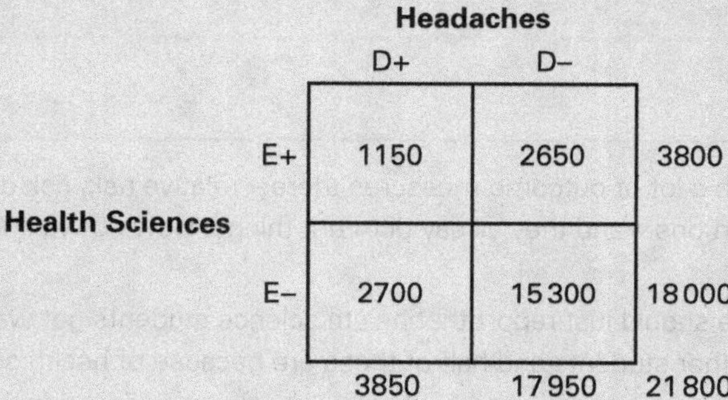

		Headaches D+	D–	
Health Sciences	E+	1150	2650	3800
	E–	2700	15 300	18 000
		3850	17 950	21 800

Figure 10.4 New headache occurrence cross-tabulated by exposure to the health sciences in two university faculties – set up to calculate relative risk (RR)

First, let's calculate the relative risk here ($I_{exposed}/I_{not\text{-}exposed}$):

$$RR = (1150/3800) / (2700/18000) = 0.30/0.15 = 2$$

This would indicate the risk for headaches in health science students is two times (double, or 100 per cent more than) the risk for arts and humanities students!

Now let's have a look at the absolute risk difference ($I_{exposed} - I_{not\text{-}exposed}$):

$$RD = 0.30 - 0.15 = 0.15$$

A figure of 150 headaches per 1000 health science students (0.15 x 1000) per month is directly attributable to their exposure to the health sciences (150 headaches would have occurred anyway). In absolute terms, the excess headache risk for health sciences is 15 per cent.

What about the attributable proportion ($RD/ I_{exposed}$)?

$$AP = 0.15/0.30 = 0.50$$

Exposure to the health sciences is responsible for 50 per cent of the headaches in health science students (0.50 x 100) each month.

WORKED EXAMPLE 10.1 CONTINUED

This is all sounding very dramatic – let's see what benefit there might be to the whole university population should we make everyone study something else instead. Because the explanatory text provides an estimate of the total university monthly headache risk (160 per 1000 students per month), we can first calculate the population risk difference ($I_{population} - I_{not\text{-}exposed}$):

$$PRD = 0.16 - 0.15 = 0.01$$

A total of 10 headaches per 1000 students per month (0.01 x 1000) can be attributed to health sciences exposure in this university.

That doesn't sound like an awful lot of headaches per 1000 students across the whole university population. Let's see what the population attributable proportion is ($PRD/I_{population}$):

$$PAP = 0.01/0.16 = 0.06$$

So, we could decrease the rate of headaches per month by 6 per cent in this university by removing health science education. I guess we would then need to carefully evaluate the costs and benefits (for the students, the university and to society) of doing something so drastic!

Rachael: There are a lot of outcome measures there – relative risk, risk differences, attributable proportions – and they all say different things. How do we know which ones to report?

Hugo: I reckon we should just report that health science students get way more headaches than other students and half of these are because of health sciences!

Author (Emma): Again, this is a completely *hypothetical* study. But you raise a very important question here. High-quality studies would report all the findings, then fully discuss their implications. However, which findings are conveyed often depends on the agenda of those doing the reporting. Relative measures always emphasise differences in risk, while absolute differences tend to minimise them. For instance, compare the RR and absolute risk differences for the two comparison faculties in Worked Example 10.1. The increased risk for health science students was 100 per cent in relative terms, but only 15 per cent in absolute terms.

Interaction

From time to time, the topic of confounding has arisen in this book and will be dealt with in more detail in Chapter 11, but it is worth mentioning again here because of the issues it can cause when we are trying to determine whether a particular relationship is the 'real deal'. As we know, confounders are variables (or factors) that are associated both with the exposure and the outcome. When they are unidentified, and therefore not controlled in some way, they can create spurious impressions of a relationship that might not even really exist. An ever-present potential confounder to watch for might be age, which is pretty much associated with most health outcomes. An apparently clear relationship between female sex and dementia, for instance, may well be confounded by age as females live longer than males and advanced age is associated with dementia.

Aside from confounding, there are other ways in which additional variables can exert an influence on relationships. As Rothman's model highlights, there is often the situation where more than one causal factor is involved on the pathway to a given outcome. Such factors may change the relationship by acting as an **effect modifier** or by truly interacting with the presumed causal factor to change the degree of the outcome. Briefly, these are factors that change the impact of an exposure so the effect of the exposure differs between groups depending on the presence of the effect modifier. For instance, age is an effect modifier for many outcomes, as is vaccination in the relationship between microbes and disease.

Effect modifier: A variable that changes the effect of a causal factor of interest (a form of interaction).

I know it sounds pretty similar, but effect modification is different from confounding. Confounding distorts the true relationship between exposures and outcomes, while effect modification simply means the association differs among categories defined by a particular factor. In a retrospective cohort study of COVID-19 outcomes in China, for instance, the researchers reported that sex was an effect modifier, with males with hypertension and coronary heart disease at greater risk of severe COVID-19 outcomes relative to females with hypertension and coronary heart disease (15). In this case, sex wasn't a variable that masked or distorted a true relationship but was identified by the authors as an important predictor of outcome.

And what about interaction? Well, the term is used in three different ways. One of these describes effect modification (as we have just discussed) – where the outcome of an exposure differs depending on the existence of another variable (the effect modifier). Another use of the term is in relation to statistical modelling of variables that all have an influence on an outcome (a story for a different book). Here, we will focus a little on what is known as *biological* interaction. This is a situation where the operation of two or more causal factors results in a different outcome than would normally be expected from the individual operation of each factor. The combined operation of these causal factors might increase the degree of the outcome (synergism), or might modify the relationship by reducing the impact of the exposure on the outcome (antagonism).

Let's consider an example that is often used to explain this concept: the interaction of asbestos exposure and smoking with lung cancer (16). Exposure to asbestos has long been linked to the development of lung cancer and, most importantly, a specific type of cancer called mesothelioma. Among other uses, asbestos was once widely used to help insulate buildings from fire but, due to a large volume of incontrovertible evidence about its health dangers, is no longer mined or used in building products (17). Just as compelling was the evidence for interaction provided by Hammond et al. (16), who followed up health and mortality outcomes in more than 12 000 men who had been occupationally exposed to asbestos at least 20 years prior to the study. The investigators proposed some sort of interaction going on between smoking and asbestos exposure that caused greater lung cancer mortality than the sum of either of these two risk factors operating alone.

Biological interaction comes in two main flavours – following additive and multiplicative models. In additive interaction, the effect of two exposures results in an outcome that is greater than just adding the independent risks attributable to each of the exposures. Multiplicative interactions are present when the combined effect of two exposures is larger than would be expected from simply multiplying the risks attributable to each of the two exposures. To illustrate these two models of interaction, let's have a look at some of Hammond et al.'s (16) asbestos and smoking data in Figure 10.5.

		Asbestos exposure: Yes	Asbestos exposure: No
Smoking exposure	Yes	601.6	122.6
	No	58.4	11.3

Figure 10.5 Lung cancer mortality rates (per 100 000 person-years) in relation to exposure to asbestos and smoking. Adapted from (16).

In Figure 10.5, we can see the various lung-cancer specific mortality rates estimated for non-smokers with no asbestos exposure, smoking but no asbestos exposure, asbestos but no smoking and exposure to both smoking and asbestos. The lowest mortality is in the non-exposed group (11.3 per 100 000) and the highest risk is in the group exposed to both risk factors (601.6 per 100 000), with different mortality rates for smoking only (122.6 per 100 000) and asbestos exposure only (58.6 per 100 000). Lung cancer mortality in doubly exposed persons seems much higher than the other rates and suggests that there might be some sort of interaction going on.

If there is interaction following an additive model, the lung cancer mortality in persons exposed to both smoking and asbestos will be greater than summing the independent risks attributable to each of the exposures. So, all we need to do is work out what the sum of the risks would be assuming no interaction, and then compare that with the observed outcomes as follows:

- Mortality in the not exposed (background mortality) = 11.3
- Absolute mortality difference for smoking only = 122.6 – 11.3 = 111.3
- Absolute mortality difference for asbestos only = 58.4 – 11.3 = 47.1
- Mortality for smoking and asbestos should be = 11.3 + 111.3 + 47.1 = 169.7

So, if the observed lung cancer mortality rate for both asbestos and smoking had been close to 169.7 per 100 000 person-years, we could have assumed there was no interaction going on between the two exposures. But the combined exposure mortality rate was actually a much larger 601.6 per 100 000 person-years. Thus, we know that interaction was present and it far exceeded an additive model.

What about the multiplicative model? Here we need to calculate the respective relative risks for each exposure category using the not-exposed group as the 'reference category' against which the other categories are compared. In Figure 10.6, the reference category is represented by the null value (null = 1).

To work out whether there is interaction following a multiplicative model, we need to find out whether the combined effect of smoking and asbestos exposure is larger than would be expected from just multiplying (finding the product of) the individual risks associated

		Asbestos exposure: Yes	Asbestos exposure: No
Smoking exposure	Yes	53.2	10.8
	No	5.2	1

Figure 10.6 Relative risks for lung cancer mortality in relation to exposure to asbestos and smoking. Adapted from (16).

with each of the two exposures. We can work out the product of the risks, assuming no interaction, as follows:

- The RR associated with asbestos exposure multiplied by the RR associated with smoking

$$= 5.2 \times 10.8$$
$$= 56.2$$

The RR for lung cancer associated with both asbestos and smoking exposure was not greater than 56.2, which means that although there was a strong interaction on an additive scale, it was not on a multiplicative scale in this example.

Hugo: What does that mean? Does the interaction exist or not?

Rachael: Yes, which model do we believe?

Author (Emma): These important questions relate to the motivation for looking at interactions in the first place. If we wanted to find out which group would benefit most from public health action, such as removing a modifiable exposure (e.g. smoking or asbestos), we might look at additive models. If we were primarily interested in looking at mechanisms of cause, perhaps to more accurately predict outcomes, we might want to look at multiplicative models. The take-home message here is to understand that interactions occur between exposures, and the combined operation of the exposures is different from what might be expected by considering the individual operation of those exposures.

A note on validity and precision

So far we have assumed we have been measuring things, exposures and outcomes accurately in the first place. In previous chapters we have talked a little bit about bias (selection and measurement) and the problematic effect it can have on interpreting findings. One of the main ways researchers can at least minimise the potential for measurement bias is by using accurate instruments to measure phenomena of interest. To take accurate measures, the instrument must be both valid and precise. ‘Validity’ is a term that you may frequently come across when reading the scientific literature and means that the instrument (e.g. blood test, questionnaire, weight scale) is measuring what it intends to measure and does so free of systematic error (i.e. without bias). 'Precision' refers to how reproducible a measure is or how it returns the same results under the same conditions, time after time. The way accuracy is influenced by validity and precision is illustrated in Figure 10.7, using the often-represented analogy of targets but here using arrow holes (being someone who prefers archery to shooting guns). In the first target, you can see a tight grouping of holes that indicates that the archer has consistent form. The arrows repeatedly reach the target and cluster in the same area, but this is not close to the true value (the bullseye) – so, precise but not valid. In the middle target, although the arrows have again all reached the target, there is a very wide grouping around and within the bullseye – valid but not precise. The arrows have clustered tightly in a group on top of the bullseye in the third target, representing both validity and precision (accuracy!).

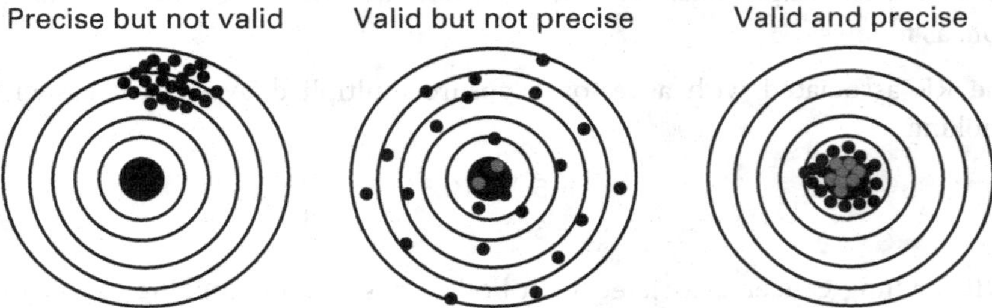

Figure 10.7 Accuracy – precision and validity

Another example from the real world might be a height chart on the wall. If you hang the chart too high, so the first centimetre marker is actually 3 centimetres above the floor, you will consistently under-estimate the height of everybody – providing a precise but invalid measure of height. If the height chart is hung correctly but only includes markers at 10-centimetre intervals, you might occasionally measure the actual height of people but not always – providing a valid but not precise measure of height. I am sure you can guess how we might measure height validly and precisely!

It is pretty important to make sure you are accurately measuring things when investigating relationships between exposures and outcomes, so researchers usually put a lot of effort into finding or designing valid measures of the phenomenon of interest. For instance, specific validity studies are often conducted to measure the validity of a newly developed survey (by testing it and comparing survey responses in a subset of the population), or only surveys that have been previously validated by other researchers are selected. This is because researchers want to be sure that the concepts the survey is designed to measure are being measured consistently, completely, accurately and in an unbiased way. In studies involving clinical measurements, instruments are often calibrated to a 'gold standard' in order to ensure precision and validity.

The other important thing to be aware of in relation to validity is whether this refers to 'internal' or 'external' validity. If you have gone to the trouble of investigating an important relationship, you might hope that your findings would be applicable to the population from which the participants were selected. This is called 'inference', applying a conclusion based on the evidence derived from your participants to the broader population from which your sample was drawn. If your participants are fairly representative of the larger population, your study might be considered to have 'external validity' – that is, they are relevant to all those in the broader population that have similar characteristics to your participants. If you have selected a specific (but probably unrepresentative) group of participants, perhaps experiencing particular circumstances, your study still may be valid (i.e. you have measured precisely what you intended to) but will be considered to have only 'internal validity'. Having internal validity is critical because this means the relationship explored in the study has been measured accurately (18). If exploring a particular relationship that only occurs in a specific circumstance is the main objective of the study, then having only internal (and not external) validity is quite acceptable. This is the aim for many qualitative studies, where the experience of a particular individual or group is explored in depth but making inferences from the findings is not a thing. In quantitative studies, internal validity only can also be totally legit if you are mainly interested in measuring the true relationship between exposures and outcomes, because it means you have ruled out confounders and effect modifiers.

Hugo: Nice bounce back to confounders and effect modifiers!

Rachael: And great segue to thinking again about the purpose of the study.

Author (Emma): Completely without value judgements, all roads lead back to the scientific question!

How meaningful is this relationship?

You see each other across a crowded room, your eyes lock together, you cross the room and chat briefly, exchanging phone numbers before you are both whisked away by your respective friends. While you are later considering sending a text to them and wondering if they will respond (could some among their friends be 'effect modifiers'), a group text message arrives with an invitation to a party at their house. You are pleased to be invited but are uncertain about the impersonal nature of the message, and ...

Okay, that's enough of that, but the romantic scene does afford us an opportunity to return to our original question: is this relationship the real deal? And, if we have established that a relationship exists, we might also question how meaningful it is. The first of these is the sort of question that epidemiologists ask themselves all the time. The second is a question that really ought to be addressed as enthusiastically as the first but is not always (as we will discuss later). In the next part of this chapter, we will review and expand on concepts underlying how statistical significance is determined and interpreted (see Chapter 9) before considering some of the issues around the relevance of findings to clinical and population health.

Statistical significance: *p* values and confidence intervals

In Chapter 7, we introduced the concept of statistical testing – the thing that researchers do to try to assure themselves that any relationships that they have identified in their analyses are not just chance findings. We have learnt that the probability of a result happening by chance can be quantified by developing a statistic called a '*p* value' (through mysterious statistical acrobatics), which can take any number up to a maximum of 1. A *p* value of 1 means there is a 100 per cent probability of an outcome occurring by chance – an unlikely prospect in the natural world. A probability of zero, however, is even more unlikely, which is why researchers always accept that there is a possibility (however small) that they may be wrong in their conclusions and report *p* values that quantify this probability. Because they don't like to be embarrassed, researchers set a threshold for the *p* value (known as 'alpha') at a level that will minimise the prospect of making claims about relationships that might not be real. Although alpha may be set at any level, the most common level for alpha is 0.05 (or 5 per cent). This means that should the *p* value be smaller than 0.05, the researchers will have more confidence that their finding did not arise by chance alone (although there is still the possibility of error – up to 5 per cent). If the *p* value is larger than 0.05, it means that there is a greater than 5 per cent probability that the observed result could have occurred by chance. From Chapter 7, a *p* value of 0.05 essentially means: *If I were to repeat this same measurement in study after study, having conducted those studies exactly as I have conducted this one, a result of this magnitude would arise on fewer than 5 per cent of occasions in a world defined by the null hypothesis.*

In Chapter 9, we heard about how researchers construct hypotheses to statistically test their results. Often, but not always, these hypotheses are set up to reflect the null world – that is, the situation where there is no relationship happening between the factors of interest. For example, if we were comparing mortality associated with different COVID-19 treatments, the following would all be considered null hypotheses (expressed as H_0):

- H_0: there is no association between outcome status and treatment strategy
- H_0: treatment strategies and outcome status are independent
- H_0: COVID-19 specific mortality is the same in each treatment group
- H_0: the relative risk of death for treatment A versus treatment B is 1.

So, we would set the null hypothesis up and test the null values against the various parameters of our study (such as the sample size and the effect size). If we had set alpha at 0.05, we would hope that our *p* value would be smaller than 0.05, so that we could then reject the null hypothesis and claim that we had found something interesting – that our result was 'statistically significant'. If our *p* value was larger than 0.05, we would have to accept that the null hypothesis was true. It is worth noting that that the alternative hypothesis, the one that says there is a relationship going on, can also be tested, but this just changes the way the *p* value is interpreted.

There is controversy about relying on *p* values to determine and communicate the meaning of relationships. At an essentially arbitrary threshold (e.g. alpha = 0.05), apparent associations are routinely dismissed, but this actually represents a common misinterpretation (19). Technically, a *p* value greater than 0.05 really just means that the null hypothesis cannot be rejected, rather than proving that the null hypothesis is true. Reporting data showing that 51 per cent of almost 800 published papers across five journals had mistakenly concluded that non-significance meant no relationship or effect, Amrhein and 800 signatories proposed that the whole concept of using *p* values to decide whether hypotheses can be accepted or rejected, associations supported or refuted, be scrapped altogether (20). Further to this, *p* values are frequently misinterpreted as measures of effect size with smaller *p* values represented as being 'highly significant', when they are usually more likely to be the product of large sample sizes (21). This is not to say that *p* values do not have their uses, but that they should be interpreted correctly on the understanding that they merely reflect, given the parameters of the study, whether a particular finding was likely to have occurred by chance alone and not whether a particular relationship is real.

In epidemiological circles, the controversy over *p* values has become so great that some journals have now banned authors from reporting them, or even using the term 'statistically significant' at all (20, 22). Many of these journals promote the use of confidence intervals instead. Introduced in Chapter 7, confidence intervals tell us a lot more about the relationships under question than the single *p* value. Comprising a lower number and a higher number that form a range of probable values around a point estimate (incidence, prevalence, relative risk, odds ratio, etc.), confidence intervals provide information about the effect size and the precision of the estimate. Like *p* values, confidence intervals are specifically set at a level of probability – conventionally at 95 per cent – and (from Chapter 7) can be interpreted to mean: *If we were to repeat the same study over and over and obtain this same measure again and again, in the long run, 95 per cent of those measures would lie between the upper and lower numbers of this confidence interval.*

Because confidence intervals tell us where the 'true' value of a relationship or outcome might lie within a range, confidence intervals can provide an idea of how precise a study estimate – such as an estimate of prevalence or the relative risk, or the odds ratio – might be. This is because the parameters of a study, including things such as the number of participants in it, hugely influence the size of the confidence interval. A wide confidence interval indicates that the study estimate has low precision, which often arises in a small study. On the other hand, a narrow confidence interval indicates an estimate with higher precision, which would usually arise from a larger study.

Much of the same information is used to calculate both *p* values and confidence intervals so, in addition to allowing a focus on effect size and precision, confidence intervals can also provide the basis of rejecting or accepting null hypotheses. If the null value appears within the range of the interval, the finding is deemed be not statistically significant. For instance, the null value of a ratio is 1, so an OR of 6 (95% CI: 0.2, 23) would be considered 'not significant' but an OR of 6 (95% CI:1.5, 9.2) would be interpreted as 'significant'. It is this dichotomous usage that is proposed by some authors to be as problematic as *p* values. Instead, Amrhein et al. suggest (20) that all the values within a confidence interval should be considered for their meaningfulness and compatibility with the data, rather than claiming there was no effect or that a relationship did not exist.

None of the above should be taken to mean that we should not bother to calculate and report *p* values and confidence intervals, or that statistical significance is not important. But these measures need to be interpreted correctly. A *p* value really just tells us the probability that a particular result would arise by chance in a world defined by the null hypothesis. Confidence intervals provide a range of probable outcomes that might arise should the same study be undertaken multiple times under the same circumstances. Both are mathematically dependent on the methods used in the study and the variation in the phenomena of interest. To completely depend on *p* values and confidence intervals to dichotomise the world into significant or not significant (read, 'real' or 'unreal') is to insist on an unwarranted level of certainty in an inherently uncertain world. High-quality, rigorous studies are those that attempt to control the uncertainties as much as possible by collecting complete and unbiased data and analysing them using robust statistical methods to describe, explain and predict outcomes from quality data. In this circumstance, as long as appropriate effect measures are calculated and findings are interpreted correctly (and without undue confidence), both *p* values and confidence intervals can help to identify 'true', if not meaningful, relationships.

Rachael: Uncertainty again? Really?

Hugo: I thought science would be a lot surer of itself!

Author (Emma): Good science will do all it can to rigorously explore relationships, but there will always be a level of uncertainty as it is not possible to control all bias, every potential confounder, effect modifier or interaction no matter how much effort is expended in the design. This is why quality research papers always include a full discussion about the limitations of the study, and authors refrain from making iron-clad conclusions. It is only when multiple good-quality studies find the same relationship that confidence is built about whether relationships really exist.

We have the power!

Most quantitative researchers spend a bit of time working out whether their proposed study would have the capacity to identify true relationships and differences between groups before they even start the project. Introduced in Chapter 9, this capacity is known as the 'power' of a study. The power quantifies how likely the study method will be able to identify differences of a specified size between comparison groups in the study. One of the main ingredients of the power calculation is the number of participants, known as the 'sample size'. A larger sample size will be able to demonstrate smaller differences between comparison groups, while a smaller sample size would mainly only be able to show larger differences. Why would anyone want to show small differences, you ask? Well, it all depends on what your research question is and what difference would be considered a meaningful one (more on this later).

The related concepts of type 1 and type 2 errors was also introduced in Chapter 9, as follows:

- Type 1 error (alpha) = rejecting the null hypothesis when it could actually be true. Typically, the probability of alpha (α) is set at 0.05 (5 per cent).
- Type 2 error (beta) = accepting the null hypothesis when it might not actually be true. Typically, the probability of beta (β) is set at 0.20 (20 per cent).

Of course, as our above discussion proposes, to speak in terms of 'true' or 'false' sets up a misleadingly certain dichotomy, but I am sure you get my drift. The beta value is actually the mathematical complement of the power, given it is calculated by subtracting the probability of a type 2 error from 1 ($1 - \beta$). So, with a beta set at 20 per cent, the power will be 80 per cent. This means that the study will have an 80 per cent probability of avoiding a type 2 error. These parameters, the alpha and the power, are used to calculate how many participants need to be in the study to show a specified difference between comparison groups. The size of the difference you want to be able to show is also one of the parameters required to calculate the sample size. Various statistical methods are utilised to actually conduct the calculation, and these vary according to the type of study design, but these days most people rely on computers to work it out. There are very many free sample size and power calculators available on the internet, and even a free program for conducting all types of epidemiological statistical analyses – 'OpenEpi' (23). Among many other useful functions, OpenEpi has a function for calculating sample sizes, and I have listed the link to it in the 'Further reading' section for those wanting to have a play.

Say I wanted to do a study to compare breast cancer outcomes in women who were exposed to daily alcohol consumption over a 20-year period. While regular alcohol intake is a known cancer risk factor, particularly breast cancer in women, breast cancer is relatively common as far as cancers go. So, I know that some breast cancer will occur in both the exposed and not-exposed groups (i.e. with or without alcohol). What I need to do first is decide just how much of a difference in breast cancer I want my study to be able to show. Let's have a play with the OpenEpi calculator to see what size of sample we might need to show differences of smaller and larger magnitude.

EXPLANATION 10.1: Sample size and study of breast cancer rates

Breast cancer rates in Australian women have tripled in the past 50 or so years, along with increasing rates of alcohol consumption over the same period (24). A dose response relationship between alcohol consumption has been consistently noted and is estimated to be around 5 per cent excess risk per each 10 gram increase of daily alcohol consumption in pre-menopausal women, rising to 9 per cent excess risk per 10 grams increase in daily consumption of alcohol in post-menopausal women (25). Overall, the excess breast cancer risk associated with regular alcohol consumption (at moderate levels) compared with no alcohol consumption has been estimated at 15 per cent (26). It is estimated that about 12 per cent of non-drinkers will develop breast cancer (27).

In our study, we want to show a difference of 15 per cent in the proportion of women who develop breast cancer among those who regularly drank a moderate amount of alcohol over 20 years and those who did not drink over the same period. We will set alpha at 5 per cent and the power at 80 per cent.

Selecting a sample size calculator for cross-sectional, cohort and RCTs (23), we have all information to calculate the sample size as follows:

Sample size calculation 1

'2-sided test' (because we might want to see if alcohol increases or decreases the breast cancer risk) = 95% *[equivalent to* $1 - \alpha$*]*

The value for power = 80% *[equivalent to* $1 - \beta$*]*

Ratio of exposed to unexposed = 1.0 *[assumes equal numbers in each comparison group, but the calculator is flexible on this]*

% of unexposed likely to have the outcome = 12%

% of exposed likely to have the outcome (includes the 15% increased risk for alcohol drinkers) = 14%

The calculator returns a required sample size of 1218 women in each comparison group, or nearly 2436 participants overall.

This sample size would give us the power to show an absolute difference of 2 per cent in risk and risk/prevalence ratio of 1.3.

What if we suspect the difference in breast cancer between alcohol drinkers and non-drinkers was actually much bigger than previous studies suggest – say double the risk (RR = 2)?

EXPLANATION 10.1 Continued

Sample size calculation 2

'2-sided test' = 95%
The value for power = 80%
Ratio of exposed to unexposed = 1.0
% of unexposed likely to have the outcome = 12%
The RR we want to demonstrate = 2

This returns a required sample size of 159 women in each comparison group, or 389 participants overall.

Rachael: In the first calculation, how can the RR show a 30 per cent increased risk but the absolute difference is only 2 per cent?

Hugo: Yeah, which one is right?

Author (Emma): Aha! Hold this thought as it brings us nicely back to those critical thinking questions (from Chapter 1), which we will be talking a little about later in this chapter: who is saying this and why are they saying it?

The calculations presented in Explanation 10.1 show how sample size and the power of a study interact depending on whether we want to show smaller or larger differences. What if we decided to go for the smaller sample size, which was designed to detect a relative difference of 2, but we only found a relative difference of 1.7? The study would probably be 'underpowered' to reach statistical significance due to the small sample size, but does that mean the relationship doesn't exist? From our discussion above, I would be wary of dichotomising reality! If we decided to undertake the larger study and found a relative difference of 30 per cent (RR = 1.3) and an absolute difference of 2 per cent, what does this mean and what are the implications for the real world? We could go on to do truly enormous studies involving millions of participants, allowing us to find tiny differences in outcomes between the exposed and not-exposed, the treated and not-treated. However, we need to question the relevance these tiny (but statistically significant) differences would have for patients being treated for a particular condition, or for the population overall. Here we are talking about the tension between statistical and clinical significance.

As we now know, 'statistical significance' refers to the probability that the results or findings would have occurred by chance. Whether this has any meaning for clinical purposes, however, will require an assessment of things such as the size of the effect, a main component of 'clinical significance'. Other factors that might affect this assessment include the overall impact of the intervention on patients' lives, duration of the effects, side-effects and ease of use, as well as cost-effectiveness. Unlike the tight rules that govern how we determine statistical significance, assessment of clinical significance is far more fluid, often relying on the individual judgement of medical practitioners or even their patients (28).

A further quandary is the tension between statistical significance and clinical/public health relevance or importance. For instance, finding statistically significant relationships between personality type and product branding may be infinitely relevant to those marketing these products, but will be unlikely to have a meaningful health impact across the population. In the ongoing context of scarce research and health resources, it is not surprising that even more resources and effort are being expended to work out ways to assess the relevance and potential public health impact of research (29). Indeed, the extent to which research outcomes will result in impacts on research and health is now a major criterion for the award of research funding from major national research institutions such as the National Health and Medical Research Council (NHMRC) in Australia, which specifically define this as research 'significance' (30).

Unlike clinical and public health significance, statistical outputs are completely dependent on the parameters entered into their calculation, and there have been examples where incorrect methods have managed to produce statistically significant results that have seriously damaged otherwise effective population health activities. An infamous example was a study on causal links between the vaccine for measles, mumps and rubella and the development of autism, which was published in the *Lancet* in 1998 (31). The study was later found to be seriously methodologically flawed and the findings widely unsupported by a vast number of much higher-quality studies, so the paper was ultimately retracted by the journal. Yet widespread media coverage of the false claims led to large decreases in vaccination coverage and the re-emergence of measles in the United Kingdom from the time of the publication to at least 2011–12 (32, 33).

The take-home message here is that designing the highest-quality quantitative studies will minimise bias and may even produce statistically significant results, but this can only move us *closer* to understanding whether a relationship is 'the real deal'. Confidence in the relationship will usually only come after many more high-quality studies. Even then, we need to consider whether the findings are clinically significant or have public health relevance. In understanding the meaningfulness of relationships, context is everything.

And 'risk'?

We have talked a lot about risk in this book, but what exactly is 'risk' and how can we define it? Well, risk is actually a statement of probability that is based on population data, so the observed incidence of breast cancer in a given population informs the assessment of risk of breast cancer for that population. Importantly, this risk is assumed for the total population and not the individuals within it. Each person will be exposed to different physiological, genetic and environmental factors that may change their risk from that of the collective. Risk also quantifies the level of association between exposures (characteristics/risk factors) and outcomes (disease/death) within a specified population. We can use epidemiological measures of health outcome (e.g. prevalence and incidence) as population risk estimates. For instance:

- The observed prevalence among South Australian prisoners tested for hepatitis C in 2005 was 42 per cent (34). The risk of hepatitis C for prisoners in South Australia is likely to be 42 per cent.
- The observed incidence of hepatitis C in Australian injection drug users in 2016–21 was 5.4 per 100 person-years, or 41 of 381 (11 per cent) injection drug users over five years (35). The risk of hepatitis C for injection drug users in Australia is 5.4 per 100 person-years. Or the risk of getting hepatitis C is 11 per cent over five years of injecting.

So, risk is a statement of probability that can be quantified using observed population measures of disease occurrence. Risk is also quantified as the level of association between exposures (risk factors) and outcomes. Through reading this book, you have become familiar with how we can compare risk between populations using both absolute measures (risk difference, excess risk) and relative measures (RR, OR and prevalence ratios). Let's have a look at how these absolute and relative measures can be used to describe and present risk.

Students are told that swapping a weekly pizza meal for hamburgers could decrease the chances of gaining weight during one year of their studies. Is it worth all students swapping pizza for hamburgers?

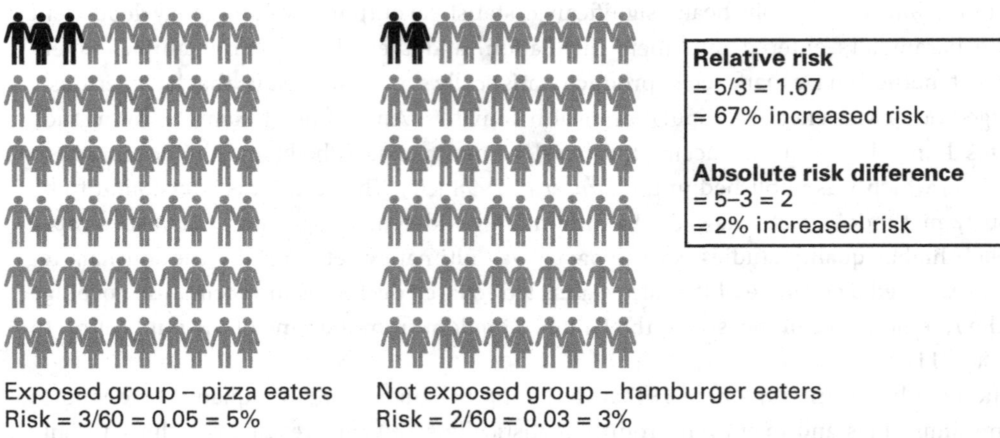

Figure 10.8 Hypothetical study of 5 per cent weight gain in 120 students. Adapted from (36).

According to Figure 10.8, the RR for 5 per cent weight gain over the year is 1.67 – a 67 per cent increase in risk seems a lot! But the absolute risk difference is only 2 per cent, so only two out of 100 students risk gaining weight if they choose pizza over hamburgers. The difference in the measures here is because the absolute risk difference excludes any background risk of weight gain that exists in both groups (remember attributable risk?). Relative risks, on the other hand, are always larger than absolute differences and will increase in magnitude along with increasing rarity of the condition of interest even if the absolute risk differences remain exactly the same. For instance, if only 3 per cent of the pizza eaters and 1 per cent of the hamburger eaters gained weight (retaining an absolute risk difference of 2 per cent), the RR would equal 3 – representing a 200 per cent increase in risk for pizza-eaters. Conversely, if 25 per cent of the pizza-eaters and 23 per cent of the hamburger-eaters gained weight (also retaining an absolute risk difference of 2 per cent), the RR would equal 1.09 – only a 9 per cent increase in risk for pizza eaters.

So, on which framing of risk should we base our pizza-eating behaviours? If I owned a hamburger franchise, relative differences might better suit my agenda. Any guesses on how a pizza shop owner might want to frame the risk? Neither representation of the risk is inaccurate, assuming this completely made-up study was of high quality, but whether relative differences or absolute differences are focused on might depend on motivation in this case. As critical thinkers, you might want a bit more information to properly consider the risk advice. If you were told there was a 67 per cent increased risk of weight gain from eating pizzas relative to hamburgers (RR = 1.67), how many people might this affect? It could mean three people with weight gain in 100 (relative to two people in 100) or 18 people in 600 (relative to 12 per 600) or 600 people in 20 000 (relative to 400 in 20 000). From the RR alone, we have no idea of the scale (or relevance) of the public health issue here.

The absolute difference of 2 per cent provides us with a clearer idea of the excess risk in numerical terms – two of every 100 students will gain 5 per cent of their baseline weight over a year if they eat pizzas rather than hamburgers (hypothetically). Whether it is worth changing university policy to prevent 2 per cent of the cohort of fast-food eating students gaining weight will need to be *weighed* (do you see what I did there?) against all the health and financial costs and benefits. The risk perception may also change according to how common pizza eating is across the whole population. And it is important to remember that risk is a property of the collective and not the individual, although it is often applied at the individual level by clinicians and lay people – so you may be on your own here in your lunch selection ...

Calculating relative and absolute measures helps to quantify any excess risk associated with particular exposures in populations, and can be framed in both relative and absolute terms. Newspaper headlines (and online news titles) often seem to prefer relative measures of risk because of the sensation they can cause (37) – we might imagine the headline: 'Pizza-eating students have twice the risk of weight gain!' High-quality research will present both measures so that risk factors can be identified, fully understood and modified where appropriate.

Hugo: Well, I think I'll be scrolling past a few more 'news' titles in future!

Rachael: This chapter showed us a lot of ways of looking at relationships, but then raised questions about all of them.

Author (Emma): Isn't questioning what critical thinking is all about?

Conclusion

In this chapter, we have explored how we can determine whether relationships between exposures and outcomes really exist, and how to work out whether those relationships are meaningful. In doing so, we reviewed many concepts from Chapter 9 and built on these to discuss some of the debate surrounding them. The way each learning objective was addressed in this chapter is summarised below.

Learning objective 1: Determine and interpret appropriate ways to measure relationships between exposures and outcomes

In these sections, we reviewed how relationships between exposures and outcomes are measured in various types, building on learning from previous chapters. The effect measures discussed included correlation coefficients, prevalence ratios, odds ratios and relative risks, with examples from published literature. Theories of causation from Bradford Hill and Rothman were also introduced.

Learning objective 2: Understand the concepts of attributable risk and interactions between variables

The concept of attributable risk was reintroduced, and we went through a worked example involving a hypothetical problem in a student population. We were introduced to the notion of interaction and the two main models of biological interaction – additive and multiplicative interaction. Also introduced were the concepts of internal and external validity and the implications for these in making inferences from study findings.

Learning objective 3: Appreciate how the meaning of relationships is interpreted and presented

Here we reviewed the concept of statistical significance and the ways *p* values and confidence intervals are used to determine it, building on previous knowledge about statistical power and sample size calculation. We discussed controversies about establishing statistical significance, whether it should determine the existence or absence of relationships and the tension between statistical and clinical/public health significance. Finally, the way 'risk' is defined and can be presented was also discussed in this section.

Further reading

Dean AG, Sullivan KM, Soe MM. OpenEpi: Open-Source Epidemiologic Statistics for Public Health. 2013. www.OpenEpi.com.

Questions

Answers are available at the end of the book.

Multiple-choice questions

1. An ecological study of soy product consumption and mortality from cancer and cardiovascular disease was undertaken in Japan (38). It reported a correlation coefficient (r) between soy protein consumption and stomach cancer mortality in males of –0.31 (*p* = 0.04). How do you interpret this finding?

A – Development of stomach cancer was directly attributable to consumption of soy protein.

B –There was a 30 per cent lower risk of stomach cancer in people who consumed soy protein.

C –The relationship between soy protein consumption and stomach cancer was not statistically significant.

D –There was an inverse relationship between consumption of soy protein and stomach cancer in males.

2. An outbreak of 52 cases of gastroenteritis was investigated at a workplace in Germany, later confirmed to be due to the bacterial *Shigella sonnei* (39). Among 25 (of 32) departments in the building, 52 cases were identified over two months. It reported an odds ratio of 3·84 (95% CI: 1·02, 14,·44) for canteen food consumption as opposed to consumption of food sourced elsewhere. Which of the below interpretations of this finding is correct?

A – Cases had an almost 400 per cent excess risk of having eaten in the canteen relative to controls.

B – It is not possible to link the canteen to the outbreak as the results were not statistically significant.

C – People who got ill had nearly four times the odds of having eaten in the canteen compared with those who didn't get ill.

D – Workers who ate in the canteen were nearly four times more likely to become a case than workers who didn't.

3. What is the necessary cause in the three sufficient causes represented in Figure 10.9?
   A – Sharing injection equipment
   B – The hepatitis C virus
   C – No clean needle program
   D – History of imprisonment.

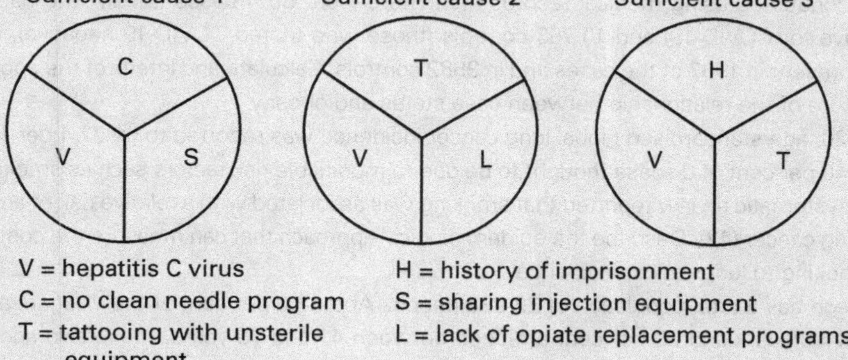

Figure 10.9 Three sufficient causes for infection with HCV. Adapted from (13).

4. People with diabetes sometimes have to use an instrument called a 'glucometer' that measures the glucose levels in a drop of their blood. The instrument is known to be very reliable (i.e. consistent in its measurement) but needs to be calibrated against a gold standard measure to ensure that the measurement of glucose is accurate. What do you think might best describe the result if the glucometer was not properly calibrated?
   A – The measurement of glucose would be neither valid nor precise.
   B – The measurement of glucose would be valid but not precise.
   C – The measurement of glucose would be precise but not valid.
   D – The measurement of glucose would be mostly accurate.
5. In a retrospective cohort study of systemic health outcomes in discharged COVID-19 patients relative to the community, the authors report that RR for respiratory disease was 10.5 in people aged under 70 years ($p < 0.001$). What would be the best way of interpreting this?
   A – Discharged COVID-19 patients under 70 years of age were more than 10 times more likely to develop respiratory disease than the general community, and the difference was statistically significant.
   B – The *p* value indicates that there was only a 0.1 per cent chance that this finding was likely to be true.
   C – The *p* value of <0.001 was 50 times less likely than a *p* value of 0.05 and this means the results were highly significant.
   D – Discharged COVID-19 patients under 70 years of age were more than 10 times more likely to develop respiratory disease than the general community, but the difference was very likely to have arisen by chance alone.

Short-answer questions

1. Researchers are collecting information about exposure to lead and health outcomes in children who live in the vicinity of a lead smelter. Every 12 months, blood tests are taken from the children to measure serum lead levels, and cognitive and physical development is measured

using validated instruments. Health status, weight, height and academic achievement are among many potential outcomes that are measured at the annual assessment. Children living in a similar geographical area but not within the lead contamination zone form the comparison group. What would be the most appropriate measure of the relationship between exposure and outcomes in this study?

2. A case-control study of factors associated with SARS-CoV-2 infection (COVID-19) in Mexico was conducted using medical records (40). There were 5074 cases (those who had tested positive for COVID-19) and 10 763 controls (those who tested COVID-19 negative). Obesity was present in 1967 of the cases and in 3582 controls. Calculate and interpret the appropriate measure of the relationship between case status and obesity.
3. In 2020, age-standardised global lung cancer incidence was reported to be 22.4 per 100 000, with 40 per cent of disease thought to be due to modifiable risk factors such as smoking (41). One systematic review reported that smoking was associated with a relative risk of around 7.5 for lung cancer (42). Describe the epidemiological approach that can measure the contribution of smoking to lung cancer incidence.
4. A village has a total population of 22 838 people. About 50 per cent of the villagers are aged below 40 years and 30 per cent are aged between 41 and 75 years. These two age groups comprise 18 270 people, 11 419 of whom were in the younger age group. Cases of 'red spot' disease have been arising regularly in the village at a rate of about 120 cases per 1000 villagers per month. In one month, a total of 4452 red spot cases were reported in villagers aged up to 75 years, and 3425 of these were reported in the younger age group. Using the information related to villagers aged up to 75 years, calculate and interpret the risk difference and attributable proportion.
5. In the 2 x 2 table in Figure 10.10 are plotted mortality rates per 100 000 population in relation to exposure to two risk factors, A and B. It has been proposed that there may be some sort of interaction going on here How would you describe the relationship between the two exposures and how could you confirm this? *Hint: could there be an additive interaction going on here?*

		Risk factor A	
		Yes	No
Risk factor B	Yes	458.2	122.6
	No	61.2	31.3

Figure 10.10 2 x 2 table of mortality rates per 100 000 population in relation to exposure to two risk factors

6. You read a study that is looking at the relationship between alcohol consumption and smoking behaviour in young people. You read that, compared with non-drinkers, the prevalence ratio for smoking in young adults who drink was reported to be 1.5 ($p = 0.051$). How do you interpret this finding? In your answer, comment on some of the controversies surrounding significance testing.

7. In the methods section of a published case-control study on breast cancer in mid-aged women, the authors state: 'We calculated that we would need to recruit 50 cases and 104 controls to be able to identify a 20 per cent exposure difference (equating to a relative risk of 2 based on an average of historical exposure prevalence) with a power of 0.80 at the 0.05 significance level' (24, p. 3). What does this mean in human language?
8. Go to the OpenEpi calculator (www.openepi.com). On the side menu, find the 'Sample size' folder, click on 'Cohort/RCT' and read the instructions that first appear. Click on the 'Enter' tab to open the interactive calculator. Let's say you want to do a study that looks at a health outcome in two populations: one that is exposed to a risk factor and one that isn't. You decide to set alpha at 5 per cent (e.g. *1 – α*) and you want to have twice as many people in the not-exposed group relative to the exposed group. The usual prevalence of the outcome in the not-exposed population is 20 per cent, and you want to have the power to show double the risk in the exposed population (RR = 2). Enter all this information and click on 'calculate'. You should see a page detailing all the information you entered into the calculation. Using the 'Kelsey' calculation (one of the three options reported after the calculation), how many participants will you need overall and in each group? And what happens if you re-enter all the same data except for reducing the RR required to 1.5?
9. You read about a study looking at a potential causal relationship between eating salads and weight gain. It is reported that among 2000 people, 12 per cent of those who gained weight over a one-month period ate salad at least once per week but only 5 per cent of those who didn't gain weight ate salad over the same time period. The authors of the study have concluded that eating salad leads to weight gain. Do you have any reason to doubt this conclusion? *Hint: think Bradford Hill.*
10. In your own words, how would you explain why relative and absolute differences in risk are so different?

References

1. Janse RJ, Hoekstra T, Jager KJ, Zoccali C, Tripepi G, Dekker FW et al. Conducting correlation analysis: Important limitations and pitfalls. *Clinical Kidney Journal*. 2021;14(11):2332–7.
2. von Frankenberg AD, do Nascimento FV, Gatelli LE, Nedel BL, Garcia SP, de Oliveira CSV et al. Major components of metabolic syndrome and adiponectin levels: A cross-sectional study. *Diabetology & Metabolic Syndrome*. 2014;6(1):26.
3. Eckel RH, Grundy SM, Zimmet PZ. The metabolic syndrome. *The Lancet*. 2005;365(9468):1415–28.
4. Badimon L, Vilahur G. LDL-cholesterol versus HDL-cholesterol in the atherosclerotic plaque: Inflammatory resolution versus thrombotic chaos. *Annals of the New York Academy of Sciences*. 2012;1254(1):18–32.
5. Blüher M. Obesity: Global epidemiology and pathogenesis. *Nature Reviews Endocrinology*. 2019;15(5):288–98.
6. Davies HTO, Crombie IK, Tavakoli M. When can odds ratios mislead? *BMJ*. 1998;316(7136):989.
7. Schmidt CO, Kohlmann T. When to use the odds ratio or the relative risk? *International Journal of Public Health*. 2008;53(3):165–7.
8. Dinede G, Abagero A, Tolosa T. Cholera outbreak in Addis Ababa, Ethiopia: A case-control study. *PLOS One*. 2020;15(7):e0235440.
9. Areri HA, Marshall A, Harvey G. Interventions to improve self-management of adults living with HIV on antiretroviral therapy: A systematic review. *PLOS One*. 2020;15(5):e0232709.
10. Rothman MS, Bessesen MT. HIV infection and osteoporosis: Pathophysiology, diagnosis, and treatment options. *Current Osteoporosis Reports*. 2012;10(4):270–7.

11. Hansen A-BE, Gerstoft J, Kronborg G, Larsen CS, Pedersen C, Pedersen G et al. Incidence of low and high-energy fractures in persons with and without HIV infection: A Danish population-based cohort study. *AIDS*. 2012;26(3). https://journals.lww.com/aidsonline/Fulltext/2012/01280/Incidence_of_low_and_high_energy_fractures_in.4.aspx

12. Bradford Hill A. The environment and disease: Association or causation? *Proceedings of the Royal Society of Medicine*. 1965;58(5):295–300.

13. Rothman KJ. Causes. *American Journal of Epidemiology*. 1976;104(6):587–92.

14. Ayoubkhani D, Khunti K, Nafilyan V, Maddox T, Humberstone B, Diamond I et al. Post-COVID syndrome in individuals admitted to hospital with COVID-19: Retrospective cohort study. *BMJ*. 2021;372:n693.

15. Liu D, Cui P, Zeng S, Wang S, Feng X, Xu S et al. Risk factors for developing into critical COVID-19 patients in Wuhan, China: A multicenter, retrospective, cohort study. *eClinicalMedicine*. 2020;25.

16. Hammond EC, Selikoff IJ, Seidman H. Asbestos exposure, cigarette smoking and death rates. *Annals of the New York Academy of Sciences*. 1979;330(1):473–790.

17. Asbestos Safety and Eradication Agency. *National Asbestos Profile for Australia*. Asbestos Safety and Eradication Agency; 2017.

18. Slack MK, Draugalis JR. Establishing the internal and external validity of experimental studies. *American Journal of Health-System Pharmacy*. 2001;58(22):2173–81.

19. Rothman KJ. *Epidemiology: An Introduction*. Oxford University Press; 2002.

20. Amrhein V, Greenland S, McShane B. Scientists rise up against statistical significance. *Nature*. 2019;567(7748):305–7.

21. Lu Y, Belitskaya-Levy I. The debate about p-values. *Shanghai Archives of Psychiatry*. 2015;27(6):381–5.

22. Lakens D. The Practical Alternative to the p Value Is the Correctly Used p Value. *Perspectives in Psychological Science*. 2021;16(3):639-48.

23. Dean AG, Sullivan KM, Soe MM. *OpenEpi: Open Source Epidemiologic Statistics for Public Health. Version 3.01*. 2013. www.OpenEpi.co

24. Miller ER, Wilson C, Chapman J, Flight I, Nguyen AM, Fletcher C et al. Connecting the dots between breast cancer, obesity and alcohol consumption in middle-aged women: Ecological and case control studies. *BMC Public Health*. 2018;18(1):460.

25. Freudenheim JL. Alcohol's effects on breast cancer in women. *Alcohol Research*. 2020;40(2):11.

26. Breastcancer.org. *Drinking Alcohol*. 2023. www.breastcancer.org/risk/risk-factors/drinking-alcohol

27. Breast Cancer Now. Alcohol and breast cancer risk. 2023. https://breastcancernow.org/about-breast-cancer/awareness/breast-cancer-risk-factors-and-causes/alcohol-and-breast-cancer-risk

28. Ranganathan P, Pramesh CS, Buyse M. Common pitfalls in statistical analysis: Clinical versus statistical significance. *Perspectives in Clinical Research*. 2015;6(3):169–70.

29. Dobrow MJ, Miller FA, Frank C, Brown AD. Understanding relevance of health research: Considerations in the context of research impact assessment. *Health Research Policy and Systems*. 2017;15(1):31.

30. Lawrence A. Ideas grants 2022: Peer reviewer briefing webinar introductions and presentation. NHMRC; 2022. www.nhmrc.gov.au/funding/find-funding/ideas-grants-2022-peer-reviewer-briefing-webinar-introductions-and-presentation. 2022.

31. Li G, Walter SD, Thabane L. Shifting the focus away from binary thinking of statistical significance and towards education for key stakeholders: Revisiting the debate on whether it's time to de-emphasize or get rid of statistical significance. *Journal of Clinical Epidemiology*. 2021;137:104–12.

32. DeStefano F, Shimabukuro TT. The MMR vaccine and autism. *Annual Review of Virology*. 2019;6(1):585–600.

33. Flaherty DK. The vaccine–autism connection: A public health crisis caused by unethical medical practices and fraudulent science. *Annals of Pharmacotherapy*. 2011;45(10):1302–4.

34. Miller ER, Bi P, Ryan P. Hepatitis C virus infection in South Australian prisoners: Seroprevalence, seroconversion, and risk factors. *International Journal of Infectious Diseases*. 2009;13(2):201–8.

35. Iversen J, Wand H, McManus H, Dore GJ, Maher L. Incidence of primary hepatitis C virus infection among people who inject drugs in Australia pre- and post-unrestricted availability of direct acting antiviral therapies. *Addiction*. 2023;118(5):901–11.

36. Noordzij M, van Diepen M, Caskey FC, Jager KJ. Relative risk versus absolute risk: One cannot be interpreted without the other. *Nephrology Dialysis Transplantation*. 2017;32(Suppl_2):ii13–ii18.

37. Williams S. Absolute versus relative risk – making sense of media stories. Cancer Research UK; 2013. https://news.cancerresearchuk.org/2013/03/15/absolute-versus-relative-risk-making-sense-of-media-stories

38. Nagata C. Ecological study of the association between soy product intake and mortality from cancer and heart disease in Japan. *International Journal of Epidemiology*. 2000;29(5):832–6.

39. Gutiérrez GI, Naranjo M, Forier A, Hendriks R, De Schrijver K, Bertrand S et al. Shigellosis outbreak linked to canteen-food consumption in a public institution: A matched case-control study. *Epidemiology & Infection*. 2011;139(12):1956–64.

40. Hernández-Garduño E. Obesity is the comorbidity more strongly associated for COVID-19 in Mexico. A case-control study. *Obesity Research & Clinical Practice*. 2020;14(4):375-9.

41. World Cancer Research Fund International. Lung cancer statistics. London: WCRF International; 2023. www.wcrf.org/cancer-trends/lung-cancer-statistics

42. Linda MOK, Gemma T, Rachel RH, Paul M, Mark W, Sanne AEP. Smoking as a risk factor for lung cancer in women and men: A systematic review and meta-analysis. *BMJ Open*. 2018;8(10):e021611.

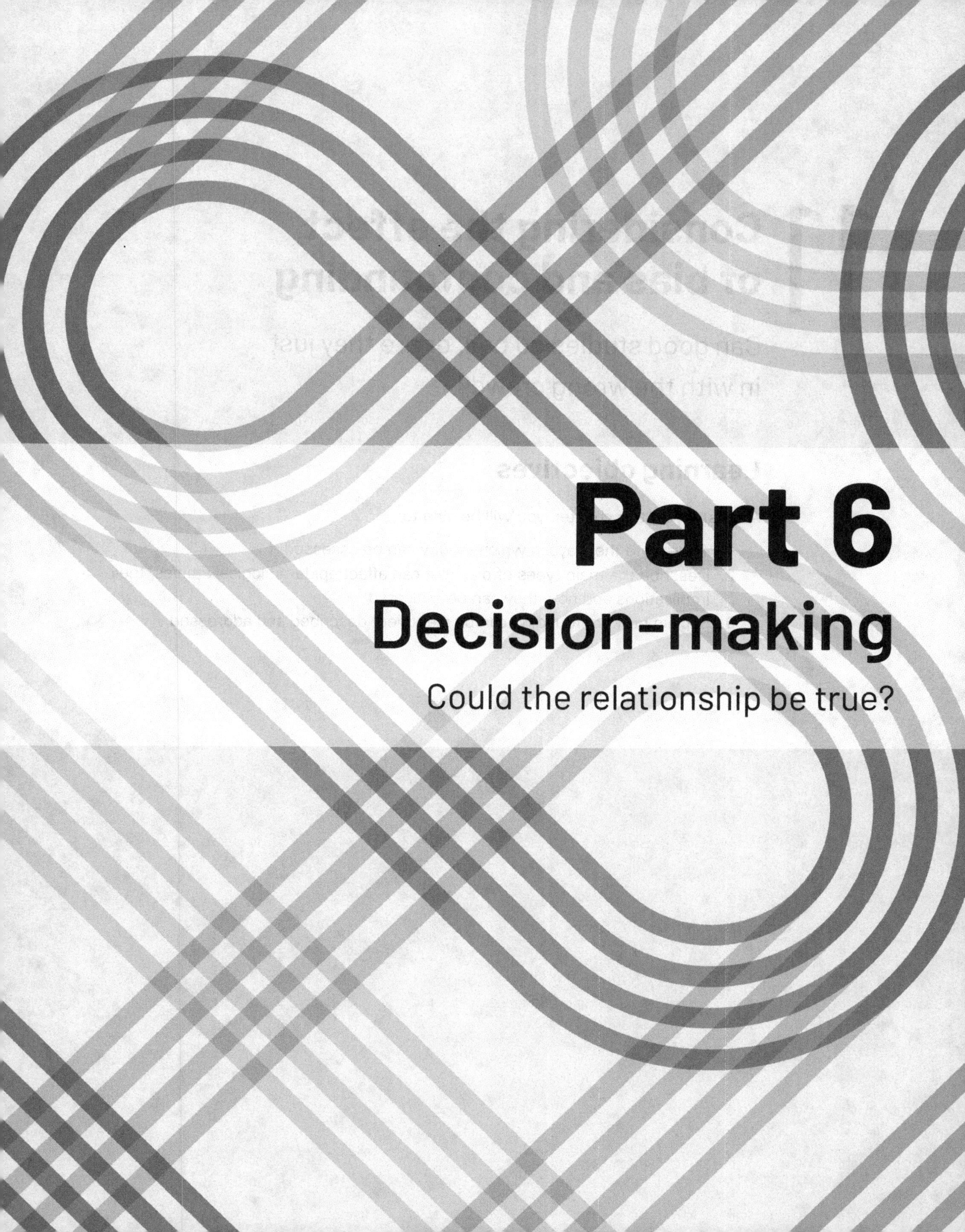

Part 6
Decision-making

Could the relationship be true?

11 Considering the effect of bias and confounding

Can good studies go bad, or are they just in with the wrong crowd?

Learning objectives

After studying this chapter, you will be able to:

1. Appreciate the ways in which validity can be assessed
2. Describe the main types of bias that can affect epidemiological studies, their implications and how they can be mitigated
3. Explain how confounding can be identified, described and addressed

Introduction

Throughout this book, we have focused on how critical thinking can be applied to responding to scientific questions. We have considered the most appropriate epidemiological study designs for different types of questions and the best ways to identify and measure relationships for specific methodological approaches. Hopefully, we have managed to convince you that arriving at evidence-based solutions requires strong evidence. Usually, this evidence will be derived from high-quality research, such as is often published in reputable scientific journals. But how do we know whether even these studies are good through and through? There is always the potential that pesky flaws, such as bias and confounding, might beset even the most (otherwise) perfect of studies. This is why the methods taken to avoid bias and confounding are always well-described in all credible published studies, as is the potential for remaining sources of error for which the design is (inevitably) unable to account, but which might still influence findings. There is always a bit of uncertainty about any evidence provided by studies and, to add to this, the very real possibility that we are not getting the full story at all times. In a phenomenon known as **publication bias**, even really high-quality studies may not be published if they report non-significant results. Yes, even in the scientific world you can feel left out if you are not one of the popular kids!

Publication bias: Occurs due to the tendency of papers that report statistically significant findings to be published more frequently in scientific journals compared with those reporting null results (a form of selection bias).

Hugo: Why would we be interested in a study that didn't find anything?

Rachael: Wouldn't a non-significant result just mean your study didn't have enough power?

Author (Emma): We will talk about this a little later, but assuming a study was of high quality and had the power to show any *meaningful* relationships, wouldn't it add something to the scientific debate to demonstrate that a treatment or preventive health action wasn't all it was cracked up to be?

In many of the preceding chapters, the concepts of bias and confounding have at least got a mention, as have some of the measures for avoiding them. In this chapter, we will revisit and extend this information to answer the question: 'Can good studies can go bad, or are they just in with the wrong crowd?' Critical to this exploration is a good understanding of the concept of 'validity', from where all wells spring, and this is where we will venture next.

Validity and its assessment

We met the concept of validity in Chapter 10. It refers to the extent to which a conclusion, concept or theory accurately reflects the true world. In relation to measuring things, validity refers to an instrument (e.g. blood test, questionnaire, weighing scale) measuring what it is intended to measure and doing so free of systematic error – that is, without bias. Together with precision (the ability of a test to repeatedly provide the same result under the same conditions), validity is about making accurate and reliable measures in research. I think we can agree that relevance and reliability are really important attributes, which is why researchers spend a lot of time and effort ensuring the instruments they develop, or adopt from previous research, can provide valid measures in their study (more on this later).

As well as applying to individual measures, the concept of validity extends to the findings of the study as a whole and, as mentioned in Chapter 10, can be defined according to whether it is 'external' or 'internal'. *External* validity refers to how well your study findings can be generalised to the population from which your sample is drawn or is intended to represent. To have external validity, the study sample must be representative of (or have similar characteristics to) the target population at the time and circumstances of the study. *Internal* validity refers to the relevance of a study to its specific sample of participants in their particular circumstance. Obviously, both types of validity are required if you want to make inferences from your findings and apply them to a broader population, but internal validity alone is quite acceptable if identifying and understanding relationships within a particular group of participants is your main objective. Critically thinking consumers of scientific literature (that's us!) require high-quality evidence; essentially, the quality of an epidemiological study equates to its validity (1).

Assessing validity

Being able to critique the validity of research is important for those in the field of health science and critical thinkers everywhere. Understanding a little of how validity can be assessed might aid in assessing the trustworthiness of research findings and how appropriately they can be applied to clinical practice and health-related policy development.

Although with much variation among scholars in different fields, the validity of a measure can be categorised into three components – content, construct and criterion validity – as summarised in Table 11.1.

Table 11.1 The three types of validity. Adapted from (2).

Content validity	How accurately a research instrument measures all components of a construct
Construct validity	How specifically a research instrument measures the intended construct
Criterion validity	How much the research instrument agrees with other instruments that measure the same (or similar) construct

Content validity refers to how well the instrument encapsulates all potential aspects of a variable or characteristic – or, if we are talking about a theoretical theme or idea, a 'construct'. A construct is usually not directly measurable but may have a bunch of associated aspects that might be measurable and that might collectively describe it. If the construct were the feeling of happiness, for example, some of the aspects that the research instrument would need to cover might include optimism, satisfaction, social engagement and positivity. Another example might be the review questions at the end of this chapter – to have content validity, the questions will need to cover all the different topics required to achieve the learning objectives of the chapter. There has been a lot of work on how to evaluate content validity (3) but, given that there isn't a great statistical method to so, determining the different aspects of a construct generally relies on research on the topic and the judgement of experts in the relevant field (4). In fact, experts in the field agreeing that an instrument is measuring the construct as intended is referred to as 'face validity', which is considered a sub-element of content validity.

Construct validity is about how well the instrument specifically measures the construct or characteristic of interest. For example, we might decide to assess knowledge of this chapter so far by asking health science students what they know about validity. Does a student who recites everything in this section have a good understanding or do they simply have a good memory? To have construct validity, we would need to know that the assessment process was specific to knowledge acquisition. Construct validity is assessed by correlating the measurement being made with a related concept. Quality of life measurements, for instance, would expect to be lower in people with chronic illnesses (4). Heale and Twycross (2) propose three types of evidence for assessing construct validity: *homogeneity* – the instrument only measures one concept; *convergence* – the instrument performs similarly to other instruments measuring related or similar concepts; and *theory evidence* – concepts measured by the instrument are consistent with other behaviours or symptoms exhibited by those being measured. So, in someone testing highly on an instrument that is meant to measure happiness, theory evidence might be observations of them frequently smiling and laughing and exhibiting a high level of social engagement.

Criterion validity is how much the research instrument agrees with other instruments that measure the same (or similar) variable or construct, assuming that the other instrument is valid itself (5). Here, statistical methods can be used to provide evidence of criterion validity by testing the correlation between the instrument findings and a 'gold standard' test (4). *Convergent* (or 'concurrent') validity would be demonstrated by a high correlation between the two instruments, but researchers might also test for *divergent* validity, where a low correlation would be preferred between instruments measuring different variables or constructs (2). An example of divergent validity might be the correlation between comprehension and memory. We would hope that an instrument measuring comprehension of this chapter would have lower correlation with an instrument for testing memory. Finally, evidence for 'predictive validity' might be found some time after the measurement was made to show that the instrument is capable of predicting future outcomes (4). For instance, testing highly for current epidemiological knowledge might predict later academic achievement (see what I did there?).

Example 11.1 shows how the three types of validity can be assessed to determine the suitability of a new instrument for measuring phenomena.

EXAMPLE 11.1

Researchers in Finland wanted to evaluate a single measure of the construct of long-term stress in the workplace (6). Their single-item measure was the five-point response (scored at 1 'not at all' to 5 'very much') to the question 'Stress means a situation in which a person feels tense, restless, nervous or anxious or is unable to sleep at night because his/her mind is troubled all the time. Do you feel this kind of stress these days?'

They statistically compared their single-item of stress symptoms to four datasets from population validation studies of different validated instruments (consisting of longer surveys) to assess the construct, content and criterion validity of their single-item measure for monitoring stress at work. The four other datasets were based on conceptually close measures such as exhaustion, sleep, vitality, mental health and optimism. They undertook correlations and factor analysis to assess validity according to convergence with similar measures, the plausibility of the relationships between health and work characteristics, and the ability of the measure to discriminate between groups.

EXAMPLE 11.1 Continued

There was convergence between the single-item measure of stress and psychological symptoms and sleep disturbances in the validated datasets. The single-item measure was found to describe aspects that were plausibly associated with health and work characteristics, and it was able to discriminate between groups based on sex, age and industrial activity as correlated with a validated scale of emotional exhaustion.

The authors conclude that the single-item stress symptom measure demonstrated satisfactory content, construct and criterion validity for group-level data and recommended that the single-item measure replace longer scales for measuring workplace stress (6).

Rachael: Do you have to do research on every question you use in a survey?

Hugo: How does any proper research get done?

Author (Emma): You would really only want to assess the validity of new instruments, or the use of previously validated instruments in population groups other than those for which the instrument was originally validated. Validation studies *are* proper research, because the process ultimately provides a trustworthy measure that can be used in many studies looking at the same phenomena and can also streamline future data collection (such as is suggested in Example 11.1). Importantly, tools that validly measure phenomena can decrease the burden for future participants by reducing the number of unnecessary questions in surveys.

While much of the above discussion, including the mention of 'constructs', seems most relevant to the measurement of psychological and social phenomena, the same schema of validity and its assessment is described, with minor modifications, in relation to epidemiological and clinical measurements. Table 11.2 presents how the three types of validity can be assessed in the world of infectious disease epidemiology.

Table 11.2 The three types of validity and their assessment in infectious disease epidemiology and its assessment. Adapted from (7).

Validity type	Description	Assessment
Content validity	Relates to the underlying biological phenomena (e.g. microbe)	Professional judgement or consensus
Construct validity	Correlates with relevant characteristics of the phenomenon (e.g. correlation with different tests of similar phenomenon)	Statistical correlation and measures of agreement
Criterion validity	Predicts an aspect of the phenomenon (e.g. tests positive or negative)	Specific test performance indices (e.g. sensitivity, specificity and predictive value)

So, whenever you read a published study that mentions using 'validated' instruments, it means someone has taken the trouble to specifically test the validity of a test, survey or scale. When planning a new study investigating a variable or a construct (or other characteristics that are difficult to directly measure), most researchers will first check that someone else hasn't already developed and validated an instrument for the measuring the same phenomenon. Being denizens of the twenty-first century (living in 'paradise for nerds', as I previously claimed in this book), we can identify and access many of these validated instruments via the internet. There are even websites where you can find out what databases you need to search to find relevant research instruments. Some websites kindly provide searching tips, such as that hosted by the University of Washington Health Science Library (8). For those wanting to explore, I have listed the University of Washington web address in the 'Further reading' section.

In the absence of pre-validated instruments, researchers might develop and validate their own instruments against criteria similar to those described above. In the case of questionnaires, researchers usually comprehensively research the factors associated with the characteristics that interest them before developing a draft survey and assessing its content validity by having their draft survey reviewed by people who are experts in a relevant field (9). A range of statistical tests can then test correlation and agreement with other similar surveys (or items within a survey) to assess construct and criterion validity, including Pearson's correlation principal component analyses and Kappa, while the content validity of instruments to measure continuous (or scale) data is most commonly assessed using the Content Validity Index (10) – all of which you may come across in your reading. While I am sure the precise statistical methods will be of interest to many of you, for the purposes of this book it is sufficient to be aware that such techniques exist and contribute to the assessment of validity. Once a survey is more or less put together, researchers may then undertake a **pilot study** in a group of people with similar characteristics to the target population (11). A pilot study is a small-scale study that is undertaken to test the feasibility and validity of an instrument or study method to evaluate and review it prior to its implementation in a larger-scale study (12). The researchers may also undertake a test–retest process, in which the instrument is tested with the same individuals at two points in time, with their responses at the two time periods correlated using statistical tests such as Kappa and Interclass Correlation Coefficients (13).

Pilot study: A small-scale study undertaken to test the feasibility and validity of a new research instrument or method to improve it prior to its use in a larger-scale study.

The process of validating laboratory-based or clinical tests, which are concerned with measuring things such as disease status or physiological function, also involves expert consensus and correlation studies. There is also a whole branch of experimental research that is about comparing the performance of new tests against a 'gold standard' (the best test available). Words such as 'sensitivity' and 'specificity' tend to get bandied around in validating new tests (revisit Table 11.2 to see which type of validity is involved here). *Sensitivity* is the ability of the test to identify a particular disease (or disease marker) in people who truly have the disease. *Specificity* is the ability of a test to identify the absence of disease in those who truly don't have the disease (or disease marker). Sensitivity and specificity are reported as percentages (or as a decimal of one), which ideally should be approaching 100 per cent (7). It is almost impossible to get all the way to 100 per cent, with the remainder being the proportion of false negatives (1 – sensitivity) and false positives (1 – specificity). Based on these parameters, another range of statistical hijinks might then ensue, including using fancy approaches such as Receiver Operator Curves (ROC) analyses. ROC analyses are about quantifying how well tests can distinguish between people who truly have disease and those who do not (14) and involves creating a graph derived from the sensitivity and specificity of tests, according to different cut-off values of the test. Cut-off values are thresholds at which a test is interpreted as positive or negative (e.g. different blood levels of glucose for diagnosing diabetes). A hypothetical **ROC curve** is presented in Figure 11.1.

ROC curve: A graphical representation of how well tests can distinguish between people who truly have disease and those who do not, based on the *sensitivity* and *specificity* of tests, according to different test thresholds.

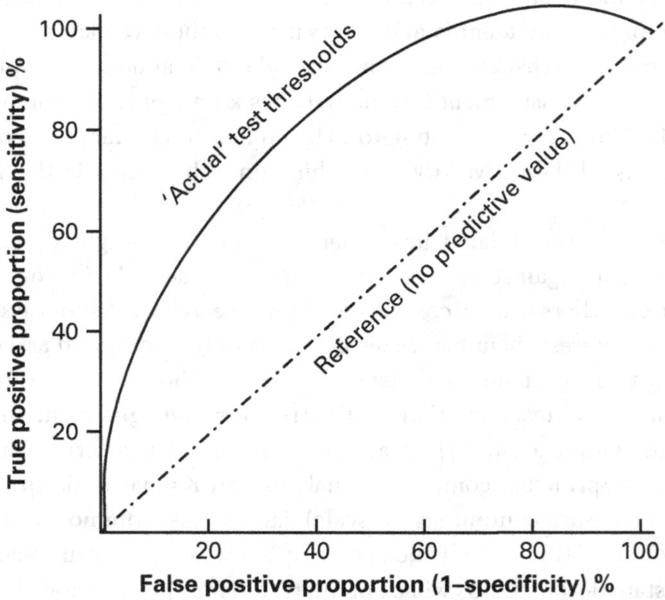

Figure 11.1 Hypothetical ROC curve for a hypothetical test. Adapted from (14).

From Figure 11.1, the hope would be that your new test results would appear in the upper left quadrant of the graph, with the best possible result being close to 100 per cent sensitivity and close to zero per cent false positives. As well as finding the optimal cut-off value for the test, a range of statistical tests can be brought to bear on the various parameters of the ROC curve to determine their statistical significance (a story for another book).

Rachael: Phew! Maybe I will need to work up to the next book!

Hugo: Yeah, totally …

Author (Emma): You don't think ROC curves rock? Well, you are going to be coming across this stuff in the literature, so it will definitely help to at least understand the various ways in which validity can be assessed.

Essentially, validity is the goal of all credible studies, which is why it is something that all researchers strive to demonstrate. Despite the good intentions, however, there is always a possibility that good studies may be led astray. In the next sections, we will consider some of the main threats to validity: bias and confounding.

Bias in epidemiological studies

In previous chapters, we heard quite a bit about the different types of bias to which case-control studies, cohort studies and randomised controlled trials are most prone. In fact, bias is an ever-present threat for all types of study designs and can be introduced at any stage of the study process, from recruitment to analysis. As we now know, bias is any unintentional systematic factor or trend in the collection or analysis of data that leads to erroneous conclusions. It can be classified into two broad categories: selection and measurement bias. *Selection bias* is a systematic error introduced in the selection of participants, or the inclusion of their information at analysis, which results in the participants having characteristics that differ from those not included in the study, but that may well be associated with different outcomes. *Measurement bias* (also known as 'information' bias) is a systematic error introduced by inaccurate and/or inconsistent measurement of study variables, or misclassification of participants according to exposure or disease status. Here we will revisit these two major categories of bias and explore their various sub-categories before considering methodological approaches that might minimise their influence on validity.

Selection bias

So, we have a pressing question on a topic of immense population health importance and we have assembled a prestigious research team to design the best study to answer it. It sounds like the makings of a perfect study – what could possibly go wrong? Well, this depends on what steps we take to also recruit the perfect sample – the most important things in all studies, the participants and their data. If we are not undertaking a whole population census, then we are talking about recruiting a sample of the population. Ideally, and depending on study design, this sample will have characteristics that are distributed in much the same way as (or be representative of) the population from which our sample is drawn. This way, whatever relationships we identify in our sample will have relevance to the broader population that interests us (the 'target population'). If we do not have a representative sample, our findings cannot be validly generalised to the target population. To avoid this possibility, our research team should try really hard to design a recruitment strategy that would maximise the representativeness of our sample. But what if there were differences among sub-groups in the population that made them harder to contact or less able to access our recruitment strategies? Without meaning to, our recruitment strategy might systematically exclude some population groups due to their inaccessibility, differences in language proficiency, or a whole range of social or cultural factors that might influence study outcomes. Essentially, we may have introduced selection bias and therefore impacted the validity of our study.

One of the more famous examples of selection bias, and the erroneous inferences to which it contributed, is described in Example 11.2.

EXAMPLE 11.2

In 1936, the *Literary Digest* published the results of their poll on who would win the next US federal election, predicting a big win for the Republican candidate Alf Landon against the Democrat Franklin Roosevelt. The magazine was confident in its findings, having successfully called the previous five elections by using very large samples of its readership (15). In its largest ever poll, in 1936 the *Literary Digest* sent out 10 million postcards to recruit survey participants from its readership, registered owners of vehicles, and people with registered telephone numbers. Approximately 2.4 million postcards were completed and returned to the magazine editors (around 20 per cent participation), who boasted that their results reflected the views of more than one in five voters in the United States.

EXAMPLE 11.2 Continued

Although the *Literary Digest* predicted a victory to Alf Landon with 57 per cent of the vote, the election was actually won by Franklin Roosevelt with a landslide of 61 per cent of the vote (16). This was a truly disastrous outcome for the credibility of the magazine, as its predictions had become a virtual landmark event in the United States and its polling had been highly respected. But this also became a watershed moment for pollsters everywhere, ultimately changing how polling was conducted from then on (17).

The most common explanation proposed for this catastrophic polling error is that the sample frame was made up of mainly wealthy persons – those who happened to read the magazine, owned cars and telephones (essentially luxury items in the 1930s) and who were most likely to vote Republican. Others have pointed out that other evidence from the time indicated that voters with cars and telephones were actually more likely to back Roosevelt, but that Democrat voters were less likely to return a completed postcard than Republican voters (18).

Whether the poll suffered from an over-representation of wealthy persons (car and telephone owners) or an over-representation of Republican voters in its readership, it is clear that its main methodological flaw was its failure to address selection bias.

The situation described in Example 11.2 shows how selection bias can seriously impact external validity. However, just as importantly, selection bias can also impact internal validity – undermining conclusions made about the very relationships in which we are interested (e.g. relationships between exposure and outcome). Elwood (19) provides the example of a study on smoking prevalence and sex in a clinic population. Surveys are sent out to all patients of the clinic, but more females respond than males. Among the males, a greater proportion of those responding are non-smokers than smokers – that is, male smokers are under-represented. So, the survey provides a valid measurement of smoking prevalence in females but not males, seriously impairing the ability of the study to explore sex-related differences in smoking.

The various study types and their different selection pathways are depicted in Figure 11.2 (19), showing how the pathways for selection become more different, with the possible influence of selection on internal validity increasing from left to right. For instance, the internal validity is likely to be highest in the randomised controlled trial (RCT), as every participant would have the same selection criteria applied right up until the moment of randomisation.

It is important to note that the very tight controls on selection in an RCT can have serious effects on *external* validity. The selection criteria are applied at an increasingly earlier point of the process for each of the subsequent designs – at the level of the eligible participants, the source of participants and the target population (left to right), allowing for differences between comparison groups to increasingly creep in. The case-control study design is likely to have the lowest internal validity as the selection criteria are applied right up at the point of the population source, where there could be important differences in characteristics between cases and controls. In a particular study, for instance, the source of cases might be a clinic population and the controls might be sourced from the local community. In the non-randomised trial, there could be differences in participants who are exposed to the intervention and those who are not, although the same selection criteria are applied up to

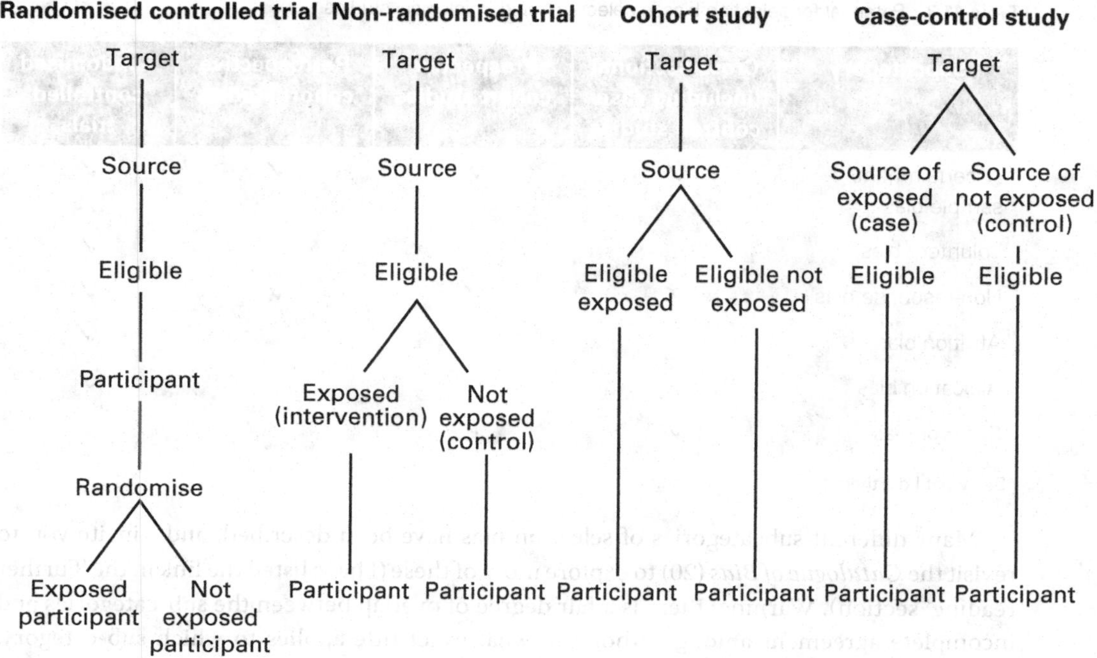

Figure 11.2 Study designs with different selection schemes. Adapted from (19).

the point of allocation. In the cohort study, we might enrol participants at the time of their first exposure, but there can be difficulties applying the same eligibility criteria to people who were never exposed. In all cases, internal validity can be compromised by selection (and the potential for selection bias) to varying degrees.

Hugo: Which is most important – external or internal validity? Can you even have external validity without internal validity?

Rachael: And even if you use validated instruments, does any selection bias could mean you might not have valid findings anyway?

Author (Emma): It really depends on the objectives of the study, but internal validity is pretty much essential. If you are exploring the relationship between two variables, then internal validity is absolutely required but is also a major determinant of external validity (assuming your sample is a representative one). And yes, bias in all forms presents the greatest threat to validity, although chance alone can also ruin the party (stay tuned for a tiny bit more on chance).

Beyond the bias that can be introduced through the process of choosing people or data to participate, which might be sub-classified as 'sample' or **ascertainment bias**, selection bias can be introduced at any point throughout a study and cause your final dataset to look different than the truth. Various sub-categories of selection bias have been described and are defined by the point in a study at which they may be introduced. Although all studies may be affected by selection bias, different study designs are more prone to different sub-categories of selection bias than others – some of the more common are listed in Table 11.3.

Ascertainment bias: (synonym 'sampling bias') Occurs when participants are recruited, surveyed or screened, but this group systematically excludes some members of the target population (a form of selection bias).

Table 11.3 Potential for selection bias in selected* epidemiological studies

Subcategory	Cross-sectional (including case-control) studies	Prospective cohort studies	Retrospective cohort studies	Randomised controlled trials
Ascertainment/ sample bias	✓	✓	✓	✓
Volunteer bias				✓
Non-response bias	✓	✓	✓	✓
Attrition bias		✓		✓
Allocation bias				✓
Survivor bias	✓	✓		

*See what I did there?

Many different subcategories of selection bias have been described, and I invite you to revisit the *Catalogue of Bias* (20) to explore more of these (I have listed the link in the 'Further reading' section). Warning: there is a fair degree of overlap between the sub-categories and incomplete agreement among authors on what exact title applies to which sub-category. From Table 11.3, we can see that *ascertainment bias* (or *sampling bias*) is a potential problem for all study types. This is the type of bias that that occurs when participants are recruited, surveyed or screened, but some members of the target population are more likely to be included than others. The *Literary Digest* 1936 poll (Example 11.2) is an example of this sub-category of selection bias. Also occurring at the time of recruitment, *volunteer bias* primarily affects clinical trials and can occur when people agree to participate, or even request to be included, in a study because they perceive it will provide a therapeutic benefit, either to themselves or others in their care. The bias is introduced when people who volunteer are different in some way (e.g. in health status, educationally, socioeconomically, in language proficiency or even in relation to the health issue of interest) from the overall target population.

Non-response bias: Occurs when people decline to participate in a study, or study participants do not provide requested information, and non-responders differ in important ways from responders (a form of selection bias).

Non-response bias can be a problem for most study types, particularly if a survey is involved. It happens when people decline to participate in a study, or study participants do not provide requested information, and non-responders differ in important ways from responders. Non-response bias can become even more problematic when the non-response may actually be associated with the phenomenon of interest. A study of ageing and health status might involve sending online survey links to residents of a community. Non-response bias could affect such a study in more than one way. Older persons are probably less likely to use internet services relative to younger persons, and people in poor health might be less likely to engage in surveys relative to healthier persons.

As we heard in previous chapters, all prospective studies can expect a certain amount of 'loss to follow-up' (also known as 'attrition'), which is when researchers lose contact with study participants for various reasons. These reasons could include moving to a new location, an error in documenting contact details or simply because people no longer want to be involved in the study. Assuming the losses to follow-up are not excessive, and it has been suggested that up to 20 per cent loss to follow-up is 'acceptable' (21), this shouldn't be the end of the world as long as sufficient numbers remain in the study to proceed with a meaningful analysis. However, if the attrition is occurring differentially between comparison groups, a bias is introduced – specifically, this is known as *attrition bias*. RCTs may find that the participants who make it all the way through the treatment differ from those who have withdrawn (perhaps due to side-effects, deterioration or even death), artificially inflating the benefits of treatment. Including only those completing the treatment in the analysis of RCTs is known as 'per protocol' analysis because the analysis only includes those participants who complied with all parts of the treatment or study protocol.

Any study that involves evaluating interventions among comparison groups can be prone to **allocation bias** – I'm looking at you, RCTs. Allocation bias can occur when researchers or clinicians are aware of which treatment or intervention eligible participants will receive, or can predict the allocation sequence. As we heard in Chapter 9, the problem with this is that, even without meaning to, clinicians may assign patients to treatment or control groups based on their prognosis. Patients who the clinician thinks really need the treatment (e.g. sicker patients) might be more likely to be assigned to the intervention group. Alternatively, patients with lots of other health problems that might negatively impact any treatment they were to receive, and thus not show the true benefit of the new treatment, may be assigned to the control group. It is important to note that such behaviours might be inadvertent or represent the natural desire of clinicians to help their patients, but the end result is an imbalance between comparison groups that masks the true effect of the intervention.

Allocation bias: Occurs when researchers or clinicians are aware of which treatment or intervention eligible participants are going to receive, or can predict the allocation sequence, resulting in an imbalance between comparison groups that may include characteristics that vary in their response to the intervention being evaluated in a clinical trial (a form of selection bias).

The final sub-category in the non-exhaustive list presented in Table 11.3 is *survivor bias*. This type of bias can result in samples of people with illnesses and/or their exposures that do not reflect the situation in reality because those with the illness or exposure have not survived to be sampled. This leads to lower measures of disease occurrence in exposed populations than expected, and therefore dilutes estimates aiming to quantify relationship between exposures and outcomes (e.g. odds ratios). Most types of studies are prone to survivor bias, but particularly case-control studies relying on interviews with cases for exposure data or studying illnesses with short survival times. Cohort studies comparing health outcomes in workers with those of the general population may under-estimate relative risk as all the sicker people may have left the workplace (decreasing workplace incidence) and now reside in the community (increasing population incidence). This is actually a variant of survivor bias known as the *healthy worker effect* (22).

Rachael: RCTs seem to be at risk for most types of selection bias!

Hugo: Yeah – what have you got against RCTs?

Author (Emma): I'm not picking on RCTs, but they are prone to most of the forms of selection bias listed in Table 11.3 by virtue of the prospective nature of the design and the fact that they involve actively assigning people to exposure groups. It is worth noting that good-quality RCTs also have a number of specific design features to minimise these potential sources of selection bias (you might want to revisit Chapter 9 to remind yourself of some of these features). However, as mentioned, RCTs adhere to eligibility and other protocols that are so tightly designed and implemented to ensure internal validity that they inevitably impact external validity.

Minimising selection bias

Although it isn't possible to be entirely free of the potential for selection bias, a number of strategies can help to minimise the threat it poses to validity. Nearly all the design features of RCTs are specifically about minimising selection bias, and include processes such as randomisation and allocation concealment, and the tight protocols that dictate them. Even at the end of the study, RCTs have strategies to reduce the potential for attrition bias by analysing data by what is known as 'intent to treat'. Intent to treat analyses includes the data of all participants of each group to which they had been allocated (after randomisation) as if they completed all parts of the study protocol, even if they withdrew or were lost to follow-up. Unlike per protocol analysis, intent to treat analysis preserves the benefits of comparability between groups conferred by the randomisation process and also provides a better reflection of the performance of the intervention in real practice (23). After all, if lots of people are dropping out of treatment, this may reflect the treatment's acceptability (or even its safety).

The main strategies to minimise selection bias for all studies are implemented during the design phase, although there are some statistical methods (such as stratified analysis and multivariate analyses) that can be employed if all else fails and assuming the potential bias is ultimately identified. Much of the potential for ascertainment bias in case-control studies can be minimised by ensuring there are really solid case and exposure definitions that are standardised and used by all the investigators on the team. It is important that both cases and controls are selected independently of their exposure status. While not really a problem for prospective studies, participants in retrospective cohort studies should be selected independently of their outcome status. Selecting appropriate comparison groups can actually be a fraught issue for all types of studies. The most important thing is that the groups being compared are as similar as possible with respect to all potentially important demographic characteristics, with the exception of the main focus of the study – for example, case status for case-control studies or exposure status for cohort studies.

Statistical approaches to sampling in observational studies include matching, which is most commonly associated with case-control studies but is also used in cohort studies (24). In individual matching, each member of a study group is matched to a participant in the comparison group according to characteristics that might have an influence on the phenomenon of interest (e.g. age, sex and socioeconomic status). Group matching can also be employed, where distributions of characteristics are similar in each group. For instance, each group will have the same proportion of females or people in certain age groups. Other statistical approaches to minimise ascertainment bias may include an element of randomness in both cohort and case-control designs (25). In relation to case-control studies, in Chapter 7 we discussed how controls might be identified from random samples of the whole population or of neighbourhoods, potentially also randomly selected samples of those with demographic similarities to the cases. In Chapter 8, we heard a about a retrospective cohort study that randomly selected a comparison group from the general population to compare with recently discharged COVID-19 cases (26).

Strategies to minimise non-response bias are mainly about making participation as easy as possible. Designing surveys with as few questions as possible can help to reduce the burden for participants, as well as using online survey techniques where appropriate. Careful wording in questionnaires is also important; using piloted instruments can greatly help with this. Establishing reminder systems that prompt participants to complete surveys or assessments can be useful as long as these approaches are not overdone (who wants to be nagged by some scientist?). Ensuring that questions regarding sensitive matters are handled sensitively is also critically important. Participants need to know that the information is confidential and will be handled with the utmost privacy and security. Even the most herculean efforts to improve response will fail to eliminate the potential for non-response bias. So, assessing any information that might have been obtained about non-responders can help to provide reassurance that non-responders and responders are similar, at least with respect to important characteristics. Alternatively, identified biases might be dealt with statistically at analysis.

Similar approaches taken to addressing non-response bias may also help reduce the potential for attrition bias in prospective studies. This is all about keeping people engaged and interested in the project. In a cohort study, frequent reminders might help with finding ways to engage participants through some sort of 'buy-in'. This might include getting participants involved in study-related blogs, using apps for ongoing communication and providing small incentives such as shopping vouchers. Keeping track, or even interviewing a few, of those who drop out and then comparing what information has been collected about them with those who remain can also provide important insights on the nature and extent of any selection bias due to attrition. Similar strategies for minimising attrition have also been proposed for RCTs, as well as using trial assistants specifically tasked with managing follow-up and the process of blinding, which helps to maintain engagement in controls in a way that open trials don't necessarily (27) achieve. As mentioned, randomisation and allocation concealment are the main methods for minimising allocation bias, though these are only a problem for clinical trials.

Finally, minimising survivor bias primarily requires the researchers to be aware of the possibility of, and closely looking for, any data or participants who may be missing or excluded from the sample. Using multiple sources of information can help here, including a review of population statistics. If looking at exposures and outcomes in occupational groups, rather than using the general population for comparison, exploring high and low exposures in the same occupational setting might minimise the potential for the health worker effect (28). As always, identifying the potential for bias in the first place makes it possible to minimise its effects at analysis.

Measurement bias

Okay, we have cleared up the selection bias problem and we are all go – important issue, prestigious research team, representative sample and strategies for recruitment and retention, validity all sorted! Well, not quite, as there remains further opportunity for a whole other category of bias to mess things up here. *Measurement bias* is introduced when the manner in which we collect information is faulty in some way, so we end up with inaccurate or misleading conclusions about exposures and outcomes. Measurement bias can be introduced at any time during the collection of data and their analyses. While all studies can be affected by measurement bias, studies that include an element of self-reporting, or any subjective judgements or discretion, or use previously documented data, or ... actually there are too many clauses, so let's just stick with 'all studies can be affected by measurement bias'. However, given that they frequently rely on self-reported phenomena, observational studies do tend to have a 'rep' for measurement bias.

Example 11.3 describes a study investigating inaccuracies in self-reported work activity, which could explain how measurement bias might be introduced in studies concerning occupational exposures (29).

EXAMPLE 11.3

A study conducted in the United States looked at work patterns and perceived task dullness (cognitive task demand), and heart rate and perceived physical exertion (physical task demand) and their influence on self-reported task duration (29). The researchers randomly assigned 24 adult male and female participants to two groups undertaking three tasks: shelving boxes, a typing exercise and a filing activity. One group undertook the tasks one after the other for 40 minutes each (continuous work pattern), while the other group worked in randomly allocated sequences of four, eight, 12 and 16 minutes of all three tasks (discontinuous work pattern). Participants' heart rates were monitored during the two hours of work, after which they completed a survey on the perceived duration, dullness and physical exertion of the three tasks.

Overall, the participants over-estimated the time they spent shelving boxes (up to 38 per cent) and filing (up to 9 per cent), while under-estimating the time they spent undertaking the typing activity (up to 22 per cent). The inaccurate estimates were most pronounced in the discontinuous work pattern group but, relative to the continuous work group, the discontinuous work group reported a higher level of dullness in relation to the shelving and filing and lower dullness for typing. The perceived dullness of the task was associated with over-estimations of the duration of time engaged in the activity. Although the least physically demanding task (typing) was associated with an under-estimation of work time, participant assessment of the duration of the task was not associated with either self-assessed or objective measures of the physical demands of the activity.

The authors concluded that the type of task and work pattern does impact on the accuracy of self-reported activity duration, which could introduce bias in epidemiological research that relies on self-reports of exposure time (30).

The study discussed in Example 11.3 could be bad news for studies looking at outcomes associated with cumulative workplace exposures of various types (chemicals, radiation, psychological stress, ergonomic and musculoskeletal stress) if they are relying on self-reported estimates of exposure duration.

Hugo: Ah! So that explains why cleaning up my room takes so long!

Rachael: And why we run out of time when we are writing a paper!

Author (Emma): To be clear – those are *your perceptions*, which could well lead to bias if relied upon to measure exposure to tidying and writing papers.

As mentioned, measurement bias can be introduced at pretty much any stage during the conduct of a study and, like selection bias, comes in multiple flavours. The specific sub-category of bias highlighted in Example 11.3 might be referred to as 'self-report' bias, a type of measurement bias that can be introduced due to inaccurate perceptions. Self-report bias is closely related to 'recall bias', which is listed in Table 11.4 along with some of the other common sub-categories of measurement bias and the types of studies with which they tend to be associated.

Table 11.4 Measurement bias in selected epidemiological studies

Subcategory	Cross-sectional (including case-control) studies	Prospective cohort studies	Retrospective cohort studies	Randomised controlled trials
Recall bias	✓	✓		
Social desirability bias	✓	✓	✓	✓
Hawthorne effect	✓	✓		
Observer bias	✓	✓	✓	
Misclassification of cases/exposure	✓	✓	✓	✓

Recall bias can arise when there is differential recall of exposures between comparison groups in epidemiological studies. All studies relying on participant memory can encounter problems with inaccurate or incomplete recall, but the design of case-control studies inherently increases the likelihood of recall bias (see discussion in Chapter 7). The problem of differential collection can occur because of the participants' known case status. Let's say you were diagnosed with a chronic disease; you would likely spend a lot of time thinking about its possible causes. You almost certainly would Google it and come across a number of cues to memory on the internet about potential risk factors and exposures – cues that someone who was not similarly afflicted would be unlikely to come across. If I recruited you as a case for my study, I might be thrilled at the level of detail in your exposure history but would probably find that few among the controls were able to remember potential exposures as clearly. Recall bias can also affect retrospective cohort studies, or any study where exposure data relies on self-reports and the outcome is already known to the participant (31).

Whenever data are collected via self-reporting, the potential for some type of measurement bias arises. The kinds of information that participants are inclined to provide may be strongly influenced by social and cultural factors and lead to a category of measurement bias known as *social desirability bias.* This can occur when participants provide responses that they perceive the researcher wants to hear or are reluctant to disclose information for fear of disapproval. For instance, survey participants might report they do more exercise or drink less alcohol than is really the case. The relationship between exposures and outcomes can be diluted by this sub-category of bias, particularly if the behaviour was socially frowned upon or legally unsanctioned (e.g. injection drug use) and the behaviour was more likely to be engaged in by the members of only one of two comparison groups. A relative of social desirability bias is the *Hawthorne effect,* in which participants change their risk behaviour due to their being observed. For example, the Hawthorne effect was noted in a study of healthcare workers, who tended to wash their hands more often when they are aware of being observed relative to when the observers were hidden (32).

Observer bias: (synonyms 'outcome' or 'detection bias') Occurs due to variation in the way outcomes are measured in study, leading to misclassification of outcomes in comparison groups (a form of measurement bias).

Observer bias can arise when there is variation in the way outcomes are measured in a study. This sub-category of measurement bias is most associated with prospective cohort studies and intervention studies such as RCTs. For instance, observer bias might arise from differences in measuring blood pressure with non-digital blood pressure monitors. Mercury-based sphygmomanometers (and no, this won't be in the test) rely on the operator's hearing to measure blood pressure using a stethoscope. Obviously, differences in hearing acuity provide an opportunity for variation here, but so do habits in documenting blood pressure readings. For instance, many clinicians round the numbers up or down when recording blood pressure measurements.

Observer bias can lead to *misclassification bias*, which occurs when people are incorrectly categorised into groups based on their exposure or outcome. We have already looked at the potential impacts of misclassification in relation to cohort studies and I invite you to revisit this in Chapter 7. In short, the impacts of misclassification very much depend on whether the misclassification is non-differential (randomly distributed between categories of exposure or outcome) or differential (affecting exposure/outcome categories unevenly). Non-differential misclassification will likely reduce the measure of association (e.g. RR or OR) towards the null value. Differential misclassification will result in bias and, depending on which category of exposure or outcome is affected and in what way, could impact the measure of association in any direction.

Minimising measurement bias

The main strategies for minimising measurement bias (it is not possible to completely eliminate its potential) are implemented at all stages of a quality study – through the selection and use of study instruments, the process of collecting data and data analysis methods. Prior to the study, an exhaustive effort should be made to identify existing validated instruments, or a process for developing and validating new instruments could be undertaken (aren't you glad we had that chat about validity earlier?). Standardised processes for utilising research instruments should be established and, when multiple people will be collecting data for the study, may involve training and education of research personnel (33).

There are a number of strategies that help to reduce recall bias, some of which were proposed in Chapter 7. When retrospective information is required from participants, selecting a shorter period of recall is likely to be more effective than a longer period. Sometimes this is difficult to arrange, particularly if you are specifically dealing with events from a long time ago (e.g. exposure to asbestos and later development of mesothelioma). In this case, providing cues to memory can prompt recall, including providing lists of the types of exposures of interest and describing the contextual information in examples. Stratifying the recall period for participants has also been proposed (34) where the participants likely to have experienced an event quite frequently are asked to report information about a shorter period of time than those who experienced the event less often. For instance, finding out how often health science students ate pizza and chips in the last month can then be used to estimate annual pizza and chip consumption, while others might be able to more accurately recall the actual number of times they ate pizza and chips in the past year. Social desirability responding can be minimised by using non-judgemental language, ensuring information is collected in a private location and reassurances of strong protocols regarding confidentiality. For all types of self-reported data, using other sources of information, such as test results and other documented data, can help to validate information provided by participants and at the very least provide a basis for its measurement and analysis.

Another type of measurement bias originating from data derived directly from participants can result from the Hawthorne effect. Considering that the Hawthorne effect may actually be in play whenever participants are directly observed, answer questions about their behaviour or are aware of even being studied (35), it may be all but impossible to rule out. The best way to deal with this type of bias is to recognise that it may be a factor in any study that involves observing or self-reporting behaviours. Using design features, such as hidden observers (32), or at least taking steps to measure its influence (36) are really the only ethical ways to minimise the potential impact of the Hawthorne effect, given knowledge of being in a study on its own is thought to be sufficient for its activation.

Many of the above strategies are required to fend off the potential for observer bias, the sub-category of bias that can result in misclassification bias. Standardised instruments and training on their use when there is more than one data collector can help to reduce variation in outcome measurement. But there is an element of subjectivity in measuring outcomes as well. Expectations of treatment response may play a part, as might expectations and beliefs regarding the impact of potential exposures. In RCTs, blinding can be applied to assure that the outcome assessor does not know who is in the intervention group. Similarly, in cohort studies, the exposure status of participants can be unknown by those assessing the outcomes. Assuming they do not have an obvious diagnosis, research personnel collecting exposure information in case-control studies could also be kept unaware of the case status of participants.

Rachael: This is all very depressing – there seem to be so many ways research can end up being biased!

Hugo: How can we trust what we are reading?

Author (Emma): Yes, the potential for bias will always be with us and represents an ever-present threat to validity. Importantly, the authors of good-quality studies always report what methods they have employed to minimise and account for bias, plus they will identify any remaining sources of bias and discuss their potential impact on the conclusions made. It is up to you, as critical-thinking consumers of the literature, to evaluate whether they have accounted for potential bias and to compare their study to the work of others before reaching your own conclusions.

Publication bias

At the beginning of this chapter, we asked whether good studies could go bad, or were just in with the wrong crowd. The above discussion shows that otherwise-good studies can indeed be led astray by bias. As it turns out, even unbiased studies can be caught hanging out with the wrong crowd, leading themselves and others down the wrong path. This can occur through 'publication bias' – a form of selection bias in which RCTs showing positive effects of interventions, or other types of studies showing statistically significant results in general, are published more frequently than those reporting negative treatment impacts of treatment or non-significant results (37). The problem with all this is that public health policy and treatment regimens tend to be based on the published evidence, and these published studies also form the basis of systematic reviews. As described in Chapter 9, systematic reviews synthesise all of the evidence presented in well-conducted studies on specified topics (predominantly RCTs, if not exclusively) and are seen as the pinnacle of scientific rigour. Particularly where the results of multiple RCTs are statistically pooled together in a meta-analysis, the existence of publication bias will lead to erroneous conclusions about the true effect size of the interventions being investigated.

Despite long awareness of it, publication bias continues to be an issue, although some journals have developed policies to minimise the rejection of null results (20). As discussed in Chapter 1, the peer-review process is good but not perfect, and peer reviewers are not infallible, so further methods are needed to address this issue. Registering trials on publicly available registers when they are first funded, or ethically approved, might be a way to check the outcome of studies that may or may not have ultimately been published. One such registry is the Australian New Zealand Clinical Trials Registry (ANZCTR) (38), which lists voluntarily registered trials and can be searched freely. The ANZCTR is one of the contributors to an international registry operated by the World Health Organization (39). I have listed the links for both registries in the 'Further reading' section. Making such registries mandatory and freely accessible (including pharmaceutical registries) is one strategy that has been proposed (37). It is important to note, however, that no such registries currently exist for observational studies.

A note on chance

Even based on the remote possibility that a study manages to eliminate all possible opportunities for measurement bias, there still remains one more threat to validity: chance. Random error due to chance is not bias but it is very difficult to prevent because, well, it happens by chance. Its main effect is to create imprecision in measuring exposures and outcomes and, if there's a lot of it, chance can cause assessments of exposures and outcomes to deviate from the truth in unpredictable ways (31). Say I wanted to know how many people in your class ate pizza and chips last week so I could extrapolate from this to estimate annual pizza and chip consumption. On the particular week chosen for the recall period, however, some of you had decided to go on a diet, come down with a gastrointestinal illness or just didn't feel like fatty foods in general. Clearly, this unforeseen and uncontrollable variation in consumption patterns would have knock-on effects for my annual estimate. The easiest way to minimise the effect of chance is to enrol large numbers of participants in order to dilute its impact or use random selection so any chance variation is evenly spread among comparison groups. The only other design element that can reduce the impact of chance variation on measurement bias is to ensure valid instruments are always used and the precise use of the instrument is adequately controlled.

Statistical tests can quantify the influence of random errors in analyses of data, which include estimating p values and confidence intervals. The pros and cons of these measures have been discussed previously (see Chapter 10), but their main purpose is to let everybody know how likely it was that the findings being reported could have occurred by chance. The mere existence of such measures indicates that chance inevitably affects all studies, and they provide a way for reporting the estimated magnitude of the potential error. Importantly, good-quality studies report all the efforts taken to minimise bias and chance as much as possible, but never claim that these have been completely eliminated.

Confounding

Completing our tour of various threats to validity, we come to the concept of confounding. Unlike bias, confounding is not something that is introduced during the process of research but reflects existing relationships between variables in the real world that can really confuse conclusions if the situation is not identified and addressed. Confounding occurs when the true relationship between a potential cause and an outcome is distorted by the existence of one or more additional factors that are associated with the potential cause and the outcome. Figure 11.3 shows the traditional model and criteria often used to describe confounding.

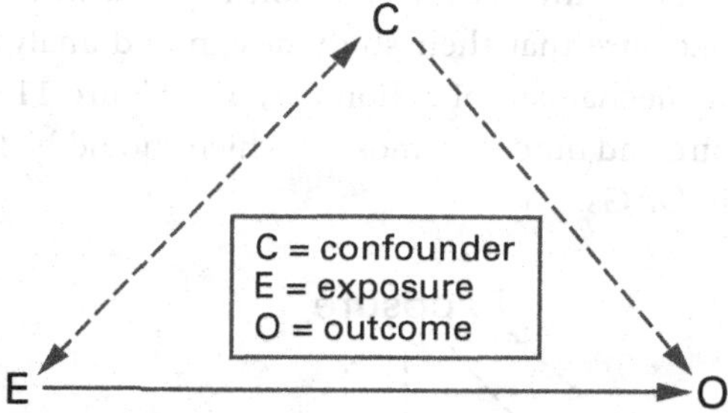

Figure 11.3 Traditional model of confounding

Note: C must be an independent risk factor for O; C must be associated with E; and C must not be on the causal pathway between E and O.

Using the model presented in Figure 11.3, say we were interested in looking at the relationship between pizza consumption (our exposure) and weight gain (our outcome). Is it possible that consumption of chips could be confounding this relationship? Let's see whether chip consumption meets the criteria for confounding: chip consumption is an independent risk factor for weight gain; chips are associated with pizza (at least in this book); and chips are not on the causal pathway between pizza consumption and weight gain – that is, eating pizza does not *cause* one to eat chips. Although, could pizza be a gateway food? Perhaps a more health science-y example might help here. Figure 11.4 shows obesity as a confounder in the relationship between high blood pressure (hypertension) and end-stage renal disease (ESRD).

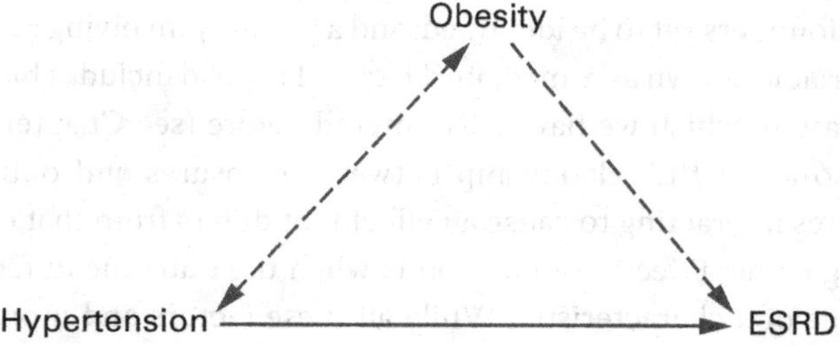

Figure 11.4 Relationship between hypertension and end stage renal disease confounding by obesity. Adapted from (40).

Figure 11.4 shows that obesity is associated with hypertension, obesity is a risk factor for end-stage renal disease and obesity is not caused by hypertension. Since obesity meets all the criteria for confounding, we can say that the relationship between hypertension and end-stage renal disease might be confounded by obesity.

Directed acyclic graphs (DAGs): A graphical depiction of unidirectional pathways between an exposure and outcome of interest, identifying all the variables that mediate or confound the causal pathway.

In recent years, more complex ways to describe confounding and causal pathways between exposures and outcomes have increasingly been used by epidemiologists. These graphical representations are called **directed acyclic graphs (DAGs).** DAGs are a graphical depiction of unidirectional pathways (the 'directed' part) between an exposure and outcome of interest, identifying all the variables on the pathway (without looping back to any variable – that's the 'acyclic' part) that may possibly impact that relationship and where this is occurring. This allows researchers to make sure that their study design and analysis account for all these possible factors and their mechanism of action (41, 42). Figure 11.5 shows some potential pathways between exposure and outcome, most of which should be familiar to you and all of which can be expressed in DAGs.

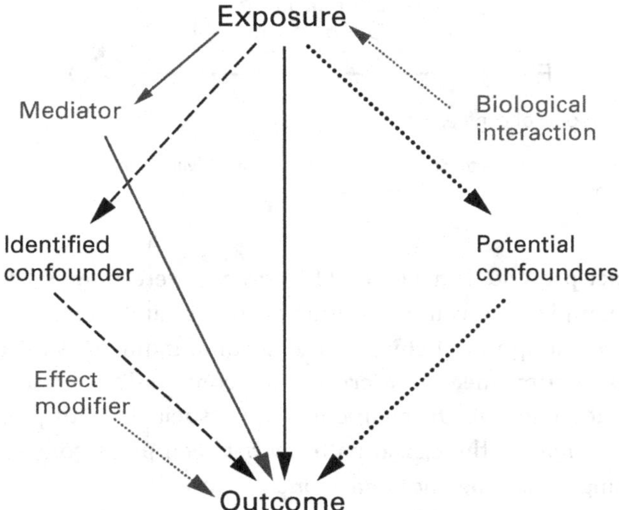

Figure 11.5 Common pathways between exposures and outcomes. Adapted from (42).

Figure 11.5 shows four possible pathways between an exposure and outcome: a direct relationship; the likely involvement of an identified confounder; the possible involvement of one or more of confounders yet to be identified; and a pathway involving an intermediate stage or presence of a variable known as a 'mediator'. Figure 11.5 also includes biological interaction and effect modification, which we have encountered before (see Chapter 10), and these are influences that also affect the relationship between exposures and outcomes. Interaction means two exposures interacting to cause an effect that differs from that expected from each exposure operating alone. Effect modification is when the outcome differs according to the presence or absence of a characteristic. While all these factors and more can be described in complex DAGs, even simple DAGs can help to identify confounders, as the example in Figure 11.6 demonstrates.

For those who would like to learn more about how DAGS are constructed, and even have a go at drawing one, I have included the link to the free program 'DAGitty'(44) in the 'Further reading' section.

The increasing use of DAGS essentially represents the scientific realisation that relationships can be complicated – rarely is there a direct pathway between exposure and outcome without other factors (physiological, environmental and perhaps even social) exerting an effect and confounding interpretations.

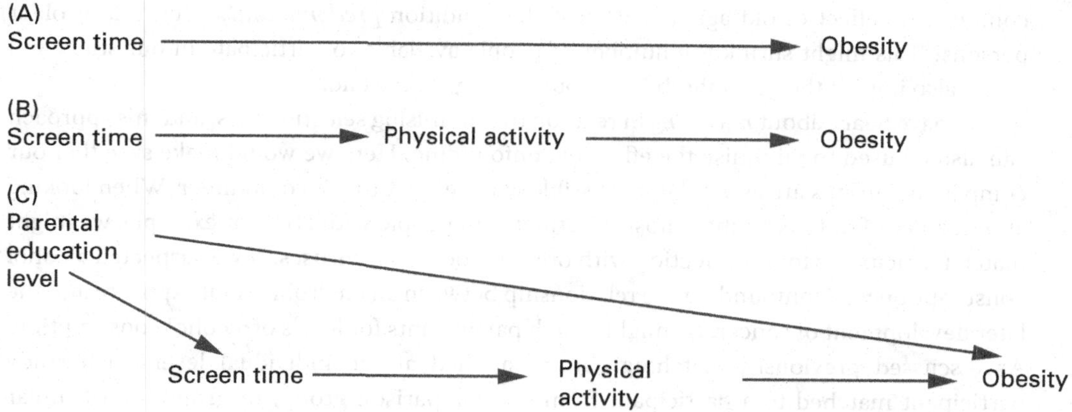

Figure 11.6 Hypothetical DAGs for screentime and obesity: (A) relationship of interest – screen time (the exposure) causes obesity (the outcome); (B) screen time acts on obesity through the mediator of physical activity; (C) low parental education increases both screen time and obesity, and is therefore identified as a confounder. Adapted from (43).

Hugo: Ha, ha, DAGs – they must have spent a lot of time coming up with that acronym!

Rachael: How do we know if the researcher making the DAG has missed something?

Author (Emma): Even scientists have a bit of fun from time to time, Hugo. As the use of DAGs has become more common, a certain lack of transparency about the assumptions underlying them has become apparent (42). But they do represent another tool for identifying confounders and it is likely that reporting associated with DAGs will become more standardised in future.

Mitigating confounding

Right then, we know that the potential for confounding is out there somewhere, so how do we deal with this threat to validity? The critical thing is to identify all potential confounders so the appropriate steps can be taken to deal with them, either in the design of studies or when analysing data collected in the study.

Addressing confounding in the design

This is where we head off confounding at the pass. We may well have a list of likely suspects identified via multiples sources, such as through comprehensive research on the topic and expert knowledge. But there are also some potential confounders that researchers almost always have to be on the lookout for, including things such as age, sex, socioeconomic status and comorbid conditions. The main design features to address confounding involve controlling the methods of selection in the first place.

Restriction might be the first design element to consider here, in which eligibility criteria specifically exclude participants on the presence or absence of the potential confounder. For instance, if increasing age is associated with the development of a condition of interest (as it nearly always is), we might limit participation to people in younger age groups. This would clearly help to study the relationship between exposures and outcomes without the confounding effect of old age, but what if the condition *predominantly* occurred in older persons? This might shrink the number of people available to participate in our study and might also impact the generalisability of our findings in the end.

We have heard about *matching* in relation to minimising selection bias, and this approach can also be used to minimise the effect of confounding. Here we would make sure that our comparison groups are as similar as possible with respect to the confounder. When looking at outcomes of different tuberculosis treatments in people with HIV, for example, we might match participants for co-infection with other blood-borne viruses. If we suspected alcohol consumption was confounding the relationship between an environmental exposure and the later development of cancer, we might match participants for levels of alcohol consumption. As discussed previously, matching can be applied at the individual level (each study participant matched to a participant from the comparison group) or group level (similar proportions of each group have the characteristic); both require specific statistical methods at analysis. One drawback of matching is the extra time and effort it might take to find suitable matches among those eligible for study. Also, matching on a variable means it is no longer possible to consider its relationship with the outcome. It stands to reason that all the variables by which we have excluded or matched participants can no longer play a part in the analysis.

Earlier in this chapter, we proposed *randomisation and random selection* as methods of minimising sampling bias in RCTs, cohort studies and case-control studies. The idea behind randomising is that the process increases the probability of having comparison groups that look pretty similar with respect to the confounder, particularly if the groups are relatively large. Another approach could be to use stratified random selection, in which the random selection occurs within groups of potential participants defined by levels of the confounder (e.g. age groups).

Addressing confounders at analysis

Of course, we may not have identified potential confounders at the outset, or they may even have emerged during the investigation. For whatever reason we didn't include design features to address confounding were not included, we need to approach this issue through analyses. One way to start is to undertake a simple analysis to check for the presence of confounding using my old favourite, 2 x 2 tables. Let's have a look at a hypothetical example first.

EXAMPLE 11.4

A hypothetical study investigated the relationship between chronic hepatitis C infection and the development of diabetes type 2. They looked at test results for the conditions of interest that were available for 4200 people who were attending drug and alcohol clinics in a major metropolitan city. They identified 378 cases of diabetes and 2800 cases of hepatitis C among the participants, with 280 participants testing positive for both conditions. We can plot these data in a 2 x 2 table and work out whether there is an excess risk for diabetes in people with chronic hepatitis C by calculating a prevalence ratio (see Figure 11.7).

PR = (280/2800)/(98/1400) = 1.4

The prevalence ratio suggests that people with hepatitis C have a 40 per cent increased likelihood of diabetes relative to people without hepatitis C.

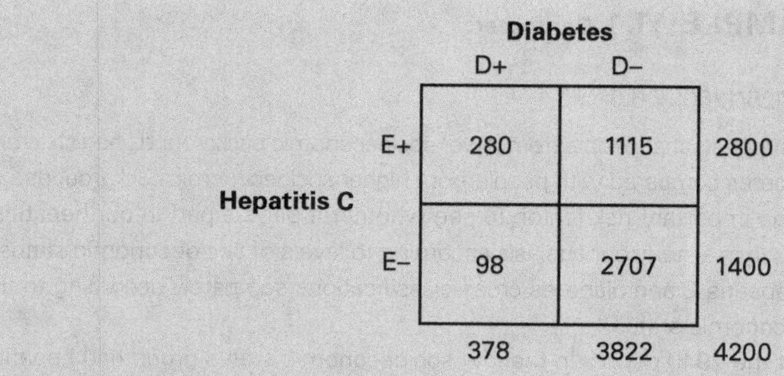

		Diabetes		
		D+	D–	
Hepatitis C	E+	280	1115	2800
	E–	98	2707	1400
		378	3822	4200

Figure 11.7 Diabetes status cross-tabulated by hepatitis C status in drug and alcohol clinic attendees – set up to calculate prevalence ratio (PR)

So, what should we conclude from our hypothetical study? That hepatitis C is a risk factor for diabetes? What if something else is confounding the relationship here? A review of the scientific literature will likely provide evidence that risk behaviours such as injection drug use are strongly associated with hepatitis C, and characteristics such as obesity are strongly associated with type 2 diabetes. In this scenario, the researchers might not have a lot of other information about the clinic attendees, but they may well have access to things such as residential postcode data that can give researchers an idea of the participants' socioeconomic status. Lower socioeconomic status has been associated with both hepatitis C and diabetes – mediated through riskier injection practices in the case of hepatitis C and body mass index (BMI) in the case of diabetes. We can use this information to find out whether socioeconomic status might be a confounder in this investigation by stratifying our analysis. Let's have a go at working through this together.

WORKED EXAMPLE 11.1

Using postcode data, we can sort our participants into 'low' and 'high' socioeconomic groups. Let's say that 2940 of the participants (about two-thirds) reside in the lower socioeconomic group, in which 353 had diabetes. Combined with all the other data we have so far, and with the magic of marginal totals, we can complete a 2 x 2 table cross-classifying socioeconomic status by diabetes and calculate the prevalence ratio (see Figure 11.8).

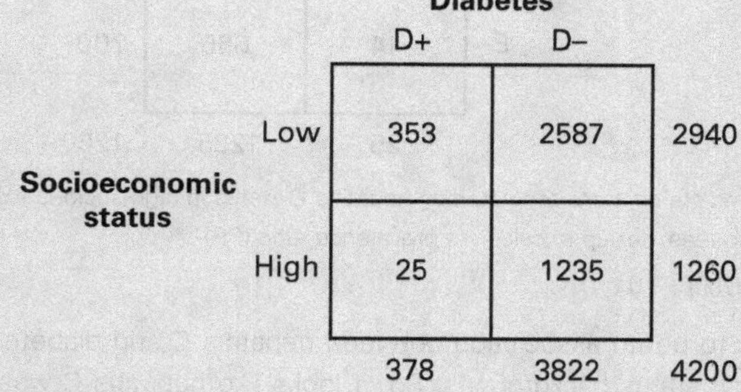

		Diabetes		
		D+	D–	
Socioeconomic status	Low	353	2587	2940
	High	25	1235	1260
		378	3822	4200

Figure 11.8 Diabetes status cross-tabulated by low and high socioeconomic status drug and alcohol clinic attendees – set up to calculate prevalence ratio (PR)

WORKED EXAMPLE 11.1 Continued

PR = (353/2940)/(25/1260) = 6.0

The prevalence ratio suggests that people from lower socioeconomic backgrounds had six times the prevalence of diabetes compared with people from higher socioeconomic backgrounds.

That seems like an important risk factor. To see whether it plays a part in our hepatitis–diabetes relationship, let's *stratify* our analysis according to levels of socioeconomic status – that is, repeat our hepatitis C and diabetes cross-classifications separately according to the two levels of socioeconomic status.

Let's say 2240 of the 2940 people in the low socioeconomic status group had hepatitis C and, of these, 269 had both hepatitis C and diabetes – 616 had neither. Using marginal totals, we can fill out a 2 x 2 table for the low-socioeconomic status group (see Figure 11.9).

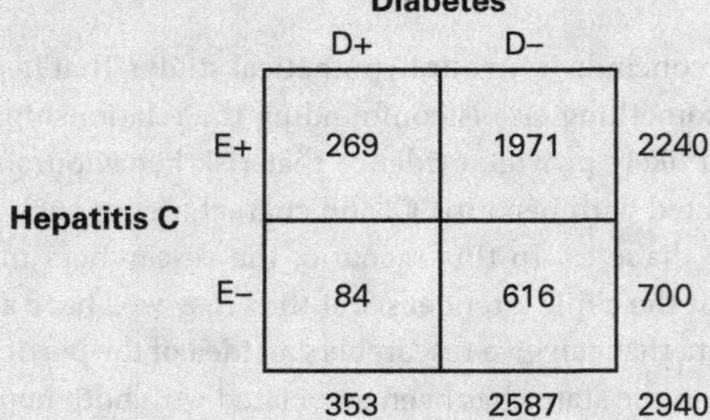

Hepatitis C	Diabetes D+	Diabetes D–	
E+	269	1971	2240
E–	84	616	700
	353	2587	2940

Figure 11.9 Diabetes status cross-tabulated by hepatitis C status in low socioeconomic status drug and alcohol clinic attendees – set up to calculate prevalence ratio (PR)

PR = (269/2 240)/(84/700) = 1.0

There is no association between hepatitis C and diabetes among people with lower socioeconomic status.

Plugging in the remaining cases for the high socioeconomic status group, we get Figure 11.10.

Hepatitis C	Diabetes D+	Diabetes D–	
E+	11	549	560
E–	14	686	700
	25	1235	1260

Figure 11.10 Diabetes status cross-tabulated by hepatitis C status in high-socioeconomic status drug and alcohol clinic attendees, set up to calculate prevalence ratio (PR)

PR = (11/560)/(14/700) = 1.0

There also seems to be no association between hepatitis C and diabetes in people from high socioeconomic status backgrounds. So, it looks like hepatitis C was not really a risk for diabetes after all – at least in these drug and alcohol service attendees. The apparent association between hepatitis C and diabetes was confounded by socioeconomic status.

Hugo: Man – that was tricky, but I think I get it!

Rachael: I'm starting to get why you like 2 x 2 tables!

Author (Emma): Yes – there are many things that can be calculated from a cross-classification and there is something very reassuring about how they always add up!

This hypothetical example is actually an example of a *stratified analysis*, which is one of the ways of dealing with potential confounders at analysis. Essentially, data are sorted into groups defined by each category of the confounder (e.g. age groups, sex, education level); the exposure–outcome relationship is then assessed separately for each level of the confounder. Having identified any confounders, we might also consider controlling for their effects through *adjustment* (or *standardisation*). We heard about adjustment earlier in this book in relation to age-standardised incidence (see Chapters 3 and 8). This is the statistical process of weighting crude incidence rates to account for changes in the age structure of populations over time. Similar statistical processes can be used to adjust for just about any variety of confounder. The Mantel-Haenszel technique is one that you may come across in your reading. It provides a summary measure of effect (e.g. RR or OR) for the relationship of interest that is weighted according to strata of a single confounding variable. If there is more than one confounder (or several suspected confounders), the analysis may include 'multivariate' statistical techniques, such as multivariate logistic regression and multivariate analysis of variance (MANOVA). Sadly, a full explanation of these and other very useful statistical techniques will have to wait for another book. For now, it is useful to recognise that statistical methods have been undertaken to control for potential confounders when you see such techniques reported in scientific papers.

Conclusion

In this chapter, we have looked at many of the ways in which good studies can go bad in considering the effect of bias and confounding. We reviewed and expanded on some of the concepts introduced in previous chapters, underscoring the importance of validity, and how bias and confounding represent its main threats. Summaries of how the learning objectives of the chapter were addressed appear below.

Learning objective 1: Appreciate the ways in which validity can be assessed

Here we revisited and expanded on the concept of validity as it applies to research as a whole (internal and external validity) as well as to instruments used in research. We described the different components of validity (content, construct and criterion validity) and how these components can be assessed to determine the validity of research instruments in various scientific fields. We also looked at how the validity of biological tests is assessed using measures such as sensitivity and specificity, and how these can be used to assess test validity using ROC curves.

Learning objective 2: Describe the main types of bias that can affect epidemiological studies, their implications and how they can be mitigated

The main types of bias (selection and measurement bias) were discussed in detail, including selected sub-categories of each type together with specific strategies for their minimisation. We also looked at publication bias and efforts proposed to address this as an ongoing concern, and briefly discussed the remaining impact of chance and the importance of quantifying its influence in research.

Learning objective 3: Understand how confounding can be identified, described and addressed

In this section, we reviewed the concept of confounding and how it can impact conclusions about relationships between exposures and outcomes. We were introduced to DAGs and how they graphically represent all types of potential influences on exposure–outcome relationships and are particularly useful for visualising potential causal pathways that include confounders. We learnt about strategies in the design of studies that might be employed to minimise the potential for confounders, had a go at stratified analysis and heard about other ways to address confounding at the time of analysis.

Further reading

ANZCTR. Australian New Zealand Clinical Trials Registry. 2023. www.anzctr.org.au

Bankhead, C, Aronson, JK, Nunan, D. *Catalogue of Bias*. 2017. https://catalogofbias.org/biases/attrition-bias

ICTPRP. International Clinical Trials Registry Platform: Search Portal. 2023. https://trialsearch.who.int

Rich J, Schnall J. Measurement tools/research instruments. 2023. https://guides.lib.uw.edu/hsl/measure/home

Textor J. DAGitty – draw and analyze causal diagrams. 2016. www.dagitty.net

Questions

Answers are available at the end of the book.

Multiple-choice questions

1. Which of the following best describes the concept of validity?

A – Allocation sequences have been adequately concealed.
B – The research tool is highly sensitive.
C – The research findings reflect the truth in the real world.
D – All of the above.

2. Which of the following best describes types of validity used in assessment?

A – *Criterion validity:* how much the research instrument agrees with other instruments that measure the same (or similar) variable or construct
B – *Construct validity:* how well the instrument specifically measures the construct or characteristic of interest
C – *Content validity:* how well the instrument encapsulates all potential aspects of a variable or construct
D – All of the above.

3. A case-control study is undertaken to explore the relationship between heart disease and long-term consumption of foods with high fat content. To what broad type and what specific category of bias might this study be prone?

A – Measurement bias: attrition bias
B – Selection bias: survivor bias

C – Measurement bias: recall bias
D – Selection bias: the Hawthorne Effect.

4. Which of the following best describes the impact of selection bias on validity?
A – Only external validity is affected
B – Only internal validity is affected
C – Both external and internal validity can be affected
D – Neither internal nor external validity is affected.

5. Confounding might be at play in which of the following relationships?
A – Frequent pizza consumption is associated with weight gain; getting older is also associated with weight gain.
B – Vaping is associated with respiratory disease; respiratory disease is also associated with mycobacterium tuberculosis infection.
C – Smoking is associated with throat cancer; alcohol consumption is associated with both smoking and throat cancer.
D – Chronic hepatitis C infection is associated with liver cirrhosis; liver cirrhosis is associated with liver cancer.

Short-answer questions

1. There are two types of validity, *external* and *internal*. In your own words, explain what these types are and why they are important.
2. I am developing a survey to use in my study but there is a construct (a variable that can only be measured by measuring a range of related factors) that I want to measure, which hasn't been measured in previous surveys. Using your own words, explain the three types of validity that I might want to assess in relation to my new measure.
3. The ageing of the population brings with it enormous implications for health planning and resources, as many chronic conditions are associated with increasing age. A study is planned to measure the health status people aged 65 years and older and compare this with the health status of younger people. The researchers will target all patients currently in residential care homes for recruitment. What sort of bias might this recruitment strategy introduce and what strategies do you think could minimise the potential for this type of bias?
4. Prison population around the world are known to have higher prevalence of infection due to hepatitis C than the communities from which the prisoners originate. As with community-dwelling populations, sharing injection equipment is the main risk factor for infection, but studies have found that prison history, in itself, is an independent risk factor for hepatitis C (45). Researchers want to untangle the relationships between injection drug use, imprisonment and hepatitis C status. They plan to undertake a case-control study among patients attending infectious disease services at a major public hospital. Cases will be those diagnosed with hepatitis C infection and controls will be other patients attending the clinic with no hepatitis C or other blood-borne virus infection. They will be asked about the exposure history, including occasions of imprisonment and continuing and past injection drug use. What specific category of measurement bias might be introduced in collecting this type of exposure information, and what strategies do you think could minimise the potential for this type of bias?
5. RCTs are famous for sitting pretty much at the top of the hierarchy for scientific rigour. What is the fundamental reason for this reputation, what are some of the specific design features they employ that facilitate this and what implications does this have for validity?

6. A study is undertaken in 200 health science students to look at the effect of coffee consumption on insomnia. Half the students drank coffee during the day and half did not. Although outcome data – more than two periods of wakefulness greater than 10 minutes – were collected from participants, the researchers were aware that people often inaccurately report their insomnia episodes, so cameras were used to assess periods of wakefulness during the night. Table 11.5 compares participant-reported episodes of wakefulness according to exposure to coffee drinking. From the table, it is clear that student reports of wakefulness differ from the real-world measurement as observed with a camera, resulting in a misclassification of outcome data. What are the two misclassification types presented in the table and which of these has introduced bias into this study?

Table 11.5 Daily coffee consumption and wakeful periods >10 minutes overnight in health science students (n = 200)

	Wakefulness (n)	No wakefulness (n)	Relative risk
Camera (true world)*			
Coffee (n = 100)	16	83	1.6
No coffee (n = 100)	10	90	
Misclassification A			
Coffee (n = 100)	12	88	1.5
No coffee (n = 100)	8	92	
Misclassification B			
Coffee (n = 500)	16	83	2.0
No coffee (n = 500)	8	92	

*Hypothetically!

7. Head to the *Catalogue of Bias* (https://catalogofbias.org/biases) and select 'Publication bias' from the 'Select a bias' menu under 'all biases'. Read through the evidence from examining 'cohorts' of trials on the same topic and also look at some of the suggested methods for preventing it. The authors also talk about the impact, but this is mainly with regard to pooled estimates of findings in systematic reviews. Given publication bias effects in both trials and observational studies, what broader implications of this type of bias might you be concerned about from a population health point of view?
8. Researchers have collected a whole lot of information on dementia and measured the extent of cognitive decline among a population of elderly persons in residential care homes. They make the startling discovery that the level of cognitive decline is negatively correlated with height. So, people with dementia had less cognitive decline if they were taller. Then one of the researchers noted that the shorter people tended to be female. All of this information is depicted in Figure 11.11. What do you think is going on here that might have created the impression of a relationship between cognitive decline and height in dementia patients? Explain your reasoning.

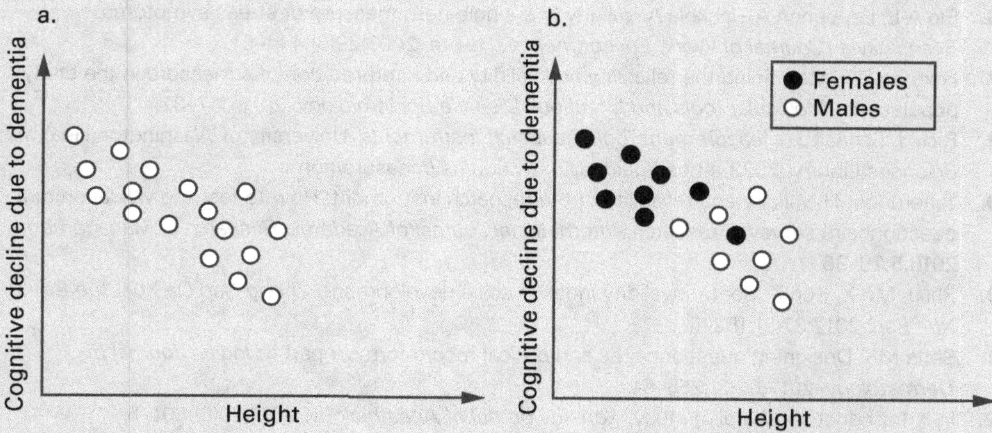

Figure 11.11 The relationship between dementia-related cognitive decline and height

9. In this chapter, we looked at an example of confounding in Figure 11.4 – the relationship between hypertension (high blood pressure) and end-stage renal disease (ESRD) – and identified obesity as a confounder. But what if we were specifically interested in looking at the relationship between obesity and ESRD? Looking at Figure 11.12, could hypertension be a confounder?

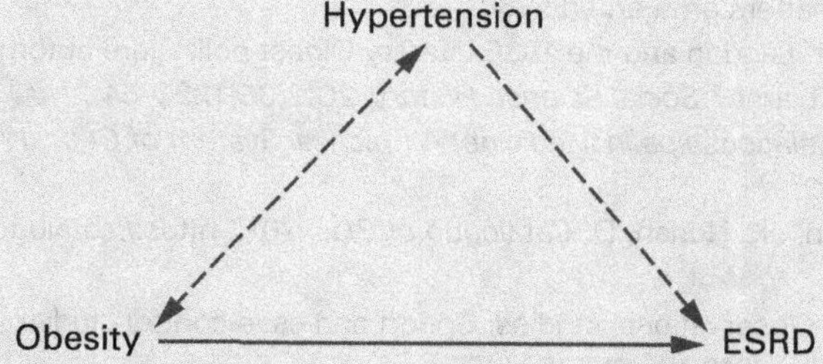

Figure 11.12 The relationship between obesity and ESRD – is hypertension a confounder? Adapted from (46).

10. If we were undertaking a case-control study, what specific strategies could we employ to address the confounding seen described in Question 9?

References

1. Zaccai JH. How to assess epidemiological studies. *Postgraduate Medical Journal*. 2004;80(941):140–7.
2. Heale R, Twycross A. Validity and reliability in quantitative studies. *Evidence Based Nursing*. 2015;18(3):66.
3. Almanasreh E, Moles R, Chen TF. Evaluation of methods used for estimating content validity. *Research in Social and Administrative Pharmacy*. 2019;15(2):214–21.
4. Kimberlin CL, Winterstein AG. Validity and reliability of measurement instruments used in research. *American Journal of Health-System Pharmacy*. 2008;65(23):2276–84.
5. Roberts P, Priest H. Reliability and validity in research. *Nursing Standard*. 2006;20:41–45.

6. Elo A-L, Leppänen A, Jahkola A. Validity of a single-item measure of stress symptoms. *Scandinavian Journal of Work, Environment & Health*. 2003;29(6):444–51.
7. Foxman B. Determining the reliability and validity and interpretation of a measure in the study populations. *Molecular Tools and Infectious Disease Epidemiology*. 2011. 117–32.
8. Rich J, Schnall J. *Measurement Tools/Research Instruments*. University of Washington Health Sciences Library; 2023. https://guides.lib.uw.edu/hsl/measure/home
9. Taherdoost H. Validity and reliability of the research instrument: How to test the validation of a questionnaire survey in research. *International Journal of Academic Research in Management*. 2016;5:28–36.
10. Shi J, Mo X, Sun Z. Content validity index in scale development. *Zhong Nan Da Xue Xue Bao Yi Xue Ban*. 2012;37(2):152–5.
11. Setia MS. Designing questionnaires and clinical record forms – part II. *Indian Journal of Dermatology*. 2017;62(3):258–61.
12. In J. Introduction of a pilot study. *Korean Journal of Anesthiology*. 2017;70(6):601–5.
13. Weir JP. Quantifying test-retest reliability using the intraclass correlation coefficient and the SEM. *The Journal of Strength & Conditioning Research*. 2005;19(1):252–6.
14. Hajian-Tilaki K. Receiver operating characteristic (ROC) curve analysis for medical diagnostic test evaluation. *Caspian Journal of International Medicine*. 2013;4(2):627–35.
15. Norman JM. The 'Literary Digest' straw poll correctly predicts the election of Woodrow Wilson. *HistoryofInformation.com*. 2023. www.historyofinformation.com/detail.php?entryid=1652
16. The American Presidency Project. *Statistics: 1936*. University of California Santa Barbara; 2023. www.presidency.ucsb.edu/statistics/elections/1936
17. History Matters. Landon in a landslide: The poll that changed polling. George Mason University; 2018. https://historymatters.gmu.edu/d/5168
18. Lusinchi D. 'President' Landon and the 1936 Literary Digest poll: Were automobile and telephone owners to blame? *Social Science History*. 2012;36(1):23–54.
19. Elwood MJ. *Causal Relationships in Medicine: A Practical System of Critical Appraisal*. Oxford University Press; 1992.
20. Bankhead, C, Aronson, JK, Nunan, D. *Catalogue of Bias*. 2017. https://catalogofbias.org/biases/attrition-bias
21. Song JW, Chung KC. Observational studies: Cohort and case-control studies. Plastic Reconstructive Surgery. 2010;126(6):2234–42.
22. Kirkeleit J, Riise T, Bjørge T, Christiani DC. The healthy worker effect in cancer incidence studies. *American Journal of Epidemiology*. 2013;177(11):1218–24.
23. Ranganathan P, Pramesh CS, Aggarwal R. Common pitfalls in statistical analysis: Intention-to-treat versus per-protocol analysis. *Perspectives in Clinical Research*. 2016;7(3):144–6.
24. Sjölander A, Greenland S. Ignoring the matching variables in cohort studies – when is it valid and why? *Statistics in Medicine*. 2013;32(27):4696–708.
25. Mantel N. Avoidance of bias in cohort studies. *National Cancer Institute Monographs*. 1985;67:169–72.
26. Ayoubkhani D, Khunti K, Nafilyan V, Maddox T, Humberstone B, Diamond I et al. Post-COVID syndrome in individuals admitted to hospital with COVID-19: Retrospective cohort study. *BMJ*. 2021;372:n693.
27. Brueton V, Tierney J, Stenning S, Nazareth I, Meredith S, Harding S et al. Strategies to reduce attrition in randomised trials. *Trials*. 2011;12(Suppl 1):A128.
28. Chowdhury R, Shah D, Payal AR. Healthy worker effect phenomenon: Revisited with emphasis on statistical methods – a review. *Indian Journal of Occupational Environmental Medicine*. 2017;21(1):2–8.
29. Barrero LH, Katz JN, Perry MJ, Krishnan R, Ware JH, Dennerlein JT. Work pattern causes bias in self-reported activity duration: A randomised study of mechanisms and implications for exposure assessment and epidemiology. *Occupational and Environmental Medicine*. 2009;66(1):38–44.

30. Chang CH, Menéndez CC, Robertson MM, Amick BC, Johnson PW, del Pino RJ et al. Daily self-reports resulted in information bias when assessing exposure duration to computer use. *American Journal of Independent Medicine*. 2010;53(11):1142–9.

31. Jager KJ, Tripepi G, Chesnaye NC, Dekker FW, Zoccali C, Stel VS. Where to look for the most frequent biases? *Nephrology*. 2020;25(6):435–41.

32. Wu K-S, Lee SS-J, Chen J-K, Chen Y-S, Tsai H-C, Chen Y-J et al. Identifying heterogeneity in the Hawthorne effect on hand hygiene observation: A cohort study of overtly and covertly observed results. *BMC Infectious Diseases*. 2018;18(1):369.

33. Pannucci CJ, Wilkins EG. Identifying and avoiding bias in research. *Plastic Reconstructive Surgery*. 2010;126(2):619–25.

34. Althubaiti A. Information bias in health research: Definition, pitfalls, and adjustment methods. *Journal of Multidisciplinary Healthcare*. 2016;9:211–17.

35. McCambridge J, Witton J, Elbourne DR. Systematic review of the Hawthorne effect: New concepts are needed to study research participation effects. *Journal of Clinical Epidemiology*. 2014;67(3):267–77.

36. McCarney R, Warner J, Iliffe S, van Haselen R, Griffin M, Fisher P. The Hawthorne effect: a randomised, controlled trial. *BMC Medical Research Methodology*. 2007;7(1):30.

37. Song F, Parekh-Bhurke S, Hooper L, Loke YK, Ryder JJ, Sutton AJ et al. Extent of publication bias in different categories of research cohorts: A meta-analysis of empirical studies. *BMC Medical Research Methodology*. 2009;9:79.

38. ANZCTR. Australian New Zealand Clinical Trials Registry New South Wales, Australia: ANZCTR; 2023. www.anzctr.org.au

39. ICTPRP. International Clinical Trials Registry Platform: Search Portal Geneva. 2023. https://trialsearch.who.int

40. van Stralen KJ, Dekker FW, Zoccali C, Jager KJ. Confounding. *Nephron Clinical Practice*. 2010;116(2):c143–7.

41. Digitale JC, Martin JN, Glymour MM. Tutorial on directed acyclic graphs. *Journal of Clinical Epidemiology*. 2022;142:264–7.

42. Tennant PWG, Murray EJ, Arnold KF, Berrie L, Fox MP, Gadd SC et al. Use of directed acyclic graphs (DAGs) to identify confounders in applied health research: Review and recommendations. *International Journal of Epidemiology*. 2021;50(2):620–32.

43. Williams TC, Bach CC, Matthiesen NB, Henriksen TB, Gagliardi L. Directed acyclic graphs: A tool for causal studies in paediatrics. *Pediatric Research*. 2018;84(4):487–93.

44. Textor J. DAGitty – draw and analyze causal diagrams. 2016. www.dagitty.net

45. Miller ER, Bi P, Ryan P. Hepatitis C virus infection in South Australian prisoners: Seroprevalence, seroconversion, and risk factors. *International Journal of Infectious Disease*. 2009;13(2):201–8.

46. Jager KJ, Zoccali C, MacLeod A, Dekker FW. Confounding: What it is and how to deal with it. *Kidney International*. 2008;73(3):256–60.

12 Bringing it together

So what?

Learning objectives

After studying this chapter, you will be able to apply critical thinking to:

1. Reading the scientific literature
2. Evaluating research methods used for answering scientific questions
3. Synthesising scientific evidence

Introduction

So, here we are at the final chapter. At this point, you might be inclined to ask 'So what?' Although some of you may have found this book to be so compelling that you have decided to become an epidemiologist, it is likely that most of you will looking for other ways for this epidemiology stuff to value-add to your health science learning and ongoing professional or academic lives. In modern life, we are deluged with health information that is provided in multiple formats, including social media, news websites, online videos, televised news bulletins and chat shows, and even academic texts and other forms of published literature. How are we to find something approaching the truth in this plethora of often-contradictory information? In its focus on epidemiology, this book has aimed to provide you with the tools for evaluating scientific information using critical thinking – a way of identifying and evaluating evidence that has wide applicability to just about every area of human endeavour.

In Chapter 1, we followed a process of critical thinking to address a claim about catching a cold from the draught of an open window. If you remember, we worked through discrete stages of critical thinking in analysing, evaluating, reasoning, problem-solving and finally reaching a decision about the claim.

Hugo: I remember it was a relief to finally sort all that out!

Rachael: Yes, and thank goodness we now know it's safe to sit near open windows!

Author (Emma): Well, we know that the evidence strongly suggests you won't catch a cold just from sitting near open windows, but there always remains room for uncertainty when it comes to science!

Critical thinking allows us to sort out all types of claims and competing arguments, to separate the wheat from the chaff, to recognise the cream of the crop and identify reality from 'feel-osophy' (see Chapter 1 for an explanation of this term). In this final chapter, we will apply critical thinking to obtaining and synthesising epidemiological evidence, using the opportunity to remind you just how far your epidemiological knowledge has grown.

The scientific literature

If there is one thing all students are likely to become very familiar with by the end of their studies, it is researching topics to prepare an academic paper or for other assessment activities. Engaged in such a task, it is to be hoped that you will not simply be writing up your opinions and then fishing around on the web for information to support them. Hopefully, you will consider the problem from multiple viewpoints, collect information from a variety of authoritative sources, synthesise this information in a well-written summary, then present an informed conclusion. In undertaking this process, which is essentially an exercise in critical thinking, it is possible that many of you would take advantage of Google Scholar (1) to find academic publications on particular topics, or visit an online national or international statistics repository to find out the latest population data, such the Australian Bureau of Statistics (2) or the World Health Organization (3). Some of you may go to academic search engines such as PubMed (4) to search for papers on specific health science topics or visit the Cochrane Library (5) to find the latest relevant systematic reviews. I have included the links to these helpful websites in the 'Further reading' section.

In fact, the same process of critical thinking is followed by all good researchers to understand what is currently known about a topic, establish research gaps, inform the design of studies, interpret and explain research findings and formulate recommendations for future practice and research. It is important to note that this process is followed regardless of the methodological approach. So, critical thinking is not just about epidemiology and not even just about your current studies, but it can be a lifelong approach to arriving at, and then acting on, informed judgements that are relevant to all personal and professional situations. To help you apply critical thinking in epidemiology, in this book we have provided you with an 'epidemiological toolbox' – a collection of epidemiological concepts and approaches suitable for specifically addressing a scientific question. Having this toolbox makes it possible to explore an epidemiological problem, understand the appropriate methods for investigating it and interpret findings related to these investigations. Let's look at Example 12.1 to put some of this into play.

EXAMPLE 12.1

In Mexico, Tobels-Pérez et al. (6) conducted a study in temporary workers who were hired by the government to specifically respond to the COVID-19 pandemic. They wanted to compare SARs-CoV-2 infection rates and COVID-19 severity among different categories of workers who had various levels of contact with COVID-19 cases.

They identified workers from the personnel database of the Mexican Social Security Institute (IMSS in Spanish). The IMSS provides social, economic and healthcare services to half the Mexican population. The identified workers were actively followed up from March to December 2020 and monitored for the outcomes: laboratory-confirmed symptomatic cases; workers without symptoms but identified as contacts of confirmed cases; and COVID-19-associated hospitalisations and deaths. The three categories of workers were those providing direct care to SARs-CoV-2 infected cases (COVID teams); other healthcare workers not directly providing care to infected cases (OAHCW); and workers who had underlying morbidity or were of an age that made them susceptible to poor COVID-19 outcomes and were authorised by the IMSS to stay at home for their own protection (HPW), who served as controls. The study analysed outcomes according to work category and also analysed mortality according to work role (e.g. ambulance driver, doctor, nurse, administrative worker).

This is a quote from the results section in the published abstract (6, p. 349):

> Among a total of 542 381 workers, 41 461 were granted stay-at-home protection due to advanced age or comorbidities. Among the 500 920 total active workers, 85 477 and 283 884 were classified into COVID teams and OAHCW, respectively. Infection rates for COVID teams, OAHCW and HPW were 20.1% [95% confidence interval (CI) 19.8–20.4], 13.7% (95% CI 13.5–13.8), and 12.2% (95% CI 11.8–12.5), respectively. The risk of hospitalization was higher among HPW. COVID teams had lower mortality rate per 10 000 workers compared to HPW (5.0, 95% CI 4.0–7.0 versus 18.1, 95% CI 14.0–23.0).

Compared to administrative workers, ambulance personnel (RR 1.20; 95% CI 1.09–1.32), social workers (RR 1.16; 95% CI 1.08–1.24), patient transporters (RR 1.15; 95% CI 1.09–1.22) and nurses (RR 1.13; 95% CI 1.10–1.15) had a higher risk of infection after adjusting for age and gender. Crude differences in mortality rates were observed according to job category, which could be explained by differences in age, sex, and comorbidity distribution. Diabetes, obesity, hypertension, hemolytic anemia, and HIV were associated with increased fatality rates.

The authors concluded that those involved in active COVID-19 care had higher rates of infection than OAHCW or HPW. Relative to doctors, respiratory therapists, nurses and ambulance personnel had higher infection rates and they recommended that greater efforts should be made to reduce transmission among these groups. Poor prognosis related to COVID-19 complications was more likely to occur in those with comorbidities such as diabetes, obesity, arterial hypertension, haemolytic anaemia and HIV (6).

Let's use our epidemiological knowledge to interpret the abstract of the study described in Example 12.1. (From here on, the concepts that we have covered in this book have been helpfully italicised.) It seems the scientific question was about COVID-19 risk for workers involved in different areas of human service activity. They wanted to see whether these risks differed according to levels of contact with people infected with SARs-CoV-2. It is pretty clear that they have used a *cohort study* design to address this question, because they have identified a cohort of workers and then categorised them into exposure groups – namely, those with a lot of contact with COVID-19 patients (COVID teams), those with less contact (OAHCW) and those with none (HPW), who were the controls. They then followed up all three groups over a period of nine to 10 months and monitored them for various outcomes – so we know this is a *prospective* cohort study. It makes sense that an *observational* study was chosen, as an experimental study, such as a *randomised controlled trial* (RCT), would be ethically inappropriate. A cohort design was a good choice because they knew what their exposure was (i.e. contact with COVID-19 patients) and wanted to know what the associated outcomes were. The large size of the cohort and the short duration of the exposure–outcome period suited a prospective approach.

In the results section, the authors reported the *cumulative incidence* of infection in each group, with the clue here being that incidence is reported as percentages of the total time of follow-up rather than per *person-time*. As might be expected, the incidence of SARs-CoV-2 infection decreased along with the level of direct COVID-19 patient contact. The narrow *95 per cent confidence intervals* reported for cumulative incidence indicates *precision* in the estimates, probably due to the large size of the sample. They do not quantify the risk in the abstract, but HPW (those staying at home due to their susceptibility to poor outcomes) had a higher risk of hospitalisation when they were infected, as 12 per cent were during this study. *Mortality* rates were reported per 10 000 workers (again, this looks to be cumulative incidence as person-time is not reported as the denominator) and the mortality rate was lower in the COVID team relative to the HPWs. The study does not report a *mortality rate ratio* (*MRR*) in the abstract, but we can use the mortality rates that they have reported to calculate an MRR as follows:

$$\begin{aligned} \text{MRR} &= \text{Mortality}_{\text{exposed}} / \text{Mortality}_{\text{not exposed}} \\ &= 5.0 / 18.1 \\ &= 0.28 \end{aligned}$$

An MRR of 0.28 indicates that COVID team members had less than one-third (28 per cent) of the risk of death compared with protected workers once all were infected with SARs-CoV-2. Of course, we would need more information to work out whether a result of this magnitude could have arisen by chance or what the influence of other variables might have been.

The authors report the *relative risk* (RR) of infection for various work roles compared with workers with administrative roles (the reference category). You will recall that RR is a ratio that is calculated by dividing the incidence (or risk) in the exposed group by the incidence (or risk) in the unexposed group. It seems that, relative to the reference category, ambulance personnel had a 20 per cent increased risk of infection, social workers had a 16 per cent increased risk and patient transporters and nurses had an increased risk of 15 per cent and 13 per cent respectively. The confidence intervals are fairly narrow (suggesting precision) and indicate that the estimates of relative risk are *statistically significant* (as they do not overlap the *null* value). The estimates of RR have also been *adjusted* for age and sex (or weighted, using statistical techniques), so it looks like these factors do not account for the differences seen between the categories of workers. Although *crude* mortality (the observed and unadjusted rate) differed according to work role, these differences disappeared once the RR was adjusted for age, sex and comorbidities such as diabetes, obesity, hypertension, haemolytic anaemia and HIV, all of which were associated with poorer COVID-19 outcomes.

Hugo: Could you say that age and comorbidities were *confounders*?

Rachael: Yes, weren't age and comorbidities why some of the workers were protected at home?

Author (Emma): Let's see whether comorbidities and age fit the criteria for confounding in the relationship between work role and COVID-19 mortality: (1) age and comorbidities are independent risk factors for COVD-19 mortality; 2) age and comorbidities could well be associated with work role; and (3) age and comorbidities are not on the causal pathway between work role and COVID-19 mortality. So it looks like some fancy statistical adjustment may have removed the effect of these potential confounders!

We heard about the ambiguities associated with *case-fatality* in Chapter 2 – is this a ratio a proportion or a rate? In Example 12.1, the authors refer to case-fatality as a rate, but I think it is also reasonable to interpret case-fatality as a proportion of the COVID-19 infected cases who died. The author's overall conclusions seem appropriate for the reported results.

And all of this epidemiology stuff that you now know was in a single abstract! Of course, we would need to read the entire paper to get an idea of the *validity* of the findings and then read more studies on the topic to reach our own conclusion about the relationships described.

Reading a scientific paper

Reading any published literature is essentially an exercise in critical thinking. It involves recalling and reflecting on your learning and understanding the terminology used (epidemiological concepts anyone!), differentiating fact from opinion, identifying the relationships between events and factors, making inferences and applying all of this to reach a judgement that makes sense in the real world (7). Most scientific papers are reported in more or less the same way, which greatly facilitates the process of thinking critically about their contents.

Commentaries, theoretical papers and *systematic reviews* have their own particular reporting formats, for which there is a little variation among journals, but *primary studies* (at least those describing quantitative studies) are usually reported using the following components:

1. title, authors' names and affiliations
2. abstract – a summary of the study that may be written in a single paragraph or structured into specific elements (e.g. objectives/aims, methods, results, conclusion)
3. introduction – provides the context, rationale and aims of the study, usually highlighting the importance of the issue being investigated
4. methods – specific detail on the study design, the participants, the instruments used and approach to data analysis. Should include any measures taken to minimise bias and confounding
5. results – all the findings in the form of text, tables and figures
6. discussion – interpretation of the findings and where they fit within the published literature, the limitations of the study (particularly any remaining potential sources of *bias*) and any recommendations for further research
7. conclusion – summarises the main findings and any recommendations of the study.

A whole bunch of reporting guidelines have been established by expert groups for reporting on different types of study designs. Many journals now subscribe to these guidelines, which prescribe the content of every component of a paper, including all those sections listed above. These reporting guidelines are available from the 'EQUATOR Network' website (8), and include the CONSORT Statement for RCTs, the STROBE checklist for observational studies and the PRISMA Statement for systematic reviews. I have included a link to the EQUATOR website in the 'Further reading' section so you can check out the guidelines (and find out what all these acronyms stand for).

When you go and search the literature on a topic, the title of the paper will generally be the very first thing you see and, in many cases, may be the only thing you read. Authors (and the journals that publish their papers) are fully aware of this, so usually take a great deal of trouble to design a concise, informative and interesting title to create a great initial impression (9). As well as stating the main topic of the study, in recent years many scientific journals have required the title to identify the specific approach used in the research (10). So a title might include a subtitle such as 'A *double-blind, placebo-controlled trial*,' 'A *cross-sectional study*,' or 'A *retrospective cohort study*.' This can be really helpful in identifying or excluding papers but, while widespread, such informative titles are yet to become the rule. So, as long as the title is of some interest, reading the abstract is the next thing to do.

Reading the abstract and introduction

A well-written abstract is usually a useful summary of the entire study, including the conclusions (warning: abstracts contain spoilers!). Different journals may vary on the exact format required for abstracts, but whether they are structured into section headings (similar to the body of the paper itself) or written as a single summary paragraph, most abstracts should contain the purpose of the study, a brief explanation of the main methods used (participants, settings, study instruments and principal analytical approach), key findings and main conclusions. The important thing is that, like titles, abstracts are indexed on many search engines (such as PubMed), which means they are fully displayed when you search for topics and may turn out to be the only part of the paper that is read. This can happen if the main paper is written in a language other than that used by the searcher, or if the paper is not easily accessible due to being published in a subscription-only journal, or simply that the publication turns out to be not particularly relevant to the topic of interest after all.

Reading the abstract of a paper is a great way to get an idea of whether the work is of interest to you and to determine whether you have the necessary knowledge to understand the epidemiological and other scientific concepts included in the paper. I would caution being deterred too easily, however, remembering that epidemiology involves lot of synonyms, so you might actually know more about the concepts than you think you do. You might also be surprised by what new knowledge you might pick up by tackling a 'tricky' publication. We can look to the reputation of the journal itself and at the institutional affiliations of the authors for some clues about the credibility of the work. To get a sense of the validity of the study conclusions, however, there is nothing for it but to read the whole paper, paying particular attention to the methods section of the study.

This is not to say that you should skip the introduction section – far from it! The introduction provides the whole rationale for the study. It provides the background of the issue being explored, summarising what is currently known and explaining the gap that the research is intended to fill through clearly stating the aims or purpose of the study. A good introduction will highlight all the questions remaining about the phenomenon of interest and clearly set out the logic of the approach taken to address these questions. If not, this is where the critical reader should easily be able recognise any inconsistencies in the logic and rationale for the study. Did the stated aims for the study flow from the rationale provided and did the authors convince you of the need for their study? From your wider reading (characteristic of the critical reader), does it look as if the research will add something new to the knowledge base, providing much-needed confirmation of earlier findings, or does it seem to be merely covering well-trodden ground? Importantly, does the summary of the research approach seem to suggest a logical way to meet the investigation aims?

Reading the methods

As well as providing evidence for the validity of study findings, the methods section of a scientific paper is about transparency and reproducibility. Essentially, this section should contain all the details required for other researchers in the field to be able to reproduce the study (11). For critical readers of the scientific literature, whether or not they are expert investigators, the methods section should at least provide sufficient detail about who the participants were and why they were included or excluded, and strategies to minimise bias and confounding (more on this later). Any research instruments should be thoroughly justified and the analytical approach should be fully explained. Example 12.2 summarises a very comprehensive methods section from a paper reporting on a study looking at sarcopenia that was published in the *American Journal of Epidemiology* (12). 'Sarcopenia' is the loss of skeletal muscle and strength that occurs when people age and is a leading cause of falls and injuries in older persons; at the time of the study, however, sarcopenia had proven to be difficult to measure precisely.

EXAMPLE 12.2

A study was undertaken in New Mexico to develop and evaluate an approach to measure skeletal muscle mass; to use the instrument to measure the prevalence of sarcopenia in Hispanic and non-Hispanic elderly people; and to look at the relationships between sarcopenia and a range of health behaviours, chronic conditions, physical function, disability and falls (12). In the methods section of their paper, the authors included the following sections.

Survey data: Conducted between May 1993 and September 1995, the New Mexico Elder Health Survey consisted of a standardised interview and comprehensive clinical examination of 808 elderly persons (426 males and 382 females). This group were part of 2200 persons initially randomly sampled from a national Medicare finance system and stratified for equal numbers of Hispanic and non-Hispanic men and women (identified via a specific ethnicity search system). Reasons for not including all of the initially identified persons were fully provided (and quantified) and included deaths, moving away, non-response or missing data, or being ineligible for the study. A random subsample of 199 participants underwent an additional body composition examination by dual-energy x-ray absorptiometry – restricted to this subgroup due to the high cost and complexity of the procedure.

Reference data: Two previous studies provided reference data. (1) The New Mexico Aging Process Study – a longitudinal study of nutrition and body composition which had data on 301 elderly people. The 1994 data from this study was used to validate equations for predicting muscle mass in the New Mexico Elder Health Survey (see above). (2) The Rosetta Study – a study looking at skeletal muscle mass and in healthy adults. Data from 229 non-Hispanic men and women aged between 18 and 40 years was used to define cut-off values for sarcopenia for young versus older people.

Survey methods: Every measure taken in the comprehensive, four-hour examination and survey was fully described and justified, and included medical and falls histories, dietary intake, lifestyle and other health behaviours, frequency of leisure activities such as jogging or tennis, physical and cognitive function, measurements of cardiac health, clinical and biochemical nutrients, chronic illnesses, diagnosed and undiagnosed non-insulin dependent diabetes, and much more. Validated scales used in the interview included the Activities of Daily Living and Instrumental Activities of Daily Living scales to measure self-reported disability and formal instruments for measuring balance and gait abnormalities. They even validated ethnicity via reported parents' and grandparents' ethnicity, country of birth, preferred language, and language fluency. The exact methods by which the physical measurements were fully described, down to the single observer who made the measurement and by whom they were trained, the standardised equipment used and how they were interpreted.

Body composition: The ways the percentage of body fat and skeletal muscle mass were quantified were detailed and included the dual-energy x-ray absorptiometry in the random subsample drawn from the Survey, data on this from the Aging Process and Rosetta studies. The authors also used the sum of lean soft-tissue masses for the arms and the legs using a previously validated system. All potential room for error in these measurements was reported as was how the measurements had been validated. The use of standardised techniques was also emphasised.

Statistical analysis: Here the authors provide a further full page of the paper (close to 700 words) on every statistical approach applied. The predictive equations used to measure muscle mass are fully presented as was the way that the equations were validated against the Aging Process and Rosetta studies, including details about the statistical correlations undertaken. The authors explained how they arrived at a definition of 'sarcopenia' (previously not quantitatively defined): 'Cutoff values for sarcopenia in each sex were defined as values two standard deviations below the sex-specific means of the Rosetta Study reference data for young adults aged 18–40 years' (12, p. 758). Finally, the authors provided details about all the variables used in multivariate logistic regressions (including age, ethnicity, obesity, income, chronic disease and disability, etc.) and how each variable was defined.

The paper from Example 12.2 is a particularly good example of a methods section because it clearly describes and justifies all methods used to a level that is sufficient for other experts in the field to replicate the study. Its quality might explain why the paper is among the top 100 cited papers in the field of public, environmental and occupational health (13). In case you were wondering, the authors did establish a valid mechanism for measuring the extent of sarcopenia, and demonstrated that sarcopenia increased with age from around 20 per cent in people under 70 years of age to about 60 per cent in people older than 80 years, with the *prevalence* being slightly higher in Hispanic persons compared with non-Hispanic persons (12).

The length of the methods section depends on the complexity of the research approach, with growing use of supplemental or additional files (available digitally) for more complex descriptions, but the requirement for meeting the principles of transparency and reproducibility is increasingly emphasised by reputable journals. Sadly, this has not always been the case and insufficient detail is a problem that affects papers based on all types of study design. Agnes et al. (14) undertook a systematic review of more than 20 000 RCTs that had been included in previous systematic reviews. This showed that inadequate reporting of things such as *allocation concealment* and *blinding* affected up to 50 per cent or more of papers on RCTs published between 2011 and 2014. Although the problem decreased over time, inadequate reporting of RCT methods was still common, particularly for papers published in low-impact journals (14). And the problem is not confined to RCTs, with the same issue impacting observational studies. For instance, in a study looking at the reproducibility of 38 published cohort studies that all used two specific health datasets to which the authors had access, seven identified studies had to be excluded – five due to very poor design and two due to 'grossly inadequate reporting' (15, p. 1). Another study evaluated the reporting of methods in 244 observational studies on cancer against the STROBE Statement (see above) and found that 70 per cent of these publications were 'satisfactory' but most did not report on essential methodological aspects, such as *matching, absolute risk differences* and how they managed missing data (16). The authors found little difference in the reporting of methods between higher and lower ranked journals. Even systematic reviews, considered to be the most rigorous of scientific studies, can lapse when it comes to reporting methods. Koffel and Rehlefsen (17) found that only 22 per cent of 272 published systematic reviews (from 25 journals) provided a reproducible search strategy – the actual 'systematic' bit of a systematic review.

Rachael: Are you saying we can't even trust publications in good-quality journals?

Hugo: Why is there always a big, fat 'but' in epidemiology?

Author (Emma): I am saying that you need to use your epidemiological knowledge and apply critical thinking when reading the scientific literature. Just because a study is published does not ensure its validity.

This whole transparency and reproducibility thing has inspired long-term projects such as the Reproducibility Project: Cancer Biology, in which researchers attempted to reproduce the study results from the reported methods of 153 papers published over a period of eight years, although they also attempted to contact some the authors for more details where necessary (18). *Nature* and *Science* are among the most highly respected science journals in the world, and a publication in either of these two journals is considered a very big deal in academic circles. Yet only about two-thirds of the 21 social sciences articles (and fewer than 30 per cent of a further 17 highly cited articles) published in these venerable tomes were able to be replicated by the Reproducibility Project (19). It is a good thing that critical consumers of the scientific literature know they need to read more than one study when they are seeking to understand issues of interest.

Reading the results

The next thing to pay attention to when reading a scientific paper is the results section. In this section, the tables, figures and diagrams present the results of all the outcomes and statistical manipulations that the authors said would happen in the methods section.

In an epidemiological paper, the results section will usually flow from the presentation of *descriptive* data, then to some general statistical analysis of one-to-one relationships between exposures/risk factors and outcomes in the data (sometimes called 'bivariate' or 'univariate' analyses), and finally move on to some more fancy statistical approaches, including things such as *multivariate* analyses. Most of the results are summarised in tables and figures, which are usually also explained in the text, but lots of people (even quite seasoned academics) can have a bit of difficulty working them out. Let's have a go at reading some right now.

You may recall a paper we looked at in Chapter 9, which described an RCT investigating tuberculosis (TB) prevention in people with HIV infection in South Africa (20). This randomised double-blind, placebo-controlled trial evaluated a drug called 'isoniazid' (commonly used to treat established TB) for preventing TB in people who were currently taking antiretroviral therapy for HIV. Of 1329 HIV patients in South Africa, 662 were randomised to receive isoniazid treatment and 667 to receive the placebo for 12 months. Across the approximately three and half years of the study, the 1329 participants contributed to 3227 person-years of follow-up. Look at Table 12.1 for a summary of the outcomes, incident cases of TB and deaths.

Table 12.1 Effect of isoniazid on rate of TB or death. Adapted from (20)

	Overall	Placebo		Isoniazid		Effect	
	No. of events	**Rate per 100 person-years**	**No. of events**	**Rate per 100 person-years**	**No. of events**	**Rate per 100 person-years**	**Unadjusted hazard ratio (95% CI)**
Tuberculosis							
All TB	95	2.9	58	3.6	37	2.3	0.63 (0.41, 0.94)
Definite	34	1.1	22	1.4	12	0.7	0.54 (0.27, 1.08)
Probable	61	1.9	36	2.3	25	1.5	0.68 (0.41, 1.10)
Deaths							
All causes	37	1.0	21	1.2	16	0.9	0.72 (0.34, 1.34)

Hazard ratio: The mathematical probability of the occurrence of an event (such as a new case of disease or death) in one group over a specified period of time relative to another group.

The first thing to do when confronted with a table is to look at what it is aiming to tell you. That is, we need to identify the structure before attempting to interpret the content. The title tells us that the table presents data reporting on how isoniazid affects the rates of tuberculosis and mortality. Looking along the columns, we can see that outcomes are reported for everyone – for people in the placebo group and for people taking isoniazid. The final column provides the measure of effect, which quantifies the difference between the placebo and intervention group. We can see that the table reports both the number of events and rates per 100 person years. The effect size is reported as an 'unadjusted **hazard ratio**'. So we know a ratio of some sort has been calculated that quantifies the risk difference between the intervention group and the placebo group, and that ratio has not been adjusted – that is, not subjected to any statistical manipulation to control for potential confounders. Turning to the rows, we can see that the two main categories for which outcomes are reported are tuberculosis and deaths. The tuberculosis rows are sub-classified into rows showing outcomes for all new TB cases, definite (or confirmed) cases and probable cases. There is a single row for deaths, which is defined as *all causes* – this would mean any deaths that occurred in the participants, not just TB-*specific* deaths.

Now we know what all the rows and columns represent, we can look at the content of the table. There were 95 tuberculosis cases (34 definite and 61 probable) and 37 deaths due to all causes. We can see that there were more tuberculosis cases and deaths in the placebo group compared with the isoniazid group, but the rates per 100 person-years make it much easier to directly compare. We haven't come across the hazard ratio in this book, but this is essentially the mathematical probability of the occurrence of an event (such as a new case of disease or death) in one group over a specified period of time relative to another group. In this case, we can roughly interpret it as depicting the effect size of the treatment, similar to a relative risk. To reassure yourself of this, you can divide the rates in the treatment group by the rates in the placebo groups. For instance, the rate of tuberculosis in the isoniazid group was 2.3 per 100 person-years and the rate was 3.6 per 100 person-years in the placebo group.

$$\begin{aligned} RR &= \text{Incidence}_{\text{exposed}} / \text{Incidence}_{\text{not exposed}} \\ &= 2.3/3.6 \\ &= 0.64 \end{aligned}$$

If you repeated the exercise, you would see that all of the hazard ratios in the table are pretty close to the relative risk and, because interpreting hazard ratios follows the same rules of all ratios (such as we have become familiar with in this book), all those reported in the table indicate a protective effect for isoniazid in relation to TB and mortality (HR <1).

Now we can have a closer look at the confidence intervals reported for the HRs and you might see that, with the exception of all TB cases, the confidence intervals include the null value. So the drug was only significantly protective for probable and confirmed TB cases combined, at least in this analysis.

Hugo: Do we have to go through all of that for every table we see?
Rachael: It does seem a bit of a rigmarole!
Author (Emma): A lot of people struggle with reading tables, so it is worth looking closely at all the rows and columns first to make sure you understand the information being presented. I assure you that the process becomes much faster the more you engage in it!

We can apply the same process of sorting out the structure first and then the content when reading figures, such as Figure 12.1, which shows a chart from the same RCT. This particular type of graph is known as a **Kaplan-Meier curve**, which is a statistically generated graph that shows the cumulative probability of survival (or any other event) at specified points in time in one or more groups. The cumulative probability curve goes up in steps, as the probability of the event will remain the same for everyone in the group until occurrence of the event is noted in a greater proportion of individuals by each measurement point. This type of curve is great for not only graphically representing probability of survival or death, but also the probability or risk of disease, disease complications or even uptake of risk behaviours (e.g. smoking or other substance use).

Kaplan-Meier curve: A statistically generated graph that shows the cumulative probability of survival (or any other event) at specified points in time in one or more groups.

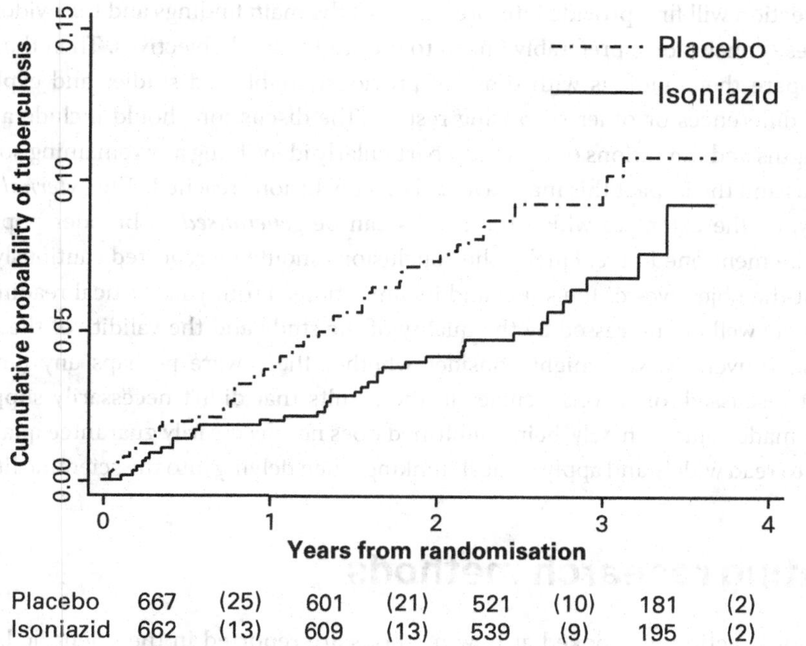

Placebo	667	(25)	601	(21)	521	(10)	181	(2)	0
Isoniazid	662	(13)	609	(13)	539	(9)	195	(2)	0

Figure 12.1 Time to death from randomisation (20, p. 685)

Note: 'Numbers show the numbers being followed at each time point, and the numbers in parentheses indicate new tuberculosis cases in each period. Logrank test *p*-value for equality of survival curves = 0.02' (20, p. 685).

Without reference to the precise mechanics of how probability curves are calculated, we can see that the one presented in Figure 12.1 is comparing the probability of TB occurring in the placebo and isoniazid groups, as indicated by the title of the figure. The y-axis (the vertical one) shows the cumulative probability of TB, ranging from 0.00 to 0.15 (zero probability to 15 per cent). The x-axis (the horizontal one) shows the time from randomisation ranging from zero to four years. As indicated in the explanatory text, the numbers under the x-axis show the actual numbers of participants who were found to have TB in each study group during each of the four years depicted on the graph and (in parentheses) the number of participants remaining in the study. Finally, we can turn our attention to the content of the figure, which shows a broken line showing the probability of TB for the placebo group across the time period and an unbroken line showing the probability of TB in the isoniazid group. The placebo group had a consistently increased probability of TB throughout the period of follow-up. The explanatory notes suggest that a statistical test compared the probability of TB in each group and was associated with a p value of 0.02. This is smaller than 0.05 and usually indicates that any differences between the groups are statistically significant (only a 2 per cent probability of the observed differences occurring by chance alone).

The main features of the data presented in tables and figures are also described in the text of the results section in scientific papers. The findings that authors specifically point out in the text here often inform their conclusions. So, closely scrutinising the tables and figures will help you in understanding whether there were any omissions in the text or inconsistencies in the reported findings.

Reading the discussion and conclusion

Here is where the authors get to summarise what they see as the key findings of their study, locating them within the existing scientific literature and explaining any that differ from what is already known, and presenting their conclusions based on these. Structurally, a good discussion section will first provide interpretations of the main findings and the evidence that supports these conclusions, preferably linked to the study stated objectives. Then the authors usually compare their findings with those of previously published studies and explain any unexpected differences or other surprising results. The discussion should include a section on the strengths and limitations of the study, particularly identifying any remaining sources of potential bias and the impact this may have had on conclusions reached. The *external validity* of the study, or the extent to which the results can be *generalised* to broader populations should also be mentioned here. Finally, the conclusions should be reported cautiously, taking into account the objectives of the study and its limitations. From your critical reading of the paper, you may well be impressed by the quality of the study and the validity of the authors' conclusions. Conversely, you might consider whether there were perhaps any limitations that weren't discussed, or inconsistencies in the results that didn't necessarily support the conclusions made. Unfortunately, being published does not necessarily guarantee quality, so it is up to you to read widely and apply critical thinking when delving into the scientific literature.

Evaluating research methods

In the previous section, we looked at how methods are reported in the scientific literature and learnt that transparency and reproducibility are really the hallmarks of a quality report. We have heard a bit about applying critical thinking to reading the scientific literature, but being a critical consumer of research also involves thinking critically about the methods employed and the conclusions that are reached from research findings. In this section, we will apply critical thinking to evaluating research methods, including how biases can be assessed, confounders identified and misinterpretations avoided.

The scientific question

Throughout this book, we have emphasised the importance of the scientific question and how it essentially dictates the type of study that is required to answer it. Naturally, being an epidemiology text, this book has focused on how to answer epidemiological questions using quantitative methods, but it is important to be aware of the limitations of quantitative approaches. Questions about people's experiences of particular circumstances and the meaning they attach to events are not the type of questions that epidemiological methods can address. As mentioned in Chapter 1, qualitative approaches use non-numeral methods (e.g. in-depth interviewing and analysis of text, audio-recording and images) to explore things such as people's attitudes and beliefs, social context and cultural realities. Qualitative approaches can be used alone, or are increasingly being used together with quantitative approaches to form different angles of inquiry in a single study (known as 'mixed methods') that allow a greater understanding of health issues and better informs the development of appropriate prevention or management strategies.

The sorts of scientific questions that can be answered by the epidemiological approaches covered in this book are summarised in Table 12.2. If our question is about how much of a condition exists in the population, who is affected and where (person, time and place), then we need the type of descriptive data that can be collected using a cross-sectional study. We can identify the prevalence of a specified condition, such as asthma, by working out the proportion of the population that is affected at a point in time. For instance, a very large study in China calculated an asthma prevalence of 4.2 per cent (95% CI: 3.1, 5.6), representing more than 45 million adults with an asthma diagnosis (21). From repeated or routine cross-sectional studies, we could also calculate cumulative incidence by estimating the proportion of a population who develop a condition over a specified period of time (e.g. the period between reports). From the data derived from two repeat surveys in Sweden, for example, the cumulative incidence of diagnosed asthma was estimated to be 1.1 per cent per year (22). We might compare the prevalence of disease between different population sub-groups by calculating prevalence ratios. In the United States, a prevalence ratio for asthma in women was reported to be 1.69 (95% CI: 1.66,1.72) relative to men (23).

Table 12.2 Types of epidemiological questions and study designs appropriate for addressing them

Question type	Study design*	Study purpose	Selected outcome measures*
How much of a condition is present? Who is affected by a condition? Where is the condition arising?	Cross-sectional (descriptive/analytic)	Quantify the distribution of a specified condition in terms of person, time and place	Prevalence, cumulative incidence, prevalence ratio, prevalence
How does the relationship between an exposure and a condition differ between different populations?	Ecological	Measures the strength and direction of the exposure – outcome relationship at the region and population level	Correlation

Table 12.1 (continued)

Question type	Study design*	Study purpose	Selected outcome measures*
What exposures/risk factors might be associated with a specified condition?	Case-control	Measures the relationships between previous exposures and an existing condition	Odds ratio
What health or other outcomes might occur after exposure to a specified risk factor?	Cohort	Measures the relationships between known exposures and multiple future outcomes	Incidence, mortality rates, relative risk
How well will this intervention manage or treat a specified condition?	RCT	Evaluates the safety and effectiveness of an intervention relative to a standard treating	Relative risk, odds ratios, mortality rate ratios, number needed to treat

*Restricted to those designs and outcome measures discussed in this book.

If we are interested in the relationship between a particular exposure and an outcome and want to see how the relationship holds across populations, we could undertake an ecological study. An example might be the relationship between obesity and breast cancer, for which population data exist in many regions of the world. Using aggregated population data from different regions or time periods, we could summarise the correlation between the exposure and outcome and measure its direction (positive or negative) and the strength of the relationship by developing a correlation coefficient ('r'). For instance, in one study the correlation coefficient for obesity and breast cancer across multiple time periods in Australia was reported to be 0.46 (p = 0.029), indicating a moderately strong, positive relationship (24).

Say we wanted to find out what risk factors might be associated with hepatocellular carcinoma (liver cancer). Although its incidence has been rising globally, this type of cancer remains relatively rare, so it makes sense that researchers might want to identify a group of cases in the first incidence and conduct a case-control study to look at all the potential exposures that might be linked with the increase in disease. One such case-control study in the United States found that chronic hepatitis C infection and obesity were among the most important risk factors associated with hepatocellular carcinoma, calculating odds ratios of 110 (95% CI: 59.2, 204) and 2.13 (95% CI: 1.52, 3.00), respectively (25).

And what if we were pretty sure about our exposures or risk factors but wanted to see what outcomes might arise from the exposure? If there was a lot of the exposure about and the outcomes were likely to occur after a relatively short period, a cohort study would probably fit the bill. During the COVID-19 pandemic, many cohort studies were conducted to investigate potential causal pathways between infection with the SARS-CoV-2 virus in multiple population groups (often defined by potentially predisposing characteristics) and disease outcomes. In a cohort study of severe COVID-19 outcomes in workers in the United Kingdom (26), the relative risk for severe disease in health workers relative to non-essential workers was 7.43 (95% CI 5.52 to 10.00). In another UK cohort study of thromboembolism in hospitalised patients (27), the incidence of thromboembolism-related hospitalisations increased during the COVID-19 pandemic (from 1090 to 1590 per 100 000 admissions over three years) and the risk for thromboembolism was higher for patients with COVID-19 (adjusted RR 1.20, 95% CI: 1.18, 1.22). The authors also report that thromboembolism-specific mortality in the community increased by 30 per cent from pre-pandemic rates but decreased by 11 per cent in hospitalised patients during the same period.

Moving away from observational studies, an RCT is the best way to answer questions about the safety and effectiveness of treatments and interventions. By strictly controlling the recruitment of participants, allocation of interventions, implementation procedures and measurement of outcomes, a well-conducted RCT will allow for the precise measurement of the actual effect of the intervention. In Chapter 9, we heard about a multicentre, open-label RCT of high- versus low-dose vitamin D in the treatment of older patients with COVID-19 in France (28). In this study, 14-day mortality due to COVID-19 was lower in the high-dose group (6 per cent) relative to the standard-dose group (11 per cent), with an adjusted hazard ratio (a measure to which we were just introduced) of 0.33 (95% CI: 0.12, 0.86) and the number needed to treat being 21 (i.e. you would need to give high-dose vitamin D supplementation to 21 people for one person to benefit). Another multi-centre RCT evaluated a drug used primarily for HIV prevention (Lopinavir–ritonavir) to treat COVID-19 patients in the United Kingdom (29) and reported a 28-day mortality ratio of 1.03 (95% CI: 0·91,1·17; $p = 0.60$), or no difference in mortality between the intervention and usual care groups.

Rachael: That actually makes sense to me!

Hugo: Now I get why you are always banging on about the scientific question!

Author (Emma): Assessing the appropriateness of the approach for addressing the study aims is an important part of critically reading the scientific literature. It is also important to keep the stated aims of the study in mind throughout your reading of the paper – are the described methods and results consistent with the purpose of the inquiry, and do the conclusions directly relate to the scientific question?

Assessing the potential for bias

As we learnt in previous chapters, all study types (including those identified in Table 12.2) can be impacted by various types of bias, which can ultimately become a threat to validity. It is not possible for even the most critical reader to determine whether bias has actually been introduced in a particular study and affected its conclusions. However, carefully looking at the methods section of a scientific paper will reveal any design features discussed by the authors that might help to minimise the potential for bias in their study. Luckily, many of these features have been discussed in relation to all the study types considered in this book. And, even more luckily, many tools have been developed to assess the potential for bias in studies and are available to you on the internet (as mentioned, we live in a time that is paradise for nerds!). For instance, a handy tool has been developed by the US National Toxicology Program (30) that has systematically reviewed tools for assessing all types of bias in all types and fields of studies. For RCTs specifically, the Cochrane Collaboration recommends the

RoB 2 tool for assessing risk of bias in randomised trials (31). For those interested, I have listed links to these resources in the 'Further reading' section.

In Chapter 11, we heard about several subtypes of selection and measurement bias that can affect all studies, and the range of subtypes to which particular study designs are most prone. Various ways to minimise the potential for each sort of bias were also described in Chapter 11, and these are the types of strategies that authors should include in their paper – and to which the critical reader will be alert. What questions should we ask ourselves to be assured that the study is as free from bias as possible? Let's look at an example.

EXAMPLE 12.3A

A paper on a cohort study investigating smoking-related lung cancer in men and women in the United States was published in *The Lancet Oncology* (32). The authors were interested in looking at whether women were more susceptible to smoking-related lung cancer than men, which was a proposition that had been raised by previous authors. The main outcomes of interest for the study were the incidence of lung cancers in men and women who never smoked and who were current smokers.

In the abstract, the authors report that, among 279 214 men and 184 623 women from eight states across the United States, the incidence of lung cancers in non-smokers was 20.3 (95% CI: 16.3, 24.3) per 100 000 person-years in men and 25.3 (21.3–29.3) per 100 000 person-years in women. Among current smokers (smoking at least two packets per day), the lung cancer incidence per 100 000 person-years in men and women was 1259.2 (95% CI: 1 035.0, 1 483.3) and 1308.9 (95% CI: 924.2, 1693.6), respectively. After adjusting for 'typical smoking dose', the hazard ratio (HR) for currently smoking women relative to men was 0.9 (95% CI: 0.8, 0.9). After adjusting for years since quitting smoking and typical smoking dose, the HR for women who were former smokers relative to men was 0.9 (95% CI: 0.9,1.0). The authors conclude that smoking was strongly associated with lung cancer in both men and women, but there was little difference in susceptibility to smoker-related cancer between them.

That sounds like a really big study and it is published in a highly respected journal. Should we accept the authors' interpretation, or could the result be biased in some way?

It is a prospective cohort study, so we know that study could be prone to the following types of bias:

- selection bias
  - ascertainment/sample bias
  - attrition bias
  - survivor bias
- measurement bias
  - social desirability bias
  - misclassification of outcome/exposure
  - observer bias.

The best thing to do here is to look at the methods section to see whether these potential sources of bias have been addressed.

EXAMPLE 12.3B

The authors explain the source of the data used for the analysis were from the database of an ongoing cohort study called the National Institute of Health American Association of Retired Persons Diet and Health (NIH-AARP) Study (32). As described in the paper, the NIH-AARP study commenced in 1995, when a risk-factor survey was posted out to 3.5 million members of the AARP who were aged between 50 and 71 years and resided in eight specified states of the United States. The NIH-AARP study annually updates addresses for their cohort using the US Postal Service change of address database, information from participants and another national change of address database.

The authors also confirmed the vital status of the participants – that is, whether they were alive or dead – by using linked data from the cancer registries, national deaths data, participant survey responses and other communications with the NIH-AARP study. At the beginning of the Results section, the authors report excluding participants who had died or had cancer at time of study baseline, proxy respondents (those whose data were provided by others), those reporting energy intake that was greater than double the interquartile range (two times the upper 25 per cent of respondents) and those with incomplete smoking behaviour data. This resulted in a cohort of 463 837 participants, of whom 279 214 were men and 184 623 were women.

The 3.5 million people invited to the NIH-AARP Study seems a lot of people, but they do not represent the entire retired person population in the United States. Estimates for around that time period put the retired population receiving social security payments in the United States at about 34 million (33). You can look up the NIH-AARP study (34) to learn that slightly more than 600 000 of those invited actually responded to the survey and returned their information. This is an impressive number of participants, but they represent only a bit more than 17 per cent of those invited. This is known as the 'participation rate' and is clearly stated by the authors at the beginning of the results section (32, p. 651). We also don't know what the attrition rate from the NIH-AARP study was, although it does seem that robust steps were taken to maintain contact with the participants.

Further reducing the size of the study sample was the authors' exclusion of those who had died or who had cancer at the beginning of the study (perhaps introducing the possibility of survivor bias), those with very high calorie consumption and those with incomplete smoking exposure information. This resulted in a cohort of around 464 000 participants – about 279 000 men and 185 000 women. This is still a very big number and this likely helps to support the internal validity of the study. However, the external validity of the study remains uncertain, as it may well be that the cohort no longer resembles the target population (American retirees). In discussing the study limitations, the authors do state that '[the] participants in our cohort were more educated, less likely to be current smokers, and more likely to be non-Hispanic white than the US population ... which might restrict the applicability of our findings to other subpopulations' (32, p. 655). In this situation, the calculated incidence of smoking-related cancer might not be generalisable to the broader population. However, the central scientific question of male and female susceptibility to smoking-related lung cancer could still be addressed by the study design (assuming the exposure–outcome relationships hold across different populations).

EXAMPLE 12.3C

Freedman et al. (32) explain in detail how the cancer cases were identified. They linked the NIH-AARP membership data with multiple state cancer registries, which they estimated would identify 90 per of the cancers occurring in the cohort. They confirmed the cases by using *International Classification of Disease (ICD) codes* (see Chapter 1) for oncology and included only those codes related to specific lung cancers of interest that were primary cancers.

All the information collected in the NIH-AARP study baseline questionnaire was also described and included data on demographics, alcohol consumption, physical activity, dietary consumption and smoking. The authors report high correlation estimates for smoking surveys with respect to reproducibility (r = 0.94) and validity (r = 0.92 for women and 0.90 for men when correlated with blood test results). Data on the number of cigarettes and precises patterns of smoking ever or currently (with those quitting <1 year regarded as current smokers) were defined, as well as how these data were summarised to maintain sufficient numbers for each stratum of cancer by histological type. Lots of information about alcohol and food consumption collected by the survey was also described, together with how these data were used to calculated total energy intake.

The authors linked participants to cancer registry data and used ICD codes to identify lung cancer cases in this study, which would greatly minimise the potential for observer bias or misclassification of outcomes, with the authors calculating that up to 10 per cent of incident cancers might have been missed using their approach. The smoking behaviour questionnaire had been previously validated and was highly correlated with objective measures of smoking, but there remained a potential for social desirability bias. As the authors later point out, however, any differential recall between men and women was unlikely to substantial given the validation tests referred to in the methods section was conducted in 'white American men and women' (32, p. 655), who predominated in their sample.

Although bias represents a threat to validity in all studies, the design strategies described by the authors of this investigation are clearly aimed at minimising its potential.

Assessing the potential for confounding

As we discovered in previous chapters, confounding is not something that is introduced by the researchers but occurs when the true relationship between a potential cause and an outcome is distorted by the existence of one or more additional factors that are associated with the potential cause and the outcome. Similar to bias, it is not possible to identify all potential confounders just by reading a paper, but we can be aware of the usual suspects to look out for, which includes things such as age, sex, socioeconomic status and comorbidities. What we really want to see when reading a paper is that the authors have identified any potential confounders and described how they have dealt with them through the features of their design and analysis.

EXAMPLE 12.3D

In the statistical analysis section of their methods section, Freedman et al. (32) listed all the tests they undertook in their analysis (e.g. Cox proportional hazards regressions) and the outcome measures they reported (e.g. age-standardised incidence rates, 95 per cent confidence intervals). The authors listed a number of potential confounders for which they had information and described the statistical models they developed that were adjusted for these potential confounders. These included age, alcohol intake, education, body mass index, physical activity level, consumption of various types of foods and energy intake.

The authors also described their efforts to uncover any statistical interactions that might be occurring by developing their models with and without factors such as time and cigarette use and evaluating differences in the relationship between smoking and lung cancer. They also used calculated multivariate adjusted population attributable risk percentages.

Methods for dealing with potential confounders at the design and analysis phases were described in Chapter 11, and many of these methods appear to have been employed here. These include identifying and collecting information on potential confounders and then controlling for their affects through statistical adjustment or standardisation. A number of potential confounders were identified in this study, so it is appropriate that the authors describe the use of multivariate statistical techniques to deal with them. Even the 'population attributable risk percentages' (known by readers of this book as *population attributable proportion* – see Chapter 10) were adjusted for multiple potential confounders.

Although we cannot be completely sure that this study was without bias or that the relationships investigated were not confounded in some unknown way, the details provided by the authors demonstrate that the study design included features likely to minimise the potential for bias and confounding. We can assess this more easily because the study is reported in a way that complies with the Strengthening the Reporting of Observational Studies in Epidemiology (STROBE) statement for observational studies (8), as stated by the authors (32, p. 651).

Hugo: I knew you were going to get back to those guidelines!

Rachael: If we read a study that doesn't comply with the reporting guidelines, does that mean we should ignore the findings?

Author (Emma): The various guidelines developed for reporting the different types of studies are very useful for evaluating the research methods of studies and, when complied with by the study authors (whether explicitly or not), add confidence that all efforts have been made to achieve valid conclusions. As we know, critical readers never rely on the findings of a single study to reach their own conclusions but synthesise the information about an issue from multiple viewpoints, hopefully attributing greater confidence in higher-quality studies relative to those of lower quality.

Synthesising the evidence

Rather than accepting the findings reported in a single paper to be truth, critical consumers of the scientific literature evaluate the body of evidence provided by multiple sources. If you have been set an assessment task, such as an essay or paper, the first thing you might do is read widely to obtain a good understanding of the topic. Let's just take a moment to consider how we might obtain the relevant resources to accomplish this. As mentioned earlier in this chapter, you might undertake a search for relevant papers using scholarly databases such as PubMed (4), or visit population data repositories such as that of the World Health Organization (3). It would be important to first develop some **search terms** to help you find the right papers – these are words or phrases that are specific to your topic, which help you narrow down the papers that are returned by the scholarly database. Many scholarly databases let you combine search terms by using **Boolean operators**, such as AND, OR and NOT. Boolean searching is named in this way because it is based on a whole algebraic system of logic developed by a nineteenth-century English mathematician called George Boole (35). Look at Explanation 12.1 to see how Boolean operators can narrow down a hypothetical search in PubMed.

Search terms: Words or phrases that are specific to a topic, used to search for relevant literature in a scholarly database.

Boolean operators: The conjunctions AND, OR and NOT, which are used to combine search terms to narrow searches for relevant papers in scholarly databases.

EXPLANATION 12.1: PubMed search strategies

I want to find papers about a new treatment for hepatitis C used in Australia – a direct acting antiviral (DAA) medication that combines two antiviral drugs, sofosbuvir and ledipasvir. I decide to search in the PubMed database, which holds citations for more than 36 million health- and medical-related papers (https://pubmed.ncbi.nlm.nih.gov).

My first search term is 'hepatitis C treatment', which returns 63 751 results. Clearly this is way too many papers for anyone to sort through, so I need to develop a more specific search strategy.

I decide to narrow down my search by adding the search term 'direct acting antivirals' and connecting this with the Boolean operator 'AND':

→ hepatitis C treatment AND direct acting antivirals.

This returns 7572 papers on DAA treatment for hepatitis C and excludes papers only focusing on other treatments. But they include a number of different types of DAA, and not just sofosbuvir and ledipasvir.

I narrow my search further by using the names of the two antiviral drugs that make up the treatment as search terms, but which Boolean operator I choose will affect my search results. If I want to see papers on either of the two DAA for treating hepatitis C, I can enter the search terms as follows:

→ hepatitis C treatment AND sofosbuvir OR ledipasvir

This returns 3445 papers on treating hepatitis C with either sofosbuvir or ledipasvir or both together. That is still a lot of papers and I am really only interested in the treatment of hepatitis C with both DAAs combined, so the following search terms might be more appropriate:

→ hepatitis C treatment AND sofosbuvir AND ledipasvir

This returns 1205 papers about treating hepatitis C with both DAAs combined.

I note that many of the papers include other DAA medications such as ribavirin, so I decide to include another Boolean operator, 'NOT':

→ hepatitis C treatment AND sofosbuvir AND ledipasvir NOT ribavirin

This search strategy reduces the number of papers to 595, all of which focus on treating hepatitis C with the two DAAs of interest but not papers that deal with ribavirin.

Now I can use the 'filters' to focus on a specific time period or a type of study, such as only searching for papers published in the past five years, and only studies concerning RCTs, which reduces the number of relevant papers to nine.

Note: Boolean operators do not have to be written in capital letters as they have been here in order to clarify the search.

From Explanation 12.1, note how the Boolean operators 'AND' and 'NOT' reduce the number of papers, while the operator 'OR' increases the number of papers returned in a search. PubMed is the database used for the hypothetical search, but the same operators can be used in many scholarly databases, each focusing on respective disciplinary fields and each with different sorts of filters for narrowing your search.

Once you have developed your search terms, interrogated the appropriate databases (hopefully using Boolean operators), found relevant sources and read widely, you are ready to synthesise the evidence. This is not the same as summarising or paraphrasing information but is a process of combining concepts and ideas from multiple sources to present a balanced argument that recognises different points of view in arriving at an informed conclusion.

Synthesising the evidence is best accomplished by following a systematic process such as that summarised in Table 12.3.

Table 12.3 Synthesising information sourced from scientific papers

Phases	Actions
1. Identify scientific papers on a specified topic	• Search scholarly databases using specified search terms and Boolean operators • Use any available filters to narrow down your search
2. Pinpoint the key points and findings	• Take notes of key findings when reading each paper • In your own words, summarise sets of common arguments/findings on a piece of paper (or document page or spreadsheet), citing the papers from which they originated
3. Identify the differences and similarity in the arguments or findings	• Group the papers based on the sets of arguments/findings already noted • It can be helpful to use different-coloured highlighters or codes to identify connections between the groups
4. Evaluate the strength of the evidence and/or the quality of the paper	As you read each paper, note: • the scientific question • the study type and main methods used • the detail provided about the participants, setting, and research instruments used • how bias and confounding are dealt with • the study size and main outcomes of interest

Table 12.3 (continued)

Phases	Actions
5. Write a balanced synopsis of the issue of interest	• Summarise the major and minor themes emerging from the literature • Highlight the agreements and disagreements between findings • Offer explanations that may account for any differences identified (e.g. the quality of the studies, variation in methods, clinical or demographic differences in study participants, diverse study settings).
6. Develop an evidence-based conclusion	• Be clear about your position and provide your rationale for it • Identify any areas of uncertainty • Consider need for future investigation if appropriate

Discerning readers of this book may have noticed that the process of synthesising information described in Table 12.3 looks a lot like an exercise in critical thinking. Certainly, this synthesis process will come pretty naturally to critical consumers of the literature. Of course, this is just one way to approach synthesising information and plenty of other systems have been proposed, including the development of a 'synthesis matrix', which is a spreadsheet that cross-tabulates a lot of the information described in phases 2 and 3 in Table 12.3. Many educational institutions provide their own online guidance to students on how to synthesise information, including providing synthesis matrix templates (36), and it is worth looking up some of these or any synthesis tips that may be offered by your own institution.

Rachael: I am going to search for 'synthesis' AND 'matrix templates'!

Hugo: To get more results, we should search for 'synthesis' OR 'matrix templates'!

Author (Emma): Very good but, depending on what database you are searching, don't forget to experiment with your Boolean operators, including a 'NOT' or two, to narrow down your search. Remember, 'OR' returns results that include *either* of your search terms, 'AND' returns results that include *both* of your search terms, while 'NOT' *excludes* results matching a further search term.

Systematic reviews

In previous chapters, particularly Chapter 9, we heard a bit about systematic reviews. This is a type of study that specifically aims to synthesise evidence from previously conducted studies. The databases the researchers searched and the search terms they used (including Boolean operators) are clearly described in the methods section of systematic reviews or are accessible from 'additional files' where more than one search was undertaken – all of which is aimed at enhancing the study's transparency and reproducibility. Systematic reviews usually synthesise the evidence from multiple RCTs, looking at the same or very similar interventions, and can include a *meta-analysis*. This is a statistical way to pool data from two or more quantitative studies to produce a single estimate of effect (e.g. a relative risk, an odds ratio, a difference in mean scores) that is weighted for the size of the studies included. Although they have traditionally synthesised RCTs to provide an unbiased evaluation of interventions, systematic reviews are increasingly used to review other types of studies to obtain more precise estimates of disease occurrence or risk. One such review synthesised 33 observational studies to obtain a pooled relative risk of the main symptoms of long COVID-19 in people infected by SARS-CoV-2 compared with symptoms experienced by uninfected people (37). From their meta-analyses of the data, the researchers report that people with COVID-19 were more likely to experience fatigue (RR = 1.72, 95% CI: 1.41, 2.10) and shortness of breath (RR = 2.60, 95% CI: 1.96, 3.44), among a range of neurological symptoms.

Systematic reviews can also be used to synthesise the results of qualitative studies. Because qualitative studies do not use numerical data, a traditional meta-analyses is not possible, but researchers often undertake 'narrative reviews' – a systematic synthesis of the data that summarises words and text to provide an explanatory summary of the reviewed literature (38). For instance, a systematic review of the qualitative literature was conducted on the lived experience of hepatitis C infection (39). The review included 46 studies and concluded that people with hepatitis C commonly felt stigmatised and unsupported when seeking care in their relationships and at work and that this was all while coping with a range of physical and psychological symptoms. Such narrative reviews are also conducted in quantitative studies when meta-analyses are not appropriate. This can happen when the included studies are very different from each other (e.g. differences in methods used, population groups or measurements taken), which is known as 'heterogeneity'. In the long COVID example discussed above, investigating health-related quality of life was one of the stated aims of the study. However, the authors report they were unable to conduct a meta-analysis on quality of life due to a high degree of heterogeneity between studies (37). Through their analysis of the text, however, they were able to report that quality of life was significantly poorer after severe hospitalised COVID relative to non-COVID patients.

Systematic reviews themselves can also be systematically reviewed in what has come to be known as an **umbrella review**. Umbrella reviews do not include primary studies, but rather review published systematic reviews conducted on the same topic. Ultimately, umbrella reviews provide a wider picture of phenomena than is possible from single systematic review because they allow for comparing and contrasting the results of different reviews (40). For instance, an umbrella review of antenatal depression (occurring during pregnancy) and its association with poor maternal and infant outcomes synthesised the evidence from 10 systematic reviews that collectively included 306 primary studies (41). The review conducted both a narrative review and meta-analyses of quantitative data. The authors report that the global prevalence of antenatal depression ranged from 15 per cent to 65 per cent and that current or previous exposure to violence or abuse, lack of social and/or partner support and family or personal history of mental health disorders were the most common risk factors for antenatal depression. From the meta-analyses, antenatal depression was associated with increased risk of infant low birthweight (RR = 1.49, 95% CI: 1.32, 1.68) and preterm birth (RR = 1.40, 95% CI: 1.16, 1.69).

Umbrella review: A systematic review that synthesises completed systematic reviews and does not include primary studies.

So, why would we want to bother with all that evaluating and synthesising stuff described above? Can't we just go to somewhere like the Cochrane Library, which is available on the internet (5), and download systematic reviews on almost any topic? After all, the 'one-stop shop' of information provided by systematic reviews means we shouldn't have to spend all that time sifting through studies if someone else has already done that for us. Although it is true that systematic reviews are incredibly valuable and time-saving resources, they do have a couple of downsides. Obviously, a systematic review cannot be undertaken unless studies have previously been undertaken and, usually, published. So, very new interventions or previously unstudied phenomena cannot be systematically reviewed. Also, because they usually rely on published studies for their source of information, you can be waiting for quite a long time for an up-to-date and relevant systematic review to become available. In the first place, the studies included in the systematic review may have taken a year or more before they can even be reported on and submitted to a journal. Then, assuming the journal will ultimately accept a submitted paper, the time to publication could be around four to six months (42). The time to publication could be very much longer if the paper is first rejected by one or more other journals. To undertake a systematic review of published papers may take a year or more, and these reviews face the same publication delays, all of which are vastly increased in the case of umbrella reviews. Because of the time lag, the Cochrane Collaboration recommends that systematic reviews be updated every two years after their initial publication. However, one analysis of 100 systematic reviews found that 23 per cent were found to have quantitative or qualitative evidence that the information was out of date by two years and 15 per cent within one year, and 7 per cent may have been out of date by the time of their publication (43). This is not to say that that systematic reviews are not incredibly useful sources of credible information. Still, even the best evidence from a study of the highest quality can only form one part of the body of evidence about a phenomenon. Critical thinkers know that evidence needs to be obtained from multiple sources and synthesised in order to reach an informed conclusion.

In this book, in addition to increasing your knowledge of epidemiological concepts, we hope we have provided you with the tools to become critical thinkers in general as well as critical consumers of the scientific literature. Some of the characteristics of critical readers of the scientific literature are presented against the characteristics of uncritical readers in Table 12.4. Which side of the table most applies to you?

Table 12.4 Critical versus uncritical readers of the scientific literature. Adapted from (44)

Critical readers	Uncritical readers
Recognise logical inconsistencies in the rationale for the study	Overlook or cannot recognise flaws in logic
Consider if the study design is the appropriate for the scientific inquiry	Assume the authors have applied the best approach without questioning
Search for the potential for bias or confounding not accounted for in the study design	Accept that bias and confounding have been accounted for without scrutiny
Check whether the authors considered the context before reaching conclusions	Accept stereotypes and inappropriate generalisations
Confirm that conclusions are justified (emerging from the findings) and well-reasoned	Accept the conclusions without challenging the authors' reasoning and the evidence
Assess the validity (as based on the study methods) of all claims	Accept claims unchallenged, without questioning their validity
Discern whether authors accounted for complexity when judging the importance of the study	Upon reading the paper, come to snap judgements about the study (oversimplify things)
Look to see whether authors have considered alternative explanations and/or come up with their own alternative explanations	Tend to confirm own personal biases (i.e. favour only evidence that reinforces their own pre-existing beliefs)

Rachael: Yay! I'm all in the left column!

Hugo: I think I might be too, but I would need to consider more information before coming to an informed conclusion.

Author (Emma): Critical thinking skills not only apply to your current and future studies but can be used in all parts of your everyday and future professional life. Critical thinkers make informed judgements about everything, so they are difficult to scam or fool, and tend to be happier in life overall than non-critical thinkers (45), so I'm glad to hear that this book has helped you both become a critical thinkers!

Conclusion

In answering the question 'So what?', in this final chapter we have aimed to show how the learning from this book can be used to provide you with the tools for evaluating scientific information. We used our epidemiological knowledge in applying critical thinking to obtaining and synthesising epidemiological evidence.

Learning objective 1: Apply critical thinking to reading the scientific literature

Here we used our epidemiological knowledge to closely examine and interpret the abstract of a scientific paper. We learnt how scientific papers are generally presented and what elements to expect in quality papers. We also revisited how to read and interpret tables and figures.

Learning objective 2: Apply critical thinking to evaluating research methods used for answering scientific questions

In this section, the relationship between the scientific question and research design was re-emphasised using examples from scientific literature. We learnt how scientific papers might be assessed for potential bias and confounding in a design-specific way by closely examining a published paper describing a cohort study.

Learning objective 3: Apply critical thinking to synthesising scientific evidence

Finally, we heard about finding and synthesising the evidence from multiple sources. As part of this, we were introduced to the idea of search terms and the use of Boolean operators, and an approach to synthesising evidence was presented. Since synthesising evidence is their main purpose, systematic reviews were revisited in this section, and their place as one part of the body of evidence available to the critical reader was emphasised.

Further reading

Australian Bureau of Statistics. Welcome to the Australian Bureau of Statistics. 2023. www.abs.gov.au
Cochrane Library of Systematic Reviews. Cochrane Library. 2023. www.cochranelibrary.com
EQUATOR Network. Enhancing the QUAlity and transparency of health research. 2023. www.equator-network.org
Google. Google Scholar. 2023. https://scholar.google.com

National Library of Medicine. PubMed. 2023. https://pubmed.ncbi.nlm.nih.gov
National Toxicology Program. Risk of bias tools. 2024. https://ntp.niehs.nih.gov/whatwestudy/assessments/noncancer/tools
RoB 2. Revised tool for assessing risk of bias in randomised trials. 2024. https://sites.google.com/site/riskofbiastool/welcome/rob-2-0-tool/current-version-of-rob-2
World Health Organization. Health topics. 2023. www.who.int/health-topics

Questions

Answers are available at the end of the book.

Multiple-choice questions

1. In recent years, there has been increasing impetus for studies published in journals to conform with certain quality standards. Which of the following qualities would best help to ensure the validity of methods?
A – Clear communication skills
B – Peer review and editorial processes
C – Transparency and reproducibility
D – Tables and figures.

2. A paper on an important health topic has been published by a well-respected research team in a very high-quality journal. Which of the following is true?
A – Publication in high-quality journals is an important academic achievement, which assures us that the findings will have validity and be free of bias and confounding.
B – There is no way to tell whether the reported study has been affected by bias or confounding, only whether steps have been taken to minimise these.
C – A hallmark of research papers published in high-quality journals is the extent to which the methods can be reproduced by other experts in the field.
D – Only systematic reviews, which are positioned at the top of the hierarchy of evidence for research designs, provide reproducible methods and valid results, regardless of the quality of the journal in which it is published.

3. In recent years, vaping (the use of e-cigarettes) has become increasingly popular among young people in many countries. This is occurring in the context of decreasing use of tobacco products in the same nations. Many in the field of public health are concerned that the gains in health from decreased tobacco use may be replaced by vaping-related harms in the future, but they don't yet fully know what the long-term health harms might be from vaping as the practice is still fairly new. Which of the following study designs might best address a question about the long-term effects of vaping?
A – Case-control study
B – RCT
C – Cohort study
D – Ecological study.

4. Critical consumers of the literature often think about the validity of the findings presented in a given paper by considering the potential for bias that might have affected the authors' conclusions. Which of the following is true about how the potential for bias might be evaluated by the reader?
A – It is not possible to assess whether valid attempts have been made to minimise bias.
B – Bias happens in all studies, and nothing can be done to minimise it.
C – The journal ranking and authority of the research team need to be considered

D – The methods section should be carefully considered for strategies discussed by the authors that would minimise bias given the design and feature of the study.

5. You have been asked to prepare a paper on an important public health issue. As part of this task, you are required to synthesise information on the prevalence of the issue and the success or otherwise of previous strategies to address it before reaching a conclusion about the best way to minimise the problem. Which of the following approaches would summarise the best way to proceed?

   A – Look up the issue on Wikipedia and paraphrase the information from that page.

   B – Investigate the view of family and friends and then look for articles and webpages that corroborate their conclusions.

   C – Undertake a search for relevant papers using appropriate search terms in scholarly databases and/or population data repositories, and compare and contrast different findings from a wide range of sources and develop an informed conclusion.

   D – Randomly search for information on the internet (including social media) and present the majority view.

Short-answer questions

1. Early in the COVID-19 pandemic, ivermectin was proposed as a treatment for infection with SARS-CoV-2. Ivermectin is actually an anti-parasitic medication used for treating intestinal worms and head lice and was later shown to be ineffective in treating COVID-19 at best and directly harmful at worst. To find out more about this, use the search terms 'COVID and ivermectin' in your web browser and describe the first 10 types of results you obtain (e.g. the source and format). Repeat the same search at Google Scholar (https://scholar.google.com.au) and describe the difference in your results.
2. Head over to the EQUATOR Network (www.equator-network.org) and view the list of different reporting guidelines for different types of studies. You would be familiar with many of the study types from reading this book, and these are listed with guidelines specific for each type. Take your time to look at some of these so you know what is there. Then click on the 'STROBE' link and download the checklist for case-control studies (it doesn't matter whether you choose the pdf or Word format). In the recommendations on what should be reported in the methods section, list any that are related to bias and nominate the type of bias to which it relates.
3. Conduct a search at PubMed (https://pubmed.ncbi.nlm.nih.gov/) using Boolean operators and filters to find primary observational studies on lung cancer in people who have never smoked that were conducted over the past 20 years. Describe the search terms and filters you used, and comment on the first 10 results that your search returned. *Hint: Filters appear on the left side, including 'Additional filters'.*
4. One of the results that could well have been returned from your Question 3 search is a study conducted in Canada by Brenner et al. (46). Read the abstract at https://pubmed.ncbi.nlm.nih.gov/20546590 and, using your own words, answer the following questions:
   a. What is the scientific question about?
   b. Comment on the appropriateness of the study design for addressing the question.
   c. Who were the participants (including any comparison groups) and what was the size of the study group(s)?
   d. What were the main outcome measures and results?
   e. What were the authors' conclusions?
5. Table 12.5 is based on data from the same study from Question 4 (46) – what is this table telling you? *Hint: Structure then content.*

Table 12.5 Demographic characteristics of lung cancer cases compared with controls. Adapted from (46)

Total	Cases – n (%)		Total	Controls – n (%)			*p* value*
	Smokers	Never smokers		Smokers	Never smokers	Total	
	289	156	445	482	466	948	
Sex							
Male	163 (56)	46 (30)	209 (47)	241 (50)	145 (31)	386 (41)	0.03
Female	126 (44)	110 (70)	236 (53)	241 (50)	321 (69)	562 (59)	
Age in years							
<35	1 (<1)	10 (6)	11 (3)	58 (12)	86 (18)	144 (15)	<0.001
35–45	9 (3)	21 (13)	30 (7)	77 (16)	89 (19)	166 (18)	
46–55	34 (12)	27 (17)	61 (14)	88 (18)	85 (18)	173 (18)	
56–65	63 (22)	28 (18)	91 (20)	101 (21)	88 (19)	189 (20)	
66–75	131 (45)	57 (37)	188 (42)	100 (21)	71 (15)	170 (18)	
>75	51 (18)	13(8)	64 (14)	58 (12)	48 (10	106 (11)	
Mean age in years	66	59	64 (±12)	56 (±16)	53 (±17)	54 (±16)	
Ethnicity							
White	255 (88)	97 (61)	352 (79)	429 (89)	346 (74)	775 (82)	0.07
Asian	21 (7)	48 (31)	69 (16)	27 (6)	78 (17)	105 (11)	
Other	13 (5)	11 (7)	24 (5)	26 (5)	42 (9)	68 (7)	
Education (years)	97 (34)	36 (23)	137 (31)	55 (11)	68 (15)	140 (15)	< 0.001
<8 years	137 (47)	52 (33)	189 (42)	212 (44)	187 (40)	399 (42)	
8–11 years ≥12 years	55 (19)	64 (41)	119 (27)	205 (43)	204 (44)	409 (43)	

*Tests difference between total cases and controls.

6. Go to the US National Toxicology Program (30), which has systematically reviewed tools for assessing all types of bias in all types and fields of studies (https://ntp.niehs.nih.gov/whatwestudy/assessments/noncancer/tools). Click on the 'Domain-tool-study design' tab and view the different biases that there are assessments under the 'domain' menu. Under the 'study design for which the tool was used' menu, select 'case-control', for which you can see that there are 36 assessment tools. Look at the domains that can be assessed by the various tools (e.g. selection, confounding, exposure) as well as the specific topics covered by the tool. The relevant assessment tools you could use are listed at the right of the page and the below right window lists the actual questions appearing in each of the listed tools. Now select 'ecological' study designs and describe and comment what you find based on your understanding of this type of study design.

7. The STROBE statement is a guideline for reporting the results of observational studies. Return to the EQUATOR website (www.equator-network.org) and download the STROBE checklist for cohort studies. Carefully read the items and then evaluate a published cohort study on any issue of interest to you, citing the page where each checklist item appears in the study. *Hint: download the pdf version of the paper to obtain the page numbers.*
8. Without referring back to this chapter just yet, discuss how you would broadly approach a synthesis of data on a scientific topic of interest.
9. Go to the Johns Hopkins Sheridan Library 'How to write a literature review' page (https://guides.library.jhu.edu/lit-review). Have a good look around to see what resources are there (for the future!), then click on 'synthesize' from the menu at the left. Download the 'Lit review pre' Excel file from the bottom left and open it. Notice that the file contains templates for summarising information from different resources, for evaluating those sources of information and for synthesising the information. Each template also has an associated example showing how to use the table. See whether you can complete the summary table (template 1) and the evaluation table (template 2) for the study you selected for Question 7.
10. Go the Cochrane library (www.cochranelibrary.com/cdsr/reviews) and find a systematic review on 'mpox'. Use the filters at the side left of the search page to find the most recently published reviews (only one was published at time of writing) and download the full content pdf (from the pdf menu at the top right). Read through the paper and establish the date of publication of the included papers. Briefly summarise what you have found, commenting on the relevance and timeliness of the review.

References

1. Google. Google Scholar. 2023. https://scholar.google.com
2. Australian Bureau of Statistics. Welcome to the Australian Bureau of Statistics. 2023. www.abs.gov.au
3. World Health Organization. Health topics Geneva. 2023. www.who.int/health-topics
4. National Library of Medicine. PubMed. 2023. https://pubmed.ncbi.nlm.nih.gov
5. Cochrane Library of Systematic Reviews. Cochrane Library. 2023. www.cochranelibrary.com
6. Robles-Pérez E, González-Díaz B, Miranda-García M, Borja-Aburto VH. Infection and death by COVID-19 in a cohort of healthcare workers in Mexico. *Scandinavian Journal of Work and Environmental Health*. 2021;47(5):349–55.
7. Tung C-A, Chang S-Y. Developing critical thinking through literature reading. *Feng Chia Journal of Humanities and Social Sciences*. 2009;19:287–317.
8. EQUATOR Network. Enhancing the QUAlity and transparency of health research. 2023. https://www.equator-network.org
9. Tullu MS. Writing the title and abstract for a research paper: Being concise, precise, and meticulous is the key. *Saudi Journal of Anaesthetics*. 2019;13(Suppl 1):S12–17.
10. International Committee of Medical Journal Editors. Preparing a manuscript for submission to a medical journal. 2023. www.icmje.org/recommendations/browse/manuscript-preparation/preparing-for-submission.html
11. PLOS. How to write your methods. 2023. https://plos.org/resource/how-to-write-your-methods
12. Baumgartner RN, Koehler KM, Gallagher D, Romero L, Heymsfield SB, Ross RR et al. Epidemiology of sarcopenia among the elderly in New Mexico. *American Journal of Epidemiology*. 1998;147(8):755–63.
13. Hernández-González V, Carné-Torrent JM, Jové-Deltell C, Pano-Rodríguez Á, Reverter-Masia J. The top 100 most cited scientific papers in the public, environmental & occupational health category of Web of Science: A bibliometric and visualized analysis. *International Journal of Environmental Research in Public Health*. 2022;19(15):9645.

14. Agnes D, Ludovic T, Ignacio A, David M, Kay D, Isabelle B et al. Evolution of poor reporting and inadequate methods over time in 20 920 randomised controlled trials included in Cochrane reviews: Research on research study. *BMJ*. 2017;357:j2490.

15. Wang SV, Verpillat P, Rassen JA, Patrick A, Garry EM, Bartels DB. Transparency and Reproducibility of Observational Cohort Studies Using Large Healthcare Databases. *Clinical Pharmacology and Therapeutics*. 2016;99(3):325–32.

16. Papathanasiou AA, Zintzaras E. Assessing the quality of reporting of observational studies in cancer. *Annals of Epidemiology*. 2010;20(1):67–73.

17. Koffel JB, Rethlefsen ML. Reproducibility of search strategies is poor in systematic reviews published in high-impact pediatrics, cardiology and surgery journals: A cross-sectional study. *PLOS One*. 2016;11(9):e0163309.

18. Center for Open Science. Reproducibility Project: Cancer biology. 2023. www.cos.io/rpcb

19. Amaral OB, Neves K. Reproducibility: Expect less of the scientific paper. *Nature*. 2021;597:329–31.

20. Rangaka MX, Wilkinson RJ, Boulle A, Glynn JR, Fielding K, van Cutsem G et al. Isoniazid plus antiretroviral therapy to prevent tuberculosis: A randomised double-blind, placebo-controlled trial. *The Lancet*. 2014;384(9944):682–90.

21. Huang K, Yang T, Xu J, Yang L, Zhao J, Zhang X et al. Prevalence, risk factors, and management of asthma in China: A national cross-sectional study. *The Lancet*. 2019;394(10196):407–18.

22. Rönmark E, Lundbäck B, Jonsson E, Jonsson AC, Lindström M, Sandström T. Incidence of asthma in adults – report from the Obstructive Lung Disease in Northern Sweden Study. *Allergy*. 1997;52(11):1071–8.

23. Zhang X, Morrison-Carpenter T, Holt JB, Callahan DB. Trends in adult current asthma prevalence and contributing risk factors in the United States by state: 2000–2009. *BMC Public Health*. 2013;13:1156.

24. Miller ER, Wilson C, Chapman J, Flight I, Nguyen AM, Fletcher C et al. Connecting the dots between breast cancer, obesity and alcohol consumption in middle-aged women: ecological and case control studies. *BMC Public Health*. 2018;18(1):460.

25. Shen Y, Risch H, Lu L, Ma X, Irwin ML, Lim JK et al. Risk factors for hepatocellular carcinoma (HCC) in the northeast of the United States: Results of a case-control study. *Cancer Causes Control*. 2020;31(4):321–32.

26. Mutambudzi M, Niedzwiedz C, Macdonald EB, Leyland A, Mair F, Anderson J et al. Occupation and risk of severe COVID-19: Prospective cohort study of 120 075 UK Biobank participants. *Occupational and Environmental Medicine*. 2021;78(5):307.

27. Aktaa S, Wu J, Nadarajah R, Rashid M, de Belder M, Deanfield J et al. Incidence and mortality due to thromboembolic events during the COVID-19 pandemic: Multi-sourced population-based health records cohort study. *Thrombosis Research*. 2021;202:17–23.

28. Annweiler C, Beaudenon M, Gautier J, Gonsard J, Boucher S, Chapelet G et al. High-dose versus standard-dose vitamin D supplementation in older adults with COVID-19 (COVIT-TRIAL): A multicenter, open-label, randomized controlled superiority trial. *PLOS Medicine*. 2022;19(5):e1003999.

29. Horby PW, Mafham M, Bell JL, Linsell L, Staplin N, Emberson J et al. Lopinavir–ritonavir in patients admitted to hospital with COVID-19 (RECOVERY): A randomised, controlled, open-label, platform trial. *The Lancet*. 2020;396(10259):1345–52.

30. National Toxicology Program. Risk of bias tools. 2024. https://ntp.niehs.nih.gov/whatwestudy/assessments/noncancer/tools

31. Sterne J, Savović J, Page MJ, Elbers RG, Blencowe NS, Boutron I et al. RoB 2: A revised tool for assessing risk of bias in randomised trials. *BMJ*. 2019;366:l4898.

32. Freedman ND, Leitzmann MF, Hollenbeck AR, Schatzkin A, Abnet CC. Cigarette smoking and subsequent risk of lung cancer in men and women: Analysis of a prospective cohort study. *The Lancet Oncology*. 2008;9(7):649–56.

33. Statistica. U.S. number of retired workers receiving social security 2010–2022. 2023. www.statista.com/statistics/194295/number-of-us-retired-workers-who-receive-social-security/#:~:text=The%20number%20of%20retired%20workers,to%2048.59%20million%20in%202022

34. National Cancer Institute. *NIH-AARP Diet and Health Study United States*. US Department of Health and Human Services; 2024. https://dceg.cancer.gov/research/who-we-study/nih-aarp-diet-health-study#:~:text=In%201995%2C%20the%20NCI%20launched,%2C%20lifestyle%2C%20and%20cancer%20risk

35. Burris S. George Boole. In: Zalta EN, Nodelman U, eds. *The Stanford Encyclopedia of Philosophy*. Metaphysics Research Lab, Stanford University; 2023. https://plato.stanford.edu/archives/win2023/entries/boole

36. Johns Hopkins Sheridan Libraries. Write a literature review: Synthesize. 2023. https://guides.library.jhu.edu/lit-review

37. Marjenberg Z, Leng S, Tascini C, Garg M, Misso K, El Guerche Seblain C et al. Risk of long COVID main symptoms after SARS-CoV-2 infection: A systematic review and meta-analysis. *Scientific Reports*. 2023;13(1):15332.

38. Popay J, Roberts H, Sowden A, Petticrew M, Arai L, Rodgers M et al. *Guidance on the Conduct of Narrative Synthesis in Systematic Reviews*. Lancaster University; 2006.

39. Dowsett LE, Coward S, Lorenzetti DL, MacKean G, Clement F. Living with hepatitis C virus: A systematic review and narrative synthesis of qualitative literature. *Canadian Journal of Gastroenterology and Hepatology*. 2017:3268650.

40. Aromataris E, Fernandez R, Godfrey CM, Holly C, Khalil H, Tungpunkom P. Summarizing systematic reviews: Methodological development, conduct and reporting of an umbrella review approach. *International Journal of Evidence Based Healthcare*. 2015;13(3):132–40.

41. Dadi AF, Miller ER, Bisetegn TA, Mwanri L. Global burden of antenatal depression and its association with adverse birth outcomes: an umbrella review. *BMC Public Health*. 2020;20(1):173.

42. Powell K. Does it take too long to publish research? *Nature*. 2016;530(7589):148–51.

43. Shojania KG, Sampson M, Ansari MT, Ji J, Doucette S, Moher D. How quickly do systematic reviews go out of date? A survival analysis. *Annals of Internal Medicine*. 2007;147(3):224–33.

44. McGregor SLT. *Understanding and Evaluating Research: A Critical Guide*. Sage; 2018.

45. Butler HA, Pentoney C, Bong MP. Predicting real-world outcomes: Critical thinking ability is a better predictor of life decisions than intelligence. *Thinking Skills and Creativity*. 2017;25:38–46.

46. Brenner DR, Hung RJ, Tsao M-S, Shepherd FA, Johnston MR, Narod S et al. Lung cancer risk in never-smokers: A population-based case-control study of epidemiologic risk factors. *BMC Cancer*. 2010;10(1):285.

Glossary

Abridged life table: The essential inputs are age-specific mortality rates and the median age of death in each age group. From this information, an artificial cohort is exposed to the implied mortality risks and the average amount of time spent at each age is determined. This is distinct from a *complete life table* in that it only requires mortality data by age groups, not single years of age.

Absolute risk difference: (synonyms 'attributable risk', 'rate difference', 'excess rate', 'risk reduction') The absolute difference in effect – may be incidence, prevalence, mortality – quantifying the direct impact of an exposure.

Aetiology: The science of causes.

Age-dependent: The risk of health-related phenomena changes with age.

Age-specific rates: Rates that are calculated after stratifying the population into specific age groups that define both the *numerator* and *denominator*.

Age-standardisation: A set of techniques developed by epidemiologists to distil raw frequency counts into a single number that accounts for both differences in population size and age structure.

Age structure: The total number of people alive at different ages at a point in time.

Aggregated data: Secondary data that have been received for the purposes of a study in some form of a contingency table.

Allocation bias: Occurs when researchers or clinicians are aware of which treatment or intervention eligible participants are going to receive, or can predict the allocation sequence, resulting in an imbalance between comparison groups that may include characteristics that vary in their response to the intervention being evaluated in a clinical trial (a form of *selection bias*).

Analytical study design: A type of epidemiological study in which the analytical intent is to explore causal relationships.

Ascertainment bias: (synonym 'sampling' bias) Occurs when participants are recruited, surveyed or screened, but this group systematically excludes some members of the target population (a form of *selection bias*).

Attributable proportion: (synonyms 'attributable risk percent', 'attributable fraction (exposed)', 'etiologic fraction') The percentage of disease occurrence (or risk) in an exposed group that can be directly attributed to the exposure.

Attributable risk: (synonyms 'absolute risk difference risk difference', 'rate difference', 'excess rate', 'risk reduction') The absolute difference in effect – may be incidence, prevalence, mortality – quantifying the direct impact of an exposure.

Attrition bias: Occurs when the study participants who are lost to follow-up have different characteristics from those who remain in the study (a form of *selection bias*).

Background rate: The rate of disease occurring in a population without direct exposure to a risk factor of interest.

Big data: Very large population-level datasets that are analysed for epidemiological trends and patterns in health, risk and human behaviour.

Bias: Any unintentional systematic factor, or trend in the collection or analysis of data, that leads to erroneous conclusions.

Blinding (synonym 'masking'): A process whereby participants and/or investigators are kept unaware of the allocation of interventions in an experimental study to prevent the introduction of bias in measuring the effect of the intervention (or outcomes).

Boolean operators: The conjunctions AND, OR and NOT, which are used to combine search terms to narrow searches for relevant papers in scholarly databases.

Case-control study: (synonyms 'case-referent' and 'retrospective' studies) An observational study that starts by identifying people with a condition of interest and a comparable group of people without the condition and retrospectively comparing their exposure histories to determine which exposures might be associated with case status.

Case fatality: A measure of *mortality* and a *frequency count* that includes the number of deaths from the phenomenon of interest over a specified period.

Case fatality risk: (synonyms 'case fatality rate', 'case fatality ratio') A measure of *mortality* that includes in the *numerator* the number of deaths from the phenomenon of interest over a specified period and in the *denominator* the incident cases of this phenomenon over the same period. Shares a numerator with *cause-specific mortality rate.*

Cause-specific mortality: A measure of *mortality* that includes the number of deaths from the phenomenon of interest over a specified period.

Cause-specific mortality rate: A measure of *mortality* and a *mortality rate* that includes in the *numerator* the number of deaths from the phenomenon of interest over a specified period and in the *denominator* the product of the number of people in the population and the period over which the numerator was observed. Shares a numerator with *case-fatality risk.*

Chronic conditions: A class of health conditions that last a long time (typically one year or more).

Cohort: A group of people who share certain characteristics, such as being in the same work environment or being born in the same year. Also now refers to the participants in a study being followed up over time.

Cohort life table: A life table that uses projected mortality trends into the future.

Cohort study: (synonyms 'concurrent', 'prospective', 'follow-up', 'incidence' studies) An observational study in which defined populations are identified on the basis of whether they have been exposed to specific health-related factors; health outcomes for exposed and unexposed groups are compared over time. Data collection may be prospective or retrospective.

Complete life table: The same as an *abridged life table* but requires mortality data by single years of age.

Concealment of allocations: A process by which the random allocation sequence of RCTs is kept secret to prevent knowledge of which participant is assigned to which study group (intervention or control).

Confidence interval: A range of values constructed around an estimate arising from an analysis (e.g. odds ratios, prevalence, incidence rate) that represents the specified probability (typically, 95 per cent) that, on repeated measurements in the same circumstances, the true value will lie between the lower and upper bounds of the interval.

Confounder: A variable that is associated with both a potential cause (*e*) and an outcome (*o*) that distorts the true relationship between *o* and *e*.

Confounding: Occurs when understanding of the relationship between one potential cause and an outcome is distorted by one or more additional factors associated with both that potential cause and the outcome.

Contingency table: A cross-tabulation of data such that categories of one characteristic are represented horizontally (in rows) and categories of another are represented vertically (in columns). In epidemiology, exposures are typically presented in the rows and outcomes in the columns.

Correlation: A relationship between variables in which the values of the variables change in relationship with each other.

Correlation coefficient: A statistical measure of the linear correlation between variables that is represented by 'r', taking the value −1 to +1 to indicate the strength of the relationship.

COVID-19: Coronavirus disease 2019, a disease caused by infection with the SARS-CoV-2 virus, first noted in 2019.

Crude rate: A rate that is calculated for all ages combined.

Data linkage: A process of combining quantitative data from multiple sources based on the common identifiers.

De-identified data: Information about characteristics of a population (or sample from a population) from which all identifying information has been removed; it is not possible to recognise particular people from whom the data have been collected.

Denominator: The number below the fraction bar.

Descriptive study design: A type of epidemiological study in which the analytical intent is not to explore causal relationships.

Dichotomous variables: Variables that have only two possible values.

Direct standardisation: Where you calculate age-specific rates and then derive a weighted sum of these rates using the age structure of a *standard population*, where each age group is expressed as a proportion of the total in that population.

Directed acyclic graphs (DAGs): A graphical depiction of unidirectional pathways between an exposure and outcome of interest, identifying all the variables that mediate or confound the causal pathway.

Disability-Adjusted Life Years (DALYs): A common health indicator used to assess the burden of disease, injury or disability in a population. It takes into account not only deaths but also the impact of non-fatal conditions on the quality of life. One DALY means the loss of one year of healthy life, and it is calculated by combining the years of life lost due to premature death and the years of life lived with illness or disability.

Duration: The average length of time someone spends as a prevalent case before leaving this group either due to getting better or dying.

Ecological fallacy: Drawing misleading conclusions about individual behaviour from group-level data.

Ecological studies: These studies are also known as correlational studies. Building upon our understanding of 'longitudinal' cross-sectional surveys, ecological studies analyse existing data at the group or population level. The quantitative measure used to determine a relationship between exposure and outcome in these studies is correlation.

Effect modifier: A variable that changes the effect of a causal factor of interest (a form of interaction).

Endemic: The persistent presence of a given disease in a specified population or area.

Epidemic: (synonym 'outbreak') An increase in the number of cases, which is beyond that normally expected for a particular region during a particular period of time.

Epidemiological studies: Discrete attempts to pursue an epidemiological question, many of which get written up and published in the scientific literature or elsewhere.

Equipoise: In clinical trials, a situation where participants understand, and experts honestly agree, that there is no evidence for the benefit of one treatment over another.

Estimated resident population: Official estimates of how many people resided in a geographic area at a point in time.

Experimental study design: A type of epidemiological study where the objective is to investigate what happens when exposure is manipulated.

Exposure: A behavioural or genetic characteristic, toxin or other substance in the environment, or a lifestyle factor that is associated with an increase/decrease in the risk of a defined outcome.

Feel-osophy: A made-up term denoting systems of belief relying on inaccurate information selected on the basis of factors such as peer influence, resentment, misunderstandings and personal agenda.

Frequency count: Number of cases of the phenomenon of interest within a specified period.

Gross domestic product (GDP) per capita: A global indicator used to measure and compare the economic growth of countries around the world. It is calculated by dividing the GDP of a country by its midyear population (World Bank Metadata Glossary: https://databank.worldbank.org/metadataglossary/world-development-indicators/series/NY.GDP.PCAP.KN). Developed countries tend to have a higher GDP per capita than developing countries.

Hawthorne effect: Where participants change their risk behaviour due to being observed in a study (a form of measurement bias).

Hazard ratio: The mathematical probability of the occurrence of an event (such as a new case of disease or death) in one group over a specified period of time relative to another group.

Health-Adjusted Life Expectancy (HALE): Extends the concept of life expectancy and reflects the average length of time a person at a specific age can expect to live in full health.

Health expectancy measures: Measures such as HALE that assess the number of years in full health for which an individual can expect to live given existing *mortality* and *morbidity* conditions. Distinct from a health gap measure.

Health gap measures: Measures such as the DALY that include an explicit value judgement about what the absence of disease burden looks like.

Healthy worker effect: A problem for studies looking at occupational exposures that results in lower incidence of disease in workers relative to the general population due to sicker persons having already left the workforce (a form of *selection bias*).

Hypothesis: A statement that proposes a relationship (or association) between two or more key variables, which the researcher intends to test in a study. In the context of an epidemiological study, a hypothesis often proposes a relationship between an exposure factor and a specific health outcome.

Incidence: Synonymous with *incident case* or *incidence rate*, depending on context.

Incidence rate: The rate at which new cases of a specified disease or health state arise in the population at risk over a specified period of time.

Incident case: A new case of the phenomenon of interest in a defined population within a specified period. A measure of *morbidity*.

Indirect standardisation: Where you compare the raw frequency count of the phenomenon of interest in a population against the number you would expect to have observed had that population experienced the same age-specific rates as a standard population.

Individualistic fallacy: Drawing misleading conclusions about group behaviour from individual-level data. Also known as the 'atomistic fallacy'.

Infectious diseases: (synomyn 'communicable diseases') A class of illnesses resulting from specific infectious agents or their toxic products.

Inference: A conclusion reached about a subset (or sample) of the population that is applied to the whole population from which the sample was drawn.

Interaction: The independent operation of two or more factors on a causal pathway that enhance or prevent an outcome. The combined operation of these causal factors might increase or decrease the degree of the outcome to an extent that exceeds the sum of their individual effects.

Interval scale: These have ordered categories with consistent intervals between them, but there is no true zero point. Temperature measured in Celsius or Fahrenheit is an example of interval scale data. While differences between temperatures are consistent (e.g. the difference between 10°C and 20°C is the same as that between 20°C and 30°C), a temperature of 0°C does not represent the absence of heat.

Kaplan-Meier curve: A statistically generated graph that shows the cumulative probability of survival (or any other event) at specified points in time in one or more groups.

Life expectancy: The average number of years an individual of a given age can be expected to live. A measure of *mortality*.

Life expectancy at birth: The average number of years a hypothetical newborn child could be expected to live if they were to experience the observed age-specific mortality rates of a population or group for the rest of their life.

Measurement bias: (synonym 'information bias') Systematic error introduced by inaccurate and/or inconsistent measurement of study variables or misclassification of participants according to exposure or disease status.

Meta-analysis: Statistical methods used to pool the data from two or more quantitative studies to produce a single estimate of effect.

Micro data: (synonym 'unit record data') Secondary data that has been received as individual records that can be aggregated into custom contingency tables using statistical software.

Morbidity: Any measure that does not include death as an outcome. Includes measures such as *incidence, prevalence, remission, duration* and *severity*.

Mortality: Death, often expressed as the rate of death occurring in a given population over a specified period of time.

Mortality rate: Any *rate* where the phenomenon of interest is death. A measure of *mortality.*

Mortality rate ratio (MRR): A ratio of the incidence of death in the exposed group relative to the not-exposed group.

Multi-level study: A study in which different units of analysis for the exposure variables are incorporated into one analysis.

Nominal scale: This is the simplest measurement scale and involves categorising data into distinct categories or groups without any inherent order. Examples include gender (male, female) and marital status (single, married, divorced). Nominal data cannot be ranked or ordered numerically.

Non-experimental design: A type of epidemiological study that utilises data on exposures and outcomes without any intervention on behalf of those conducting the study, other than to analyse the data in some way. 'Observational study design' is another term used here.

Non-response bias: Occurs when people decline to participate in a study, or study participants do not provide requested information, and non-responders differ in important ways from responders (a form of *selection bias*).

Normative value: A value judgement about how the world *should be,* rather than how it actually is.

Number needed to treat (NNT): The number of patients who need to be treated to prevent one specified outcome (e.g. death, stroke, improvement, cure).

Numerator: The number above the fraction bar.

Observer bias: (synonyms 'outcome bias', 'detection bias') Occurs due to variation in the way outcomes are measured in a study, leading to misclassification of outcomes in comparison groups (a form of measurement bias).

Odds ratio: (synonyms 'cross-product ratio' and 'relative odds') A ratio of the odds of exposure in cases (or an affected group) relative to the odds of the same exposure in cases (or an unaffected group).

Operationalisation: Turning an abstract conceptual idea into something that is measurable. In so doing, researchers seek to define specific criteria, measurements or procedures that capture the essence of the concept in a tangible and measurable form. This process is essential for ensuring that the variables under investigation can be observed, measured and analysed reliably and consistently across different settings and studies.

Ordinal scale: In this scale, data are categorised into distinct groups with an inherent order or ranking, but the differences between categories are not consistent or quantifiable. Examples include survey responses indicating levels of agreement (strongly disagree, disagree, neutral, agree, strongly agree). While there is a clear order, the intervals between categories are not meaningful.

Outbreak (synonym 'epidemic'): An increase in the number of cases, which is beyond that normally expected for a particular region during a particular period of time.

Outbreak investigation: The process of gathering information to identify the cause and aetiology of a disease epidemic within a community and a specific timeframe, as well as to implement control measures to limit the spread of the disease.

Outcomes: The different health states that a person might experience.

***p* value:** The long-run probability that a statistical finding of a particular value would have arisen by chance in a world defined by the null value.

Period life table: A life table that uses mortality rates for a given period (usually a year) and assumes these apply without change into the future.

Period prevalence: Existing cases of the phenomenon of interest in a defined population over a period of time.

Person-time: The combined time study participants are observed to be at risk of a particular outcome from the beginning of the observation period to developing the outcome, leaving the study (e.g. loss to follow-up, death) or the end of the study. Each person contributes only the time they spent under observation. May be defined as any period (days, weeks, years) and is used in the denominator of calculations of person-time incidence or *mortality rates.*

Pilot study: A small-scale study undertaken to test the feasibility and validity of a new research instrument or method to improve it prior to its use in a larger-scale study.

Placebo: An inactive or inert medication or procedure that simulates an experimental medication or procedure being evaluated in a trial.

Placebo effect: When people receiving a placebo experience an improvement in physical or mental health despite receiving an inactive treatment.

Point prevalence: Existing cases of the phenomenon of interest in a defined population at a specified point in time.

Population attributable proportion: (synonyms 'etiologic fraction/proportion', 'attributable risk percent (population)') The percentage of disease occurrence (or risk) in the population that can be directly attributed to a particular exposure.

Population pyramid: A type of graph that depicts the age structure of a population where the x-axis (the horizontal axis) represents the size of the population, and the y-axis (the vertical axis) indicates the different age groups, starting with the youngest at the bottom. Males are typically represented on the left, females on the right.

Potential Years of Life Lost (PYLL): Calculated by summing up deaths occurring at each age in a population and multiplying this by the number of remaining years that could have been lived up to an agreed limit.

Prevalence: The proportion of a specified population affected by a specified disease or health state at a specified point in time.

Prevalence odds ratio (POR): Another measure of association commonly used in cross-sectional studies. It can be measured in two different ways: (1) by dividing the odds of outcome in the exposed group by that of the unexposed group; or (2) by dividing the odds of exposure in the diseased group by that of the non-diseased group.

Prevalence proportion: the number of *prevalent cases* divided by the whole population. Cannot be less than 0 or greater than 1. A measure of *morbidity*.

Prevalence ratio (PR): A quantitative measure used to determine the strength and direction of association between exposure and outcome in cross-sectional studies. It is computed by dividing the prevalence of disease in the exposed group by that of the unexposed group.

Prevalent case: An existing case of the phenomenon of interest in a defined population at a specified point in time (*point prevalence*) or over a period of time (*period prevalence*). A measure of *morbidity*.

Primary data: Data that are collected by those conducting a study for the purposes of that study.

Probability sampling: A sampling method used in quantitative studies that involves randomly selecting a sample from a large population in a way that ensures that every member of the population has an equal chance or a pre-determined probability of being selected for the sample. Common random sampling techniques include simple random sampling, systematic random sampling, stratified sampling and cluster sampling.

Protective factor: A factor/variable that decreases the chance of having a particular disease or health condition among the people who are exposed to this factor.

Publication bias: Occurs due to the tendency of papers that report statistically significant findings to be published more frequently in scientific journals compared with those reporting null results (a form of *selection bias*).

Quantitative methods: Those methods dealing with counting, measuring and comparing things.

Randomised controlled trial (RCT): An experimental study design in which participants are randomly allocated to intervention (or study) groups or control group to receive a treatment or therapy or not. The outcomes are rigorously compared (performance, cure or improvement, deaths, safety, side-effects, etc.).

Randomisation: A process of allocating participants to intervention and control groups by chance to ensure the similarity of study groups at the start of the study, in order to minimise the potential for *selection bias* and validly measure the impact of the intervention being investigated.

Rate: The occurrence of an event (e.g. counts of disease or death) divided by the number of a specified population at risk over a specified period of time.

Ratio scale: Like the interval scale but with a true zero point, meaning that a value of zero represents the absence of the measured attribute. Examples include measurements of height, weight and time. On a ratio scale, it is meaningful to calculate ratios and perform mathematical operations like multiplication and division.

Recall bias: Occurs when there is differential recall of exposures or experiences between comparison groups, which is most likely to occur in studies using self-reported data (a form of measurement bias).

Relative risk: (synonym 'rate ratio') A ratio of the risk of an event in those exposed to a specified risk factor to the risk of the same event in those not exposed. In a *cohort study,* the observed incidence in the exposed group is divided by the observed incidence in the unexposed group to calculate the relative risk.

Remission: A measure of *morbidity* concerned with the speed with which people recover from the phenomenon of interest.

Representative sample: A subset of a large population that accurately reflects the sociodemographic characteristics of the target population. The selection process of a representative sample often involves a probability sampling method (e.g. random sampling) to select members from the target population to form the study sample.

Research protocol: A detailed plan of your study, including how you will recruit participants, what data you will collect from them and how you will analyse these data.

Risk difference: (synonyms 'rate difference', 'excess rate', 'risk reduction', 'attributable risk'). The absolute difference in effect – may be incidence, prevalence, mortality – quantifying the direct impact of an exposure.

Risk factor: In the context of epidemiology, a factor/variable that increases the chance of having a particular disease or health condition among the people who are exposed to this factor.

ROC curve: A graphical representation of how well tests can distinguish between people who truly have disease and those who do not, based on the *sensitivity* and *specificity* of tests, according to different test thresholds.

Sampling error: A type of random error that occurs when the characteristics of the selected study sample differ from those of the target population. As such, the data collected from this sample does not truly represent the population data. It arises at random as people we select into each sample may be slightly different (e.g. with slightly different sociodemographic distributions).

Sampling frame: A tangible source of material that provides individual identification, geographic locations and contact information to allow researchers to access and select persons in a predetermined way for their studies.

Sampling unit: The minimum unit of observation. Ranges from an individual person, household, animal or specific microbe to an environmental hazard. In this book, the sampling unit refers to an individual person in the target population.

SARS-CoV-2: Severe Acute Respiratory Syndrome Coronavirus 2, the virus that causes COVID-19.

Scales of measurement: The different ways in which variables or data are categorised, ordered or measured in statistical analysis. These scales define the level of measurement and the properties of the data, influencing the types of statistical analyses that can be applied. There are four scales of measurement: nominal, ordinal, interval and ratio.

Scatter plot: A graph in which each individual is presented by a single dot that demonstrates their position in relation to two variables shown on the x- and y-axes. Graphically represents the relationship between the two variables across multiple individuals.

Scientific rigour: The application of the highest standards of the scientific method, particularly with reference to minimising bias.

Search terms: Words or phrases that are specific to a topic, used to search for relevant literature in a scholarly database.

Secondary data: Data used in a study that already exist because they have been collected for other purposes, usually by other people.

Selection bias: Systematic error introduced by the selection of participants, or inclusion of their information, with characteristics that differ from those not included in the study.

Sensitivity: The ability of a test to identify a particular disease (or disease marker) in people who truly have the disease. Measured as a proportion against a 'gold standard' test.

Severity: The impact of a health phenomenon.

Single-level study: A study in which the analysis is restricted to exposure and outcome variables measured at the same level.

Social desirability bias: Occurs when participants provide information in a manner they perceive will be favourable to the researcher; this is more likely to occur differentially between comparison groups (a form of measurement bias).

Specificity: The ability of a test to identify the absence of disease in those who truly don't have the disease (or disease marker). Measured as a proportion against a 'gold standard' test.

Standard population: The reference population used in age-standardisation procedures.

Stratification: The separation of a population into different groups on the basis of one or more attributes.

Study design: The way an epidemiological study has been executed.

Surveillance: Continuous monitoring of diseases or health conditions in a defined population or geographic location. Involves systematic and ongoing data collection, analysis, interpretation and dissemination to detect potential outbreaks and inform timely control measures.

Survivor bias: (synonym 'survivorship bias') Occurs when a sample of participants (or their data) includes only those who still exist (are alive, or are still in the setting of interest) and omits those who are no longer alive or available. This is a particular problem when their absence is related to the phenomenon of interest (a form of *selection bias*).

Systematic review: A review that aims to identify, evaluate and synthesise all available evidence from quality-assessed studies, using pre-determined explicit and systematic methods to address specific research questions (may or may not involve a meta-analysis).

Temporal: Synonymous with time.

Umbrella review: A systematic review that synthesises completed systematic reviews and does not include primary studies.

Unit of analysis: The 'who' or 'what' for which information is analysed and conclusions are reached.

Unit of observation: The 'who' or 'what' for which data are measured, collected or acquired.

Validity: The extent to which a conclusion, concept or theory accurately reflects the true world. In studies, whether findings accurately reflect the characteristics of a study population (internal validity) or can be generalised to a broader population (external validity). In measurement, the extent to which the instrument measures what it intends to measure (involves content, construct and criterion validity.

Volunteer bias: Occurs when persons volunteering to participate in a trial have clinical and other characteristics that may differ from those of non-volunteers (a form of *selection bias*).

Answers

Chapter 1

Multiple-choice questions

1. C
2. A
3. C
4. D
5. C

Short-answer questions

1. Your answer may not be the same as below, but hopefully you would have been able to find some competing claims.
   - *Proponents:* Mandating vaccines will decrease the number of infections in healthcare settings, reduce health staff shortages and protect vulnerable patients.
   - *Opponents:* Mandating vaccines represents an assault on civil liberty, will deter staff from working in healthcare and can disproportionately affect minorities in countries where vaccines are not paid for by the state.
2. I searched for a paper on COVID-19 vaccination and found the following author affiliations: AIDS Healthcare Foundation, Durban, South Africa; Massachusetts General Hospital, Boston, USA; RAND Corporation, Santa Monica, USA; Harvard University, Center for AIDS Research (CFAR), Boston, USA; and Harvard Medical School, Boston, USA. The study was funded by the National Institutes of Health and the Weissman Family MGH Research Scholar Award. The authors declared no conflicts of interest.
3. Epidemiologists identify and quantify health-related events in populations to determine the importance of the issue. They collect and analyse data (analysis) to determine associated risk or causal factors (evaluation) and reach conclusions about their findings (reasoning) that can inform interventions to address the health-related issue (problem-solving and decision-making).
4. I selected 'diabetes', which produced a range a list of different types of diabetes with different codes, all under the broad ICD category '05-Endocrine, nutritional or metabolic diseases'. There were lots of different types of diabetes listed, but the code for diabetes type 1 was 5A10 and the code for diabetes type 2 was 5A11.
5. I looked at the drop-down menu on the left side of the page and found the nine targets: 3.1 Maternal mortality; 3.2 Neonatal and child mortality; 3.3 Infectious diseases; 3.4 Noncommunicable diseases; 3.5 Substance abuse; 3.6 Road traffic; 3.7 Sexual and reproductive health; 3.8 Universal health coverage; and 3.9 Environmental health (1).
6. This is an example of how a passive surveillance system helps to identify changes in the occurrence of disease and prompts public health action. The features of a passive

system include the routine collection of data in the form of notifications sent in by health-related agencies when cases of notifiable diseases are suspected or identified. The data are always collected in the same way in the same population, which makes it possible to compare notifications from one year to the next. When changes occur in the pattern of notification – frequency and/or location – this can prompt investigation and appropriate public health action.

7. Epidemiology is involved in identifying and describing new and existing health-related issues in specified populations, which can help to determine health issues of importance to specific countries. Epidemiology is about determining risk factors and potential causes, characterising the relationships of these factors with health outcomes. This helps to inform the development of interventions aimed to address health issues. Epidemiology is also involved in the actual development and evaluation of diagnostic tests, vaccines and therapies. Epidemiology is involved in the surveillance and monitoring of disease states in the population, which can help to assess the progress of actions to address health priorities once they are set.
8. The chart shows the number of deaths occurring per week for the first six months of the year in Australia – comparing 2020, 2021 and 2022. Across the x-axis are the first 25 weeks of the year and the y-axis is the scale representing the number of deaths. The deaths occurring in 2020 are represented by the dotted line, 2021 deaths are represented by the dashed line and the solid line represents deaths occurring in 2022. It looks like more deaths were experienced in Australia in all weeks in 2022 than in the same period in previous years. Deaths in 2022 peaked in the first few weeks of the year, which did not reflect the pattern observed in 2020 and 2021. An increasing number of deaths occurred in all years from about week 13, decreasing again by week 24; however, the numbers were higher and the increase steeper in 2022 relative to earlier years.
9. This could be answered in lots of ways, as long as the scientific question can be answered using the broad approach you have suggested.
   - For example, is there a difference in health status in people who tend to have days off on Mondays relative to those who don't? This is a non-experimental design in which we might quantitatively assess the health status of all people and compare the assessment between those taking Mondays off and those who don't.
   - For example, are more Mondays taken off in my office than in a similar workplace across town? Again, this is a non-experimental design in which the sick days are compared across workplaces.
   - For example, will more cakes provided for Monday morning tea reduce Monday absenteeism? This is an experimental design in which my office work group is provided with cakes and a similar office group across town is not. Then we compare sick-day patterns between the two groups.
10. This term has been used to describe how the world has shifted from a situation where communicable disease, famine, and infant and neonatal illnesses were the principal causes of mortality to world in which diseases of the aged, non-communicable diseases, over-nutrition and lifestyle diseases contribute most to death. This change is associated with increased sanitation, improved nutrition and public health advances. It is now known that much of this change has occurred in wealthier countries and is uneven across and within populations.

Chapter 2

Multiple-choice questions

1. B
2. C
3. C
4. C
5. C

Short-answer questions

1. Counting incident cases involves measuring the number of new occurrences or onset of a disease or condition within a specified time period. This measure provides insights into the speed of new occurrences, temporal trends and patterns of the disease. Incident cases are particularly useful for studying risk factors, identifying potential causes and evaluating the effectiveness of prevention and intervention strategies. Counting prevalent cases involves measuring the total number of existing cases of a disease or condition within a population at a given point in time, regardless of when the cases initially occurred. This measure provides a snapshot of the overall burden and distribution of the disease within the population. Prevalent cases are useful for understanding the overall prevalence, assessing the need for healthcare resources and estimating the disease's impact on society.
2. An approximation method will have to be used when choosing the denominator since it is not feasible to follow everyone in the population to determine the exact amount of time they were at risk of being included in the numerator. An estimate of the resident population at the mid-point of the three-year period would be an appropriate source. This would need to be multiplied by 3 to represent the three years, on average, for which everyone in the population is assumed to have been at risk of being included in the numerator.
3. A ratio in epidemiology involves dividing one quantity (the numerator) by another such as quantity (the denominator); the result has no dimensions and can take any value. Unlike a proportion, the numerator does not need to be a subset of the denominator. For example, the ratio of male to female patients in a clinic could be 3:2, meaning there are three male patients for every two female patients. Conversely, this can also be expressed as 0.67 females for every male patient in the clinic.
4. The choice of denominator affects whether we interpret this transformation as a rate or a proportion. If a time-based denominator is used, such as total population over time, we calculate a cause-specific mortality rate. If a case-based denominator, such as the number of incidence cases over a period, is used, we calculate a case fatality rate. A cause-specific mortality rate measures the frequency of deaths from a specific cause in the entire population, while a case fatality rate measures the proportion of deaths among diagnosed cases of a specific disease.
5. The three levels of prevention outlined are primary, secondary and tertiary. Primary prevention aims to prevent the onset of disease altogether, with a focus on reducing incidence. Secondary prevention involves early intervention to limit disease progression, focusing on achieving remission or recovery. Tertiary prevention focuses on improving survival or quality of life after a disease has occurred, with an emphasis on reducing case fatality. While not every level may be applicable in every situation, all prevention activities aim to impact at least one of these levels.

6. A proportion is a ratio in which every entity counted in the numerator is also included in the denominator. A common example is the proportion of prevalent cases, calculated by dividing the number of prevalent cases by the total population. This expresses the prevalence as a fraction or percentage. However, epidemiologists disagree on what label to attach to such a number. While 'prevalence proportion' is strictly correct, it is rarely used. Instead, terms such as 'prevalence' or 'prevalence rate' are more common. 'Prevalence' can be ambiguous as it is also used to refer to the simple frequency count of prevalent cases. 'Prevalence rate' implies a time dimension, which doesn't apply to prevalent cases because they represent a moment in time.
7. Mortality and morbidity are terms used to distinguish between two broad classes of measures in epidemiology. Any ratio, proportion, or rate involving death is a measure of mortality. Examples include mortality rates and case fatality rates. Morbidity measures, on the other hand, relate to outcomes other than death and include attributes like illness, periods of illness, and illness duration. Incidence, prevalence, and duration are examples of morbidity measures.
8. The bathtub analogy is commonly used by epidemiologists to illustrate the relationships between incident cases (water running from the tap), prevalent cases (water in the bathtub), recovery and mortality (water running down the drain). While the analogy is helpful, it overlooks some important nuances. First, for many causes of ill-health, individuals can become sick more than once, as seen with COVID-19 or influenza. Second, for some conditions, such as diabetes or dementia, individuals may never fully recover, challenging the notion of recovery in the analogy. Finally, mortality is inevitable, but not necessarily from the specific cause being studied.
9. The equation $p \approx i \times d$ provides an approximation for quantifying the relationships between incident cases, prevalent cases and duration in descriptive epidemiology. It calculates the number of prevalent cases (p) by multiplying the number of incident cases (i) by the duration (d) expressed in the same unit of time over which incident cases were observed. This equation is useful when only two of the three parameters are known, and you want to determine the third. However, it is important to note that it is applicable only for conditions of relatively short duration – typically less than a year.
10. The three levels of prevention are primary, secondary and tertiary prevention.
    - *Primary prevention:* This level focuses on preventing the onset of disease altogether by reducing incidence. It involves measures that avoid the development of a disease. An example of primary prevention is vaccination programs, which are particularly effective for preventing infectious diseases such as influenza or measles.
    - *Secondary prevention:* This level is concerned with early intervention to limit disease progression, focusing on remission or recovery. It involves early detection and prompt treatment to halt the progress of a disease at an early stage. An example of secondary prevention is regular screenings for breast cancer, which can detect the disease early and significantly improve the chances of successful treatment.
    - *Tertiary prevention:* This level aims to improve survival or quality of life once a disease has occurred by reducing case fatality. It involves managing and rehabilitating patients to minimise complications and support optimal functioning. An example of tertiary prevention is cardiac rehabilitation programs for patients who have experienced a heart attack, which help improve their quality of life and reduce the risk of subsequent cardiac events.

Chapter 3

Multiple-choice questions

1. C
2. B
3. A
4. A
5. B

Short-answer questions

1. The challenges in descriptive epidemiology stem from the need to transform raw data (e.g. incident and prevalent cases, deaths) before making comparisons. While simple transformations such as rates suffice for comparing individual attributes (e.g. mortality), integrating multiple attributes demands more elaborate techniques.
2. The raw frequency count of a health-related phenomenon is influenced by both the size and age structure of a population. Using a disease of old age such as dementia as an example, a population with an older age structure (more older individuals) will have a higher incidence of new cases and more individuals living with the disease compared with a population that has a younger age structure, even if the overall size and dementia risk are the same. Rescaling frequency counts by population size alone fails to reveal this underlying similarity in dementia risk between populations with different age structures.
3. Crude rates incorporate data for all ages combined, while age-specific rates are calculated after stratifying the population into specific age groups. Age-specific rates can lead to a larger number of figures to compare, making it challenging to synthesise the information into a cohesive overall picture.
4. Age-standardisation is a set of techniques in epidemiology designed to distil raw frequency counts of health-related conditions into a single number that accounts for differences in both population size and age structure. This is useful for assessing trends in one population over time or comparing the susceptibility of different populations.
5. An age-standardised rate using the direct method is where you calculate age-specific rates from raw frequency counts and population data, then derive a weighted sum of these rates using the age structure of a standard population, where each age group is expressed as a proportion of the total in that population. The choice of the standard population must be explicitly stated for replicability.
6. Indirect standardisation is an alternative approach to age-standardisation where the raw frequency count of the phenomenon of interest is compared with the expected count if the population had experienced the same age-specific rates as a standard population. It is useful in situations where direct standardisation may not be feasible, such as when there is incomplete or unstable information about the populations being compared.
7. An abridged life table differs from a complete life table by requiring calculations by age groups rather than single years of age. The essential inputs include age-specific mortality rates and the median age of death in each age group. Using this information, an artificial cohort is exposed to the implied mortality risks and the average amount of time spent at each age is determined to create estimates of life expectancy at each age.

8. The first row of the last column of a period life table represents the average number of years a hypothetical newborn child could expect to live, based on a population's age-specific mortality rates. However, if there are declining mortality trends in the population, this approach may over-estimate mortality risk and under-estimate life expectancy for an actual child born when the data were collected. Conversely, if mortality trends are expected to increase, the opposite holds true.
9. Health-Adjusted Life Expectancy (HALE) is an extension of the life expectancy concept, originating from the need for more comprehensive assessments of population health, especially in an ageing world. HALE reflects the average length of time a person at a specific age can expect to live in full health. It aims to provide a more nuanced understanding of population health beyond mere longevity by incorporating information about time spent in states of less than full health.
10. The Disability-Adjusted Life Year (DALY) is a composite measure that combines the mortality and morbidity experience of a population into a single number, representing the 'burden of disease' in that population. Unlike Health-Adjusted Life Expectancy (HALE), DALY is a health gap measure, explicitly including a value judgement about the absence of disease burden (0 DALYs). The DALY comprises a mortality component called Years of Life Lost (YLL) and a morbidity component called Years Lived with Disability (YLD). YLL involves multiplying deaths at each age by a measure of premature mortality, while YLD incorporates a comprehensive list of possible causes of illness and injury, applying severity weights and multiplying them by estimates of prevalence and average duration for each cause. The resulting DALY is a versatile measure that can be aggregated and disaggregated by various dimensions.

Chapter 4

Multiple-choice questions

1. C
2. D
3. B
4. C
5. C

Short-answer questions

1. The thalidomide tragedy of the 1960s involved a surge in severe limb defects among newborns, known as phocomelia. The work of both Dr Lenz and Dr McBride throughout 1961 was pivotal in uncovering the cause of the tragedy. Dr Lenz used a case-control study design that, by November 1961, convinced him of the association between thalidomide exposure and birth defects in parts of Western Germany. Separately, Dr McBride conducted a detailed case series investigation of three pregnancies in Sydney, Australia, which by June 1961 had convinced him that thalidomide was the common factor. Both studies reinforced the urgency for action, prompting the cessation of thalidomide use and its subsequent global withdrawal by the end of 1961.
2. The primary objective of the COMMIT study was to assess the effectiveness of community-wide interventions in reducing smoking rates. Led by the National Cancer Institute (NCI), COMMIT involved multiple communities across the United States and aimed to implement

and evaluate comprehensive tobacco-control programs. The study adopted a community-randomised trial design, enlisting intervention and control communities, and involved collaborative efforts between researchers, health professionals and community leaders. The interventions included mass media campaigns, school and workplace programs, healthcare delivery changes and policies to create smoke-free environments. The study emphasised community involvement and tailored interventions to specific community needs, collecting extensive data on smoking prevalence, cessation rates and changes in community norms regarding tobacco use to assess the impact of interventions.

3. The primary objective of the British Doctors Study was to investigate the relationship between smoking and lung cancer. Conducted by researchers Richard Doll and A. Bradford Hill, the study involved the analysis of smoking habits and health outcomes among British physicians. Over 40 000 male doctors aged from 35 to 70 years were recruited and their smoking habits were meticulously documented through questionnaires. The study aimed to provide compelling evidence of the link between tobacco consumption and an increased risk of developing lung cancer.

4. The Broad Street Pump study is significant not only due to its lasting impact on epidemiology but also because it exemplifies a single-level study where individuals serve as the unit of analysis. In such studies, both exposure and outcome variables are analysed at the individual level, as demonstrated by Snow's investigation into factors such as people's residences and water sources.

5. In the context of cross-sectional surveys, the distinction between analytical and descriptive study designs lies in how the collected data are analysed. For example, if data from a cross-sectional survey are analysed to examine the relationship between inadequate ventilation and the common cold to understand potential causal links, the study would be classified as analytical. However, if the same data were analysed to compare the prevalence of the common cold in different populations without exploring causal relationships, the study would be classified as descriptive.

6. The systematic review is a study design that involves systematically collecting data from existing studies and sources on a particular topic, followed by making inferences about the state of knowledge based on these data. Although the topic of the review can relate to aetiology, it is not limited to it and numerical findings can be pooled across studies through meta-analysis when appropriate. However, the unit of analysis in a systematic review is other studies, rather than individuals or groups, posing challenges in its classification within conventional taxonomies. Despite this, systematic reviews are often considered to be at the top of the evidence hierarchy in discussions about causation and have a significant impact on epidemiology by providing comprehensive summaries of existing evidence.

7. The burden of disease study is a synthesis study design that integrates data from various sources such as mortality and disease registers, health surveys, epidemiological studies and systematic reviews to provide a comprehensive understanding of disease burden and its causes within a population. A central aspect of this study design is the incorporation of aetiological research to determine the proportion of disease burden attributable to different hazardous exposures. Although results are often presented for specific population groups, the unit of analysis focuses on causes of disease and injury rather than individuals or groups, challenging its classification as traditional epidemiology despite being recognised as the gold standard for descriptive epidemiological inquiry.

8. Primary data collection is essential for certain epidemiological study designs, such as case reports, case series, randomised controlled trials (RCTs) and systematic reviews. However, other study designs, such as ecological studies and burden of disease studies, heavily rely on secondary data. Additionally, study designs such as cross-sectional surveys, case-control studies, cohort studies and community intervention trials can utilise either primary or secondary data, or a combination of both, to achieve their objectives.

9. A multi-level study in epidemiology involves combining different units of analysis for exposure variables into a single study. It is gaining popularity because it helps to unravel the relationship between individual and group factors, and their impact on individual-level outcomes.
10. The cautionary lesson from Robinson's paper and subsequent research is to avoid drawing misleading conclusions about individual behaviour from group-level data, known as the ecological fallacy, as well as the reverse mistake of drawing misleading conclusions about group behaviour from individual-level data, referred to as the individualistic or atomistic fallacy.

Chapter 5

Multiple-choice questions

1. B
2. D
3. D
4. C
5. D

Short-answer questions

1. Person, place and time.
2. CVD rate is higher in males than females; the burden of communicable diseases are higher in developing countries than in developed countries; there has been an overall increasing trend in life expectancy since the beginning of the twentieth century.
3. The majority of the cases (small dots and clusters, with five and more cases) were concentrated around the Broad Street Pump (Pump A), while areas served by other pumps (Pumps B and C) had fewer cases. In addition, the areas around those pumps without any labels had no cases.
4. They are selected using a probability sampling method (such as simple random sampling, systematic sampling, stratified sampling or cluster sampling) from the target population to ensure they form a 'representative' sample of the population.
5. The trends in lung cancer mortality rates reflected the long-term prevalence of smoking in both males and females, with a time lag of around 20 to 30 years. The prevalence of smoking among males reached a high level in 1945 (2) and has been declining steadily, while the smoking rate in females rose from the early 1960s and started to drop in the mid-1980s. As a result, the mortality of lung cancer in males peaked in the late 1980s and has since fallen sharply, almost paralleling the trend of smoking (with a lag of 20+ years). Similarly, female lung cancer mortality gradually increased until 2010 and has since started to decline.
6. We can evaluate the effectiveness of a population-based vaccination program by examining the long-term patterns of the incidence of the vaccine-preventable disease and the changes in the trajectory of the disease incidence following the vaccination program.

7. Place and time characteristics.
8. **Place**: In 1990 and 2000, under-5 mortality was the highest in the African region followed by the South-East Asian region, Eastern Mediterranean, Western Pacific regions and the lowest in the Americas and Europe; however, the rate comparisons in 2020 were slightly different from the highest to the lowest: the African, Eastern Mediterranean, South-East Asian Regions, Americas, Western Pacific Region and Europe. **Time**: The under-5 mortality rates in all WHO regions showed a declining trend over time and the most significant reduction in under-5 mortality was observed between 2000 and 2020.
9. DALYs is a common indicator used to assess burden of disease, injury or disability. It takes into account not only deaths but also the impact of non-fatal conditions (such as illness or disability) on the quality of life. We can use the data of DALYs (e.g. WHO Global Health Observatory data) to compare the patterns of disease burden between two sub-populations (e.g. males and females, personal characteristic) in the same countries, or between two or more countries (place characteristic), or in the same population over time (time characteristic).
10. Descriptive epidemiology allows us to examine the patterns of disease or health-related issues, leading to the formulation of hypotheses for determining aetiology of disease or underlying factors associated with the variations in disease occurrence; it can be used to detected potential disease outbreak and help public health officials to respond quickly to control the spread of the disease; it also can be used to inform decision-making for introducing or modifying disease prevention and control measures; and to evaluate the effects of these measures.

Chapter 6

Multiple-choice questions

1. C
2. D
3. A
4. D
5. B

Short-answer questions

1. (1) The data on exposure and outcome (and other potential confounding factors) are both collected and measured at a given time point (no follow-up is required). (2) They involve one study sample and the subjects in the sample have no knowledge of either their exposure or outcome status. (3) They can be used to assess an association between exposure and outcome.
2. They are less expensive and easy to do when compared with other types of analytical studies; they can be used to generate and test hypotheses important to identifying disease aetiology; they can be used to establish an association between exposure and outcome, which can further analytical studies.
3. Cross-sectional studies cannot determine the temporal sequence of exposure and outcome events, making it difficult to assess causality; they are not suitable for studying rare diseases or health conditions; we cannot measure incidence in cross-sectional studies, so we are unable to assess the 'risk' of developing a disease; these studies are prone to various types of bias and confounding.

4. Cross-sectional studies are considered descriptive if we use them to provide a general understanding of a population, including the sociodemographic characteristics and the prevalence of specific diseases (evaluating the burden of disease) and health issues/risk factors. They are useful for informing health planning and policy. They are classified as analytical studies when they are used to assess an association between exposure and outcome of interest.
5. Prevalence of mental health issues in the vaping group = 230/900 = 0.256 = 25.6%. Prevalence of mental health issues in the non-vaping group = 615/4100 = 0.15 = 15.0%. The prevalence of mental health issues among the students who use electronic vapor products is higher than those who do not use the products (25.6% >15.0%).
6. The prevalence ratio (PR) of mental health issues between exposure (+) and (–) is:

$$PR = \frac{a/(a+b)}{c/(c+d)} = \frac{230/900}{615/4100} @ 1.70$$

The result of PR = 1.70 indicates a positive association between vaping and mental health problems, meaning that those students who use electronic vaping products are 1.7 times as likely to suffer from mental health issues compared with those who never use the products.
7. We can use the POR formula for this calculation:

$$POR = \frac{a \times d}{b \times c}$$

Prevalence odds ratio (POR) of mental health issues between vaping (+) and (-) is:

$$POR = \frac{a \times d}{b \times c} = \frac{230 \times 3485}{670 \times 615} @ 1.95$$

The result of POR = 1.95 indicates a positive association between vaping and mental health issues – that is, students who use electronic vaping products are 1.95 times more likely to suffer from mental health issues than those who do not use the products. POR shows a stronger association than PR (in Question 6).
8. The ecological fallacy arises when a correlation is found in an ecological study where the data of exposure and outcome variables are collected at the group/population level, but the result is interpreted at the individual level.
9. Ecological studies are easy to conduct and relatively inexpensive; they can be used to generate hypotheses (a feature of descriptive study) and assess population-level correlations to guide further analytical studies; they are suitable for studying rare outcomes.
10. Sampling in a cross-sectional study involves selecting a representative sample from our target population. We first need to identify an available sampling frame and choose a specific probability sampling technique (e.g. simple random sampling, stratified random sampling) to select the subjects of an intended number.

Chapter 7

Multiple-choice questions

1. C
2. B
3. D
4. C
5. C

Short-answer questions

1. This question could really be answered in two ways, with the reasoning being the important bit. You might say that a case-control study would be appropriate because the outcome is clear (chronic asthma) and multiple potential exposures could be identified. You might say that a case-control study is not appropriate as information on childhood exposures derived from adults would be difficult to verify and would be subject to potential recall bias.
2. This sounds like a case-control study, because it is retrospective – starting with identifying the cases (high academic achievers) and comparing them with controls (lower academic achievers) then comparing their exposure histories. While there is only one outcome of interest (higher academic achievement), there is more than one exposure of interest (volunteer reading and writing program, homework engagement and family support).
3. I looked up the existing case definition of obesity and found that most sources rely on the 'body mass index' (BMI) to define obesity. BMI is calculated by dividing the person's weight in kilograms divided by the square of their height in metres (kg/m^2). Adopted by most sources, the World Health Organization defines overweight as a BMI between 25 and 29 and obesity as BMI 30 or above. As this is a world-recognised definition, I will define obesity as BMI ≤30.
4. Hopefully, here you would have thought about clinic populations, community populations, hospitalised populations or notifications to state surveillance systems to source your cases. Controls should be selected independently of their exposure status, should not meet the case definition and should be sourced from as similar as possible a population as those that gave rise to the cases. If you have chosen controls that are diagnosed with another condition, hopefully you would have chosen a condition that is not known to have the same potential causes or factors as your cases (e.g. diet is a risk factor for both diabetes and obesity), or that systematically excludes people who might not be exposed to the same risk factors (e.g. people with chronic asthma might actively avoid practices known to increase transmission of influenza).
5. Cases seem to be younger than controls; there are more male controls than cases; more cases are reported to be able to read; fewer cases are partnered relative to controls.
6. Table 7.5: Characteristic of study participants with multi-drug resistant TB at a TB specialised hospital in India, 2011 – 90 cases and 90 controls.

	Cases – n (%)	Controls – n (%)	OR
Age in years			
≤30	66 (73.3)	38 (42.2)	3.76
>30	24 (26.7)	52 (57.8)	
Sex			
Male	41 (45.6)	52 (57.8)	0.61
Female	49 (54.4)	38 (42.2)	
Literacy			
Unable to read	11 (12.2)	22 (24.4)	0.43
Able to read	79 (87.8)	68 (75.6)	

	Cases – n (%)	Controls – n (%)	OR
Relationship status			
Partnered	62 (68.9)	43 (47.8)	2.42
Single	28 (31.1)	47 (52.2)	

7. The ORs for age and relationship status are greater than 1 (OR >1), which suggests that being 30 years of age or under and having a partner are associated with increased odds of having multidrug-resistant TB. The ORs for sex and literacy are less than 1 (OR <1), suggesting that being male and illiterate is associated with decreased odds of having multidrug-resistant TB. Relative to controls, cases have more than 3.7 times the odds of being younger and nearly 2.5 times the odds of being partnered. However, relative to controls, cases have just over half the odds of being male (39 per cent greater odds of being female) and less than half the odds of being illiterate (57 per cent greater odds of being able to read).
8. Whatever the OR you calculated for literacy (and hopefully it was something like 0.43), the 95 per cent confidence interval of 0.19 to 1.95 indicates that the result was not significant. If we were to repeat the study exactly the same way over and over again, taking the same measurement each time, 95 per cent of the time the OR would fall within the range of 0.19 to 1.95. This interval includes the OR of 1 – so repeated attempts could find that the true OR could be anywhere from <1 to >1. This means the OR we calculated for literacy is probably not valid.
9. Hopefully you would have noticed that the already small number of cases in total became even smaller when they were redefined into their different complication categories (deaths, ICU, ventilation). The small numbers, which greatly influence the precision of confidence intervals, may explain why the confidence interval associated with the OR for periodontal disease and death was quite wide and included the null value of 1. In contrast, because nearly all of the cases were admitted to the ICU, the confidence intervals associated with the OR for periodontal disease and ICU admissions were much narrower. You might note also that demographic, medical and behavioural factors were controlled for (through magic statistical means) in the analysis, which means they presumably have not confused the results. Overall, it would seem the that the study indicates that periodontal disease seems to be associated with poor outcomes in hospitalised COVID-19 patients.
10. Hopefully you would have thought about the advantages and disadvantages of case-control studies here. We have a relatively uncommon disease, about which we have a lot of information. We have a clear and specific case definition and we know its incidence in the population. Unless we have a lot of time and money, we couldn't simply wait for the cases to appear after exposure, since we would need to recruit a very large number of people and follow them up for up to 60 years. Losses to follow up would be high over that period of time. The disease is rare but asbestos in older buildings and home renovations are fairly common in the population, as are office and school renovations. We would definitely have to be very careful about selection and measurement bias, but a case-control study might be the best design in the first instance here!

Chapter 8

Multiple-choice questions

1. C
2. B
3. D
4. C
5. C

Short-answer questions

1. This looks like a retrospective cohort study. The direction of study was from exposure (premature birth or not) to outcome (all-cause and cardiac-specific mortality). Infants who were admitted to the NICU were identified as exposed and full-term infants at the same hospital and time were identified as not exposed. The data were all historically recorded at the hospitals and deaths registries. Outcomes per comparison groups were then compared to identify any excess cardiac-specific deaths and deaths from all causes.
2. I selected lung cancer mortality. In 2020, the crude mortality rate for lung cancer was 32.9 deaths per 100 000 population in Australia. The age-standardised mortality rate for cancer in 2020 was 26.2 per 100 000. The lower age-standardised mortality rate is because the standard population used to adjust the crude rate had a smaller proportion of people in the older age groups than the actual Australian population in 2020 (the standard used was actually the 2001 Australian population). Since deaths are associated with age, the unadjusted or crude rate reflected that greater proportion of older people with lung cancer in the 2020 population whose deaths were also likely to be attributable to age.
3. There are a few very interesting items on the list, and I have selected 'social mobility', the term used to describe how people move up and down in social status, with previous evidence showing that the United Kingdom is one of the least socially mobile countries in the developed world. The NCDS data have shown that social mobility in men is mostly unchanged over the study, while social mobility in women has increased slightly. Those born into 'working-class families' were less likely to move up into professional jobs than middle-class children were to move down. In terms of income mobility, the researchers report that mobility had decreased over the study period (60 years), with people more likely to remain in the same income groups as their parents than in previous generations.
4. We can see five causes of death listed in rows, and the number of deaths (the counts) in the first column. Columns two to five show age-standardised mortality rates for non-smokers and for smokers according to average amount of smoking per day (so we know that any increased deaths did not occur as a feature of age). There were 1714 total deaths recorded, and the standardised rates of deaths were lowest in non-smokers and highest in the smokers consuming 25 gram or more per day. For all causes of death, the highest category of smoking was associated with the highest mortality relative to non-smokers. The clearest trend in mortality was for lung cancer, which showed a clear dose-response relationship with increases in smoking amounts.
5. The absolute difference would be calculated by: $M_{exposed} - M_{not\ exposed}$. All-cause mortality rate in smokers was 13.25 per 1000 and all-cause mortality in the highest category of smoking

was 18.84 per 1000 (18.84 – 13.25 = 5.59). So, 5.59 deaths per 1000 heavy smokers were directly attributable to their heavy smoking.

6. Relative risk = Incidence (in this case incidence of death) in the exposed divided by the incidence in the not exposed. RR = 18.84/13.25 = 1.42. The relative risk of 1.42 is greater than the null (null = 1), so there was an increased risk of death in heavy smokers relative to non-smokers. The RR of 1.42 indicates that the risk of dying was 42 per cent higher in heavy smokers relative to non-smokers.

7. A completed Table 8.4:

Cause of death	Non-smokers	Daily average smoking (grams)		
		1–14	15–24	≥25
Lung cancer	1 [reference]	6.7	12.3	23.7
Other causes	1 [reference]	1.1	1.0	1.2
All-cause death	1 [reference]	1.2	1.1	1.4

So, there is a considerably increased risk of mortality from lung cancer for smokers relative to non-smokers that almost doubles for each increase in the level of smoking. Smaller increases are associated with deaths due to other causes (that are selected for this exercise) and there is increased relative risk of death from all causes for all levels of smoking relative to non-smokers.

8. Person 1 = 17 months; person 2 = 20 months; person 3 = 20 months; person 4 = 10 months; person 5 = 20 months; person 6 = 7 months; person 7 = 13 months; person 8 = 9 months; person 9 = 2 months; person 10 = 16 months. Total = 134 person months. Total cases = 3. Incidence = (3/134) x 1 000 = 22.4 per 1000 person-months

9. This is clearly a prospective cohort study with a long period of follow-up, and so will be particularly prone to a specific type of selection bias known as *attrition bias*. There are always losses to follow up in prospective studies and when this is differentially distributed between comparison groups, a systematic bias is introduced. The groups may have started out as very similar (all undergraduate) but with loss to follow-up from students withdrawing from their own study, maybe even due to stress or for health/personal reasons, we could end up with the 'healthy student effect', which could initially cause the whole cohort to be unrepresentative of the original target group. Over the many years of follow-up, attrition will start to affect the cohort and bias could be introduced for many reasons, but particularly if there was differential attrition. For instance, those who were identified as 'high-stress' types (our exposed groups) may be more likely to withdraw from the study or be lost to follow-up.

10. Hopefully you would have thought about some of the advantages and disadvantages of prospective cohort studies here. We have a relatively uncommon exposure about which we have a lot of information. We have a well-defined exposed population in which we want to explore a range of potential outcomes that are likely to occur in relatively early life. We would definitely have to be very careful about selection and measurement bias but a prospective cohort study might be an appropriate study design in this instance.

Chapter 9

Multiple-choice questions

1. C
2. C
3. C
4. C
5. D

Short-answer questions

1. Hopefully, you would have seen that this was a single-blind, placebo-controlled, parallel RCT. The patients were randomised to one of three treatment groups and were blinded to which of the three treatments they received: placebo, HC or HC plus antibiotic. They were all then followed up for 12 days, and the outcomes of interest were viral clearance (cured) or viral reduction. There was no difference in the viral clearance between the three treatment groups, with non-significant *p* values reported at both follow-up assessments. Fortunately, nobody seemed to be harmed by this experiment!
2. I used the search terms 'COVID' and 'antiviral' and returned eight completed systematic reviews each looking at different treatments. Only one study reviewed ivermectin and one reviewed hydroxychloroquine. Looking at the dates of the reviews, given that they concerned COVID-19 treatments, they were all recently published (from 2021) onwards. There were 1109 primary trials registered with Cochrane – 767 of which were on hydroxychloroquine and 218 were on ivermectin. That's a lot of time and money preoccupied investigating what may have been political rather than scientific questions! It also indicates the time lag in registering and completing these RCTs, and the further time that elapses before a systematic review can be completed.
3. Stratified randomisation might be the best way to go here. This way we could make sure that our two comparison groups look as similar as possible from the outset of the study. Making sure that there is a balance of age groups, people with additional conditions and smoking history will help to avoid factors that could potentially impact assessment (measurement bias) and confound the findings.
4. These processes are designed to prevent selection and measurement bias. Blinding in RCTs is done to prevent people's (participants, investigators, outcomes assessors) expectations influencing their assessments of outcomes. Allocation concealment has the special purpose of concealing the actual sequence of randomisation so the investigators or clinicians that are enrolling patients have no idea what group the next participant is to be assigned to.
5. This may be an example of an aspect of the placebo effect, which has been described as a psychological response to participant expectations of treatment effects triggered by the deception represented by administration of the placebo. In this example, which mainly concerns the negative aspect of the phenomenon, it may be considered a 'nocebo' effect, when participants report side-effects to treatment despite having received only the placebo.
6. At 14 days, mortality in the exposed = 6.2% and mortality in the not exposed = 11%. MMR = 6.2/11 = 0.56. The MMR of less than 1 indicates a protective effect for high-dose vitamin D at the 14-day point. The MMR of 0.56 suggests a relative reduction in mortality risk of 44%. At 28 days, mortality in the exposed = 15% and mortality in the not exposed = 16.5% MMR = 15/16.5 = 0.91. The MMR of less than 1 also indicates a protective effect for high-dose vitamin D at the 28-day point. The MMR of 0.91 suggests a slight relative reduction in mortality risk of 9 per cent.

7. Mortality in the exposed was 6.2 per cent and mortality in the non-exposed was 11 per cent. Risk difference = 0.11 – 0.062 = 0.048. NNT = 1/0.048 = 20.83. 21 older COVID-19 patients would need to be treated with high-dose vitamin D to prevent one additional death by 14 days.
8. Some of this you may have had to think about, but what the authors are saying is that they used a fancy formula to work out they needed to recruit 750 participants (including 350 HIV patients), randomised equally to two groups (i.e. randomisation ratio of 1:1) to be able to show an absolute difference of 10 per cent in mortality between groups (40 per cent vs 30 per cent). This is based on assumptions that the usual (standard) treatment would have a mortality of 40 per cent and there would be 30 per cent mortality in the intervention group, with relative reduction in risk of 30 per cent for the intervention group (hazard ratio of 0.7). These numbers would mean their study would have an 80 per cent probability of avoiding the type 2 error of accepting the null hypothesis when it is false (i.e. they would be prepared to be wrong 20 per cent of the time, or one in five). They have set a 5 per cent probability of making the type 1 error of rejecting the null hypothesis when it is true (i.e. they would be prepared to be wrong 5 per cent of the time, or one in 20).
9. Hopefully you thought about things such as the harms associated with the deception itself; withholding of treatment that might lead to a deterioration in health, or even death; and the tension between the potential risk to the participant versus the potential benefit to future patients through identifying safety and efficacy of new treatments.
10. **a.** This would clearly show the absolute difference between the two treatments but, given the patients are sick enough to be hospitalised, there is an unacceptable risk to the participants in the control group, who could become seriously ill or die.
    b. This is also a good way to show the difference between groups without leaving people untreated (assuming the safety and therapeutic benefit of the new treatment), but you would need larger numbers of participants to have sufficient power to demonstrate superior results.
    c. This is possibly the most ethical approach, but it would also require larger numbers to show a difference as, assuming the standard treatment usually confers a treatment benefit), there would probably be a limit on how much improvement could be expected with the addition of a new treatment.

Chapter 10

Multiple-choice questions

1. D
2. C
3. B
4. C
5. A

Short-answer questions

1. This sounds like a prospective cohort study, in which the known exposure is specific and data on multiple outcomes are collected. The most appropriate measure of the effect would be to compare incidence of outcomes in each comparison group through calculating relative risks and risk differences.

2. Here, the best measure of effect would be an odds ratio, which is calculating by dividing the odds of exposure in cases by the odds of exposure in controls. A 2 x 2 table of the information provided would look like this:

		COVID-19	
		Cases	Controls
Obesity	E+	1967	3582
	E–	3107	7181
		5074	10763

OR = (1967/3107)/(3582/7181) = 1.27

The odds of being obese was 27 per cent higher in cases relative to controls.

3. The concept of attributable risk could help here. Calculating attributable risk is a way to remove the background rate of disease to determine the incidence that can be directly attributable to the exposure. It works by finding out the absolute and proportional risk differences for disease between exposed and not-exposed groups and can provide information such as the disease in the exposed group that is directly attributable to their exposure or the disease in the population that is directly attributable to the exposure.

4. The first thing to do is plot the information in a 2 x 2 table like this one:

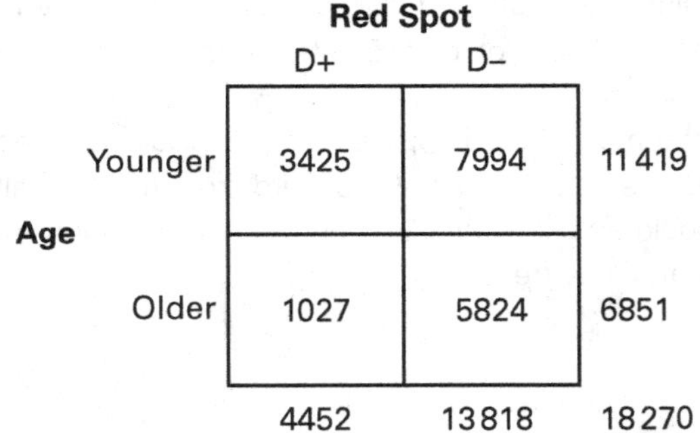

		Red Spot		
		D+	D–	
Age	Younger	3425	7994	11 419
	Older	1027	5824	6851
		4452	13 818	18 270

Let's calculate the relative risk here ($I_{exposed}/I_{not\ exposed}$):

RR = (3425/11419) / (1027/6851) = 0.30/0.15 = 2

So, the risk for red spot in people under 40 years of age is two times (double, or 100 per cent more than) the risk for people aged from 40 to 74 years of age.

Now let's have a look at the absolute risk difference ($I_{exposed} - I_{not\ exposed}$):

RD = 0.30 – 0.15 = 0.15

The 150 cases of red spot per 1000 people under 40 years (0.15 x 1000) per month are directly attributable to their age (150 cases were due to other causes). In absolute terms, the excess headache risk for younger people is 50 per cent above that of older people.

And the attributable proportion ($RD/ I_{exposed}$)?

AP = 0.15/0.30 = 0.50

Being under 40 years is responsible for 50 per cent of the red spot cases in young people (0.50 x 100).

5. If this interaction follows an additive model, mortality in those exposed to both risk factors A and B will be greater than summing the independent risks attributable to each of the exposures. We can work this out by finding out what the sum of the risks would be, assuming no interaction, then compare that to the observed outcomes as follows:
   - Mortality in the not exposed (background mortality) = 31.3
   - Absolute mortality difference for risk factor A only = 61.2 – 31.3 = 29.9
   - Absolute mortality difference for risk factor B only = 122.6 – 31.3 = 91.3
   - Mortality for risk factor A and B should be = 31.3 + 29.9 + 91.3 = 152.5. The observed mortality for exposure to risk factor A and B is 458.2 per 100 000, which is far greater than 152.5 per 100 000, so this confirms an additive interaction.
6. The OR suggests young adults who drank had 50 per cent higher odds of smoking, but the *p* value suggests that was not significant. Do we say there is no relationship between smoking and drinking behaviour because $p > 0.05$? Or do we simply need to know a bit more about the size of the sample here to see whether the study might have been under-powered to find a difference of this size? Perhaps we could consider what other studies have found about the relationship between alcohol and smoking behaviours?
7. The authors worked out that they needed to recruit 154 participants, 50 cases and 104 controls to be able to show a difference of 20 per cent in exposure history between the people with breast cancer and those without breast cancer (based on assumptions of the usual levels of exposure in middle-aged women). These numbers would mean their study would have an 80 per cent probability of avoiding making the type 2 error of accepting the null hypothesis when it is false (i.e. they would be prepared to be wrong 20 per cent of the time, or one in five). They have set a 5 per cent probability of making the type 1 error of rejecting the null hypothesis when it is true (i.e. they would be prepared to be wrong 5 per cent of the time, or one in 20).
8. For RR = 2, you would need 173 participants in total, of whom (on a 21 ratio) you would need 58 in the exposed group and 115 in the comparison group. For RR = 1.5, you would need 639 participants in total, of whom (on a 2:1 ratio) you would need 213 in the exposed group and 426 in the comparison group.
9. Well, the difference in effect was large (strength of the effect size) and the exposure seemed to precede the outcome (temporality), but none of the other Bradford Hill criteria has been met. For instance, we would need to see consistency (across repeated observations) to have faith in the conclusion, and we don't know whether the outcome is specific to these participants. Most of all, there doesn't seem to be any biologically logical mechanism (plausibility) or other types of evidence that might explain the observation (coherence).
10. Here you might explain that relative differences are always larger than absolute differences. This is because relative differences do not exclude the background risk, which absolute differences do. This means that the higher the background risk (i.e. the more common the risk is), the larger the relative difference will be, even if the absolute difference remains the same. Both relative and absolute risk measures can help to guide health policy or practice by characterising modifiable risk factors in the population. The way risk is framed, in absolute or relative terms, is often linked to the motivations for reporting risk in the first place.

Chapter 11

Multiple-choice questions

1. C
2. D
3. C
4. C
5. C

Short-answer questions

1. External validity refers to how findings from studies match what is really on in the real world. To have external validity, the study sample must be representative of (or have similar characteristics to) the target population at the time and circumstances of the study. This means the findings can be generalised to the broader population. Internal validity refers to the extent to which a study is relevant to a particular study population. Internal validity is important for identifying and understanding relationships between exposures and outcomes.
2. The types of validity that I might assess would be: content validity – have I captured all of the aspects associated with the construct?; construct validity – how specific is the measure or could I actually be measuring something else rather than the characteristic I'm interested in?; and criterion validity – how well does the measurement correlate with other instruments designed to measure a similar phenomenon?
3. If we want to be able to generalise our findings to the broader population, we need to recruit a sample that has similar characteristics to it. Most older people are not living in residential care homes; these residents usually have sufficiently poor health or cognitive status to require residential care. If we recruit only these residents, we will introduce the potential for selection bias. The main points to intervene with here would be in the design of the study. For instance – and you might come up with many more ideas – we might select people from both groups that are as similar as possible with the exception of age – so only people dwelling in the community, preferably with similar socioeconomic status, education level and so on. We might achieve this by using large samples, maybe even thinking about matching according to important characteristics that might influence outcomes. If all else fails, we might consider stratifying the analysis according to levels of those important characteristics.
4. As injection drug use is illegal in most countries, and both this practice and prison history can be stigmatised, it is possible that this study could be affected by a type of measurement bias known as social desirability bias. This can occur when participants are reluctant to provide responses that they perceive the researcher might disapprove of. The relationship between exposures and outcomes can be diluted by this subcategory of bias, and greater bias can result if the behaviour was more likely to be engaged in by the members of only one of two comparison groups. Using non-judgemental language, collecting information in a private location and describing how the participant's confidentiality will be protected may help to minimise socially desirable responding. Using other sources of data – such as information from as medical notes, may also help to confirm some information provided.
5. The main reason that RCTs are seen as the 'gold standard' are due to their efforts to minimise bias. Some of the features to minimise selection bias include strict eligibility criteria, randomisation and allocation concealment. Measurement bias is minimised

by blinding – participants, those providing the intervention and sometimes even those assessing the outcome. These processes all greatly increase the internal validity of RCTs, but the tight eligibility criteria can seriously impact external validity. This is why multiple RCTs in different populations can sometimes be required to fully assess the effectiveness and safety of a new intervention.

6. Misclassification A is actually a non-differential classification, in which both exposed and non-exposed groups have misreported their wakefulness, but in a relatively random sort of way. This has had the effect of diluting the effect size slightly but has not introduced bias. Misclassification B is a differential misclassification that only impacts non-coffee drinkers, who have reported less wakefulness than observed with the camera. This differential misclassification has introduced a bias that has provided an inflated measure of effect.
7. Hopefully you would think about the impact of publication bias on both clinical management and health policy development and resources for prevention. These areas are informed by the cumulative evidence of published studies as well as formal systematic reviews. If studies showing null results or lack of associations between exposures and outcomes are systematically excluded from publication, this would clearly result in ineffective treatments and public health interventions being recommended and resourced at the expense of more effective approaches. (I also wanted to make sure you had a look at the *Catalogue of Bias*!)
8. It looks like the relationship between cognitive decline and height may have been confounded by sex. To be a confounder, the variable must be associated with both the exposure and the outcome, and must not be on the causal pathway between the exposure and the outcome. Here, females are associated with high levels of cognitive decline in dementia (by virtue of living longer than males among other factors) and being female is not on the causal pathway between height and cognitive decline.
9. Hypertension is an independent risk factor for ESRD and is also associated with obesity. However, hypertension can also be *caused* by obesity, which means it may be on the causal pathway between obesity and ESRD. In this case, hypertension does not meet the criteria for a confounder.
10. There are two places to intervene here: in the design and at the point of analysis. We could develop a tight case (with ESRD) and control (no ESRD) criteria that restricted selection to people without hypertension. We could also match controls to ESRD cases according to the extent of any hypertension. At analysis, we could examine the prevalence of hypertension according to case status to see whether it was differentially distributed between groups. If so, we might conduct a stratified analysis – looking at the relationship between obesity and ESRD according to levels of blood pressure. Finally, we could control for the confounder through statistical techniques such as the Mantel-Haenszel technique that would provide a summary of the relationship between obesity and ESRD that is weighted according to strata blood pressure.

Chapter 12

Multiple-choice questions

1. C
2. B
3. C
4. D
5. C

Short-answer questions

1. I used Chrome as my web browser which returned nearly six million results. The first 10 listed results included a range of links to academic papers, government and non-government health-related organisations (such as the US Food and Drug Administration and the Cochrane Collaboration), as well as some books and university web pages. Repeating the search at Google Scholar returned about 25 000 results, and the first 10 results were links to academic publications. The titles indicated that the study types included systematic and other reviews, clinical trials and RCTs. Both search strategies provided information that would be helpful, depending on the purpose of the inquiry. To find out what the scientific literature is saying about ivermectin, Google Scholar would be most helpful; whereas Chrome uncovered more about health and government policy regarding its use.

2. There is one recommendation that specifies bias (item 9) in which authors are required to describe any efforts made to minimise bias. However, other items also allude to bias and would help critical readers to determine if the study might have been affected by bias. In item 6a, the authors are required to report what the eligibility criteria were, where cases and controls were sourced and how they were identified, and the rationale for their selection. This item could provide the reader with information about whether there was any potential for selection bias. In item 8, the authors are required to describe the sources of data for all variables of interest, how the variables were assessed and how the assessment methods were developed in each assessment group (cases and controls). This item relates to the potential introduction of measurement bias.

3. I entered the search terms 'lung cancer AND never smokers', which returned 2946 results. I used the 'custom range' for the publication date and entered only the years 2004 to 2014. This only reduced the number of studies to 2648. I then opened the additional filters box and, on the 'Article Type' page, selected 'Observational studies'. On the 'Species' page, I selected 'Human' and then clicked on 'Show' (this brought the filters out to the left side of the results screen, where they could then be selected). This reduced my results to 38 studies, the first 10 of which included three cohort studies, one cross-sectional study, two studies on cancer survival, two on genetics and one review. The 'Observational studies' filter may have limited the results to studies that had specifically used those words in the title or as additional 'key words'. *Note: Thrill-seekers might want to use the 'Advanced' search option, which could help to build more specific search strategies.*

4. **a.** The question was about risk factors associated with lung cancer in people who never smoked.

b. The study design was a case-control study, which is appropriated because cancer is a rare disease, and even rarer in those who have never smoked, but has clear case criteria and the case-control design allows the investigation of multiple risk factors.

c. A total of 445 cases with lung cancer identified in four major hospitals: 35 per cent were never smokers. The controls were 425 population-based people and 523 hospital-based people who were matched to the cases for frequency (i.e. not individually matched) of sex and ethnicity.

d. Outcomes included environmental tobacco smoke (ETS) exposure, family history of cancer, indoor air pollution, workplace exposures, previous respiratory diseases and smoking status. Relative to controls, cases had 60 per cent greater odds of previous exposure to occupational exposure and the odds were higher when comparing cases with controls among those who had never smoked (more than twice the odds). Cases had nearly five times the odds of previous emphysema diagnosis than controls overall, while never-smoking cases had nearly twice the odds of having had a first-degree relative with a cancer diagnosis made before the age of 50 years than never-smoking controls.

e. The authors concluded that occupational exposures and family history of early cancer were important exposures associated with lung cancer in those who had never smoked.

5. The title tells us that this table is comparing a range of demographic details for cases and controls. Looking at the structure of the table, it has three main columns presenting cases, controls and a *p* value that, according to the footnote, indicates some statistical testing of the differences between the total cases and total controls has occurred. The case and control columns have been further subdivided into smokers, never smokers and total of each comparison group. The rows present the demographic characteristics, age groups and 'mean' age (i.e. the arithmetic 'average' of the sum divided by the number of participants), categories of ethnicity and years of education according to three categories of duration in years. Turning now to the content, it looks as if there was a greater proportion of smokers among the cases relative to the controls. This is not reported in the table, but I calculate that smokers make up 65 per cent of the cases (289/445) but only 51 per cent of the controls (482/948). There was a greater proportion of male smokers among the cases relative to the controls, and the *p* value indicates that the total difference was statistically significant. The cases had more people in the upper age groups, while the spread of age was more even in controls. Mean ages were younger in controls for smokers and never smokers and the overall difference in mean age was significant ($p < 0.001$). Never-smoking controls appear to have been more highly educated than never-smoking cases (also statistically significant). So, compared with controls, cases tended to be more likely to be smokers, male, older and less educated.

6. There is only one tool listed for assessing bias in ecological designs. The tool covers nine domains, such as selection, exposure, outcome, confounding, etc. The tool referenced is the 'Navigation Guide' by Woodruff and Sutton (2014) (3), which contains eight questions in areas such as blinding, conflict of interest, confounding, exposure assessment and incomplete data. Given that ecological studies use only aggregated population data and not participants, it would seem reasonable that relatively few tools for assessing bias are available, with the main components dealing with the data quality and completeness.

7. The study I found was a cohort study on the effects of comorbidities on lung cancer outcomes. The STROBE checklist items that were complied with were: items 1a and 1b on page 1; item 2 on pages 1–2; item 3 on page 2; item 4 on page 2; item 5 on page 2; item 6a on pages 2–3; item 6b not relevant; item 7 on pages 2–3; item 8 on pages 2–3; item 11 on page 3; item 13 not relevant to the specific retrospective design; item 14 on page 5; item 15 on pages 4–6; items 16 and 17 on pages 4–6; item 18 on page 4; item 19 partly met on page 7 (but no discussion of bias); item 20 on page 7. Item 9 on bias was not specifically discussed in the methods section; item 10 on how the sample size was arrived at was not discussed; item 12 did not discuss confounding or how it was addressed; item 21 on generalisability was not specifically discussed; item 22 on funding source was not referred to. The study mostly complied with the STROBE checklist, and many of the structural features described would have met some of the items not specifically ticked off. For instance, the use of validated case criteria (such as the ICD) and specified inclusion and exclusion criteria would have addressed some questions about bias and the very large sample size (more than 100 000) might have increased the generalisability at least in the external target group (those with lung cancer).

8. After engaging in some preliminary reading, you might first design a search strategy to find authoritative resources on the topic. You would identify the databases to search, which might include Google Scholar, PubMed, relevant government and non-government websites (including a health department, the World Health Organization and cancer-related non-government organisations) and the Cochrane Library of Systematic Reviews. You would devise search terms connected by appropriate Boolean operators and narrow your search as appropriate for each database. Then you would read the papers and note down key points and themes, making connections between them. After this, you would write a balanced synopsis of the various viewpoints, evaluating the strengths and weaknesses of the evidence, before reaching your own informed conclusions.

9. This is more of an exercise than a short-answer question, but hopefully in completing this activity you will see the usefulness of using a systematic approach for synthesising information in future.

10. The review I found was published in 2023 and the authors state that they searched for papers published up to the beginning of 2023. The review was undertaken following a global outbreak of mpox when there was no specific mpox treatment, although other viral agents were used for this purpose during the outbreak. The reviewers found only five eligible ongoing RCTs (and no completed RCTs) and three non-randomised trials. Ultimately, the reviewers concluded that there wasn't yet any evidence for any treatment under investigation, but the non-randomised studies showed that one specific treatment might be unsafe to use. Systematic reviews are valued but have been criticised for being out of date by the time they are published. This review was undertaken before the publication of sufficient studies could be synthesised (although it is likely to be updated as new evidence emerges), but this still highlights that timing is everything when it comes to systematic reviews!

References

1. World Health Organization. Targets of Sustainable Development Goal 3. 2024. www.who.int/europe/about-us/our-work/sustainable-development-goals/targets-of-sustainable-development-goal-3
2. Greenhalgh EM, Bayly M, Jenkins S, Scollo MM. Prevalence of smoking—adults. In *Tobacco in Australia: Facts & Issues*. Cancer Council Victoria; 2023. www.tobaccoinaustralia.org.au/chapter-1-prevalence/1-3-prevalence-of-smoking-adults
3. Woodruff TJ, Sutton P. The Navigation Guide systematic review methodology: A rigorous and transparent method for translating environmental health science into better health outcomes. *Environm ental Health Perspectives*. 2014;122(10):1007–14.

Index

Printed in the United States
by Baker & Taylor Publisher Services